ESSENTIAL PROCEDURES

Acute Care

ESSENTIAL PROCEDURES

Acute Care

Anthony M. Angelow, PhD, APRN, ACNPC, AGACNP-BC, CEN, FAEN, FAANP

Assistant Clinical Professor
Chair, Advanced Practice Nursing
Co-Chair, Division of Graduate Nursing
College of Nursing and Health Professions
Drexel University
Philadelphia, Pennsylvania

Dawn M. Specht, MSN, PhD, RN, APN, CEN, CPEN, CCRN, CCNS, AGACNP-BC

Associate Professor Nursing
American Sentinel University
Aurora, Colorado

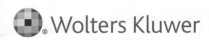. Wolters Kluwer

Philadelphia • Baltimore • New York • London
Buenos Aires • Hong Kong • Sydney • Tokyo

Acquisitions Editor: Jonathan D. Joyce
Product Development Editor: Robin Levin Richman
Editorial Assistant: Molly Kennedy
Marketing Manager: Brittany Riney
Senior Production Project Manager: Alicia Jackson
Manager, Graphic Arts & Design: Stephen Druding
Artist/Illustrator: Jennifer Clements
Senior Manufacturing Coordinator: Beth Welsh
Prepress Vendor: S4Carlisle Publishing Services

Library of Congress Cataloging-in-Publication Data

ISBN-13: 978-1-9751-2028-3

ISBN-10: 1-9751-2028-0

Library of Congress Control Number: 2021916488

shop.lww.com

Dedication

First and foremost, I dedicate this book to the two most influential people in my life, my late mother (Marie Angelow) and grandmother (Grace Domenico). Without their love, guidance, and support, I would not be the person that I am. They instilled in me the importance of hard work, dedication, commitment, and, most importantly, family. They encouraged me to reach for the moon, and if I only landed among the stars, that was always good enough; but don't ever be afraid to try again and push harder. I also dedicate this book to the many mentors, colleagues, and students who have inspired me over the years and continue to inspire me every day.

—ANTHONY M. ANGELOW

–This book is dedicated to all the frontline providers who seek to improve the care delivered to patients at the bedside. It would not have been possible without the love and support of my family. My husband, brother, and son rally to support me in every project I tackle. Thank you Chris, Chas, and CJ; without you life would be mundane. Finally, thank you Dad for instilling in me the belief that I can accomplish all things with hard work.

—DAWN M. SPECHT

Contributors

Thomas Alne, MSN, CRNP
Nurse Practitioner
Mechanical Circulatory Support Program
Hospital of the University of Pennsylvania
Philadelphia, Pennsylvania

Patrick C. Auth, PhD
Department Chair Physician Assistant
    Program (Retired)
Drexel University
Philadelphia, Pennsylvania

Steven Bocchese, MSN, CCRN,
    AGACNP-BC
Critical Care Nurse Practitioner
Thomas Jefferson University Hospital
Philadelphia, Pennsylvania

Brooke Carpenter, MS, AGACNP-BC
Critical Care Nurse Practitioner
Medical-Surgical Intensive Care Unit
California Pacific Medical Center—Van Ness
    Campus
San Francisco, California

Jennifer Coates, DNP, MBA, ACNPC,
    ACNP-BC
Adult Gerontology Acute Care Nurse
    Practitioner Track Director
Drexel University
Philadelphia, Pennsylvania

Kristina Davis, DNP, ENP-C, FNP-C,
    AGACNP-BC
Emergency Nurse Practitioner Program
    Director
College of Nursing
Rocky Mountain University of Health
    Professions
Provo, Utah

Wesley Davis, DNP, ENP-C, FNP-C,
    AGACNP-BC, CEN, FAANP
Dual Family/Emergency Program
    Coordinator
College of Nursing
University of South Alabama
Mobile, Alabama

Janice K. Delgiorno, MSN, ACNP-BC,
    CCRN, TCRN, RRT
Lead Nurse Practitioner
Department of Surgery: Division of Trauma,
    Surgical Critical Care and Acute Care
    Surgery
Cooper University Medical Center
Camden, New Jersey

Troy Derose, RN, MSN, CRNP,
    RNFA, CORLN, BC-ACGNP,
    BC-FNP
Nurse Practitioner
Department of Otorhinolaryngology—Head
    and Neck Surgery
Thomas Jefferson University Hospital
Philadelphia, Pennsylvania

Diana Filipek-Oberg, BSN, MSN
Trauma Surgery Nurse Practitioner, Clinical
    Adjunct Faculty
Trauma Surgery
Cooper University Hospital
Camden, New Jersey
Drexel University
Philadelphia, Pennsylvania

Angela Grochowski
Physician Assistant
Mackell Cody & Burrows Orthopedics
Doylestown, Pennsylvania

Ella Hawk, MSN, RN, AGACNP-BC
Thoracic Surgery Nurse Practitioner
Cooper University Hospital
Camden, New Jersey

Kristopher Jackson, MSN, AGACNP-BC, CCRN
Acute Care Nurse Practitioner
University of California San Francisco (UCSF)
    Medical Center
San Francisco, California

Dana McCloskey, MD
General Surgery Resident
Cooper University Hospital
Camden, New Jersey

Angela McGill, BS, MMS
Physician Assistant
Department of Orthopedic Surgery
Thomas Jefferson University
Philadelphia, Pennsylvania

William Pezzotti, DNP, CRNP, AGACNP-BC
Clinical Adjunct Instructor
Critical Care Nurse Practitioner at Penn
    Medicine Chester County Hospital
Department of Graduate Nursing Studies
Drexel University
Philadelphia, Pennsylvania

Allison Rusgo, MPH, MHS, PA-C
Assistant Clinical Professor
Physician Assistant
Drexel University
Philadelphia, Pennsylvania

Megan E. Schneider, MMS, MSPH, PA-C
Assistant Clinical Professor and Curriculum
    Coordinator
Physician Assistant
Drexel University
Philadelphia, Pennsylvania

Jennifer Schweinsburg, MD
General Surgery Resident
Cooper University Hospital
Camden, New Jersey

Audrey Snyder, PhD, RN, ACNP-BC, FNP-BC, FAANP, FAEN, FAAN
Nurse Practitioner
Transitional Care
Cheyenne Regional Medical Center
Cheyenne, Wyoming

Dawn M. Specht, MSN, PhD, RN, APN, CEN, CPEN, CCRN, CCNS, AGACNP-BC
Associate Professor Nursing
American Sentinel University
Aurora, Colorado

Joshua Thornsberry, DNP, ANP-BC
Cardiovascular Nurse Practitioner
Cardiovascular Medicine
Wellstar Health System
Marietta, Georgia

Damon Toczylowski, RN, MSN, CCRN, ACNPC, CCNS
Acute Care Nurse Practitioner
SICU
Rocky Mountain Regional VA Medical Center
Aurora, Colorado

Elizabeth Tomaszewski, DNP, CRNP, CCRN, ACNP-BC, ACNPC
Track Director and Assistant Clinical Professor
College of Nursing and Health Professions
Drexel University
Philadelphia, Pennsylvania

Starr Tomlinson, MSN, ACNP-BC, CCRN
Acute Care Nurse Practitioner
University of California San Francisco (UCSF)
    Medical Center
San Francisco, California

Kudret Usmani, MD
Orthopedic Surgery Resident
Cooper University Hospital
Camden, New Jersey

Salina Wydo, MD, FACS
Assistant Professor of Surgery, Program
    Director, Surgical Critical Care
Division of Trauma, Department of Surgery
Cooper University Hospital
Camden, New Jersey

Preface

The purpose of writing *Essential Procedures: Acute Care* was to provide advanced practice professionals with a tool to access the most common procedures performed in the acute care setting. While procedures require ongoing credentialing and training/evaluation, this book provides readers with the resources necessary to guide them to perform essential acute care procedures. This book enhances patient care by increasing the advanced practice provider's evidence-based knowledge while safely performing procedures. An organized, systematic approach to performing procedures is essential to ensure safe patient care.

This spiral-bound book is organized to ensure that each procedure follows a consistent, clear process that provides the reader with an organized, systematic approach to performing procedures. Each chapter includes: (1) indications for the procedure, (2) contraindications for the procedure, (3) equipment needed, (4) steps to performing the procedure, (5) potential complications of the procedure, (6) postprocedure care, and (7) evidence-based research bibliographies at the end of each chapter. This comprehensive outline delivers a succinct resource for providers to use when performing procedures. Full-color photographs and illustrations provide visual clarity to enhance and support procedure steps. There are also reference chapters that enhance acute care provider knowledge in interpreting diagnostics and responding to emergencies. Finally, in some procedures, the following three Standard Steps are assumed to be included:

1. Obtain correct identification of patient.
2. Obtain informed consent from the patient or appropriate surrogate decision maker.
3. Perform hand hygiene.

This book has been a collaborative effort written by individuals who specialize in acute care procedures. The interprofessional approach to this book provides different viewpoints and allows for applicability among various advanced practice providers. The contributors of this book include Nurse Practitioners, Physician Assistants, and Physicians who are experts in their field and in performing acute care procedures. We hope that you find this book a helpful tool that deepens your knowledge of evidence-based procedural performance.

Anthony M. Angelow, PhD, APRN, ACNPC, AGACNP-BC, CEN, FAEN, FAANP
Dawn M. Specht, MSN, PhD, RN, APN, CEN, CPEN, CCRN, CCNS, AGACNP-BC

Acknowledgments

We want to acknowledge all the contributors to this book. Without their willingness to share their expertise, this book would not have been possible. They were very timely with their submissions and approached their work with dedication and determination. Many of our contributors offered to go above and beyond to ensure the success of this book.

We would also like to acknowledge all advanced practice providers and physicians who have dedicated their lives to caring for patients in need. As a team, we collaboratively provide patients with the best possible evidence-based care. You are all frontline heroes who work diligently to serve individuals at their most vulnerable moments. To current and future advanced practice and medical students, we applaud your dedication to further developing your knowledge and engaging in a profession that touches the lives of so many people.

We would also like to acknowledge the editorial staff of Wolters Kluwer for all their assistance and support through this process.

Contents

SECTION 5   NEUROLOGICAL AND MUSCULOSKELETAL PROCEDURES

SECTION 6   HEMATOLOGICAL PROCEDURES

SECTION 7   REFERENCE MATERIALS

CHAPTER

1

Arterial Line Insertion

Kristopher Jackson
Starr Tomlinson

INDICATIONS FOR THE PROCEDURE

Arterial line insertion is a commonly performed procedure in the critical care environment. The arterial line provides real-time hemodynamic data and access to frequent blood sampling that can guide the minute-to-minute management of the critically ill patient. Often considered more accurate than the noninvasive blood pressure (BP) measurements taken with a BP cuff, arterial line readings allow providers to titrate vasoactive medications with greater precision. Because these hemodynamic measurements are obtained via a transducer connected to a catheter commonly resting in the radial or femoral artery, this line offers providers convenient access to arterial blood samples. Additionally, this makes the arterial line particularly useful when managing patients requiring serial blood draws or serial arterial blood gas (ABG) analyses.

CONTRAINDICATIONS FOR THE PROCEDURE

Relative Contraindications

There are relatively few contraindications to arterial line placement; however, thought and consideration should be given before placing these catheters in patients with marked coagulopathies or thrombocytopenia. In these patients, the bleeding risk associated with repeated arterial puncture for individual samples may actually make the arterial line a safer alternative.

The primary contraindication to the procedure is:

1. Increased risk of bleeding because of coagulopathy

Absolute Contraindications

There are three absolute contraindications to arterial line placement that should influence the insertion site selection process:

1. If the radial artery is selected as the desired insertion site, one must first perform a modified Allen test (described later in this chapter) to ensure that there is sufficient circulation through the ulnar artery so as not to impair blood flow to the hand. In the event of impaired collateral flow through the ulnar artery, an alternative insertion site should be selected.

1

2. Sites affected by suspected or confirmed soft-tissue infection or full-thickness burns should be avoided and an alternate insertion site selected.
3. Sites affected by a traumatic injury proximal to the insertion site should be avoided and an alternate insertion site selected.

EQUIPMENT NEEDED

Before beginning this or any procedure, gain familiarity with the equipment available at your institution. Many hospitals and medical centers have prepackaged arterial line insertion kits that contain all or most of the equipment necessary for this procedure, regardless of the selected insertion site:

1. Ultrasound with vascular probe and sterile, disposable probe cover
2. Monitor with available transducer port
3. Intravenous (IV) pole, transducer cable, and, if available, transducer holder
4. Eye drape
5. Pressure bag and appropriate size bag of 0.9% NaCl solution
6. Sterile gown, sterile gloves, mask, and eye protection
7. 2% chlorhexidine gluconate swabsticks (or acceptable alternative in the event of documented or suspected allergy to chlorhexidine)
8. 3 to 5 mL of 1% lidocaine without epinephrine
9. 21 gauge (or similar size needle)
10. Sterile 3 to 5 mL syringe
11. Sterile 4 × 4″ gauze
12. Sterile transparent dressing and antimicrobial patch, if required, based on institutional policy
13. Suture material

Radial Insertion Site

The radial artery is more superficial and requires a shorter needle and catheter than the femoral artery. The radial artery can be accessed successfully using either a 1¾″ 18 or 20g IV catheter and suitable sized spring wire or a commercially available 1¾″ 20g integrated catheter and wire system.

Femoral Insertion Site

The femoral artery is deeper and requires a longer needle and catheter than the radial artery. The femoral artery is typically accessed using the contents of a commercially available femoral artery insertion kit, which should include a 16 to 18g introducer needle approximately 3″ in length, an indwelling catheter approximately 6″ in length, and a 45 cm spring wire.

PERFORMING THE ALLEN TEST

If the radial artery is the intended site of insertion, one must first perform a modified Allen test to determine whether there is sufficient collateral circulation to the hand through the ulnar artery in the event of occlusion or thrombosis of the radial artery. The test is conducted by compressing both the radial and ulnar arteries to obstruct blood flow to the hand for approximately 30 seconds. If done properly, the fingers and palmar surface of the hand should appear pale. With the palmar surface of the hand visible, release pressure to the ulnar artery. The hand should flush within 5 to 15 seconds of relieving pressure to the ulnar artery, indicating sufficient collateral circulation, and is considered a positive Allen test. If the palmar surface of the hand and fingertips do not flush within 5 to 15 seconds, this suggests impaired collateral flow through the ulnar artery and is considered a negative Allen test. In the event of a negative Allen test, an alternative site should be selected. The findings of the Allen test should be included in any procedural documentation upon conclusion of the procedure; however, the documentation should avoid the use of the words "positive" or "negative" as there are discrepancies surrounding the meaning of positive or negative. If the palm remains blanched when the radial artery is occluded at 5 seconds then do *not* use the site. There is a predictive value of 0.8% for a lack of sufficient circulation. Remember that a color Doppler may be used to confirm collateral flow from the ulnar artery. If the palm becomes flushed or the pulse oximetry picks up a waveform in less than 5 seconds when the radial artery is occluded, then collateral ulnar flow is considered patent.

STEPS TO PERFORMING THE PROCEDURE

1. Perform standard steps (see Preface).
2. Perform Allen test, as above.
3. Position the patient:
   a. If inserting a radial arterial line, support the arm with pillows or on a bedside table. If necessary, immobilize and support the wrist using a commercially available wrist immobilizer.
   b. If inserting a femoral arterial line, place the patient in a flat, supine position. Ensure the patient will tolerate remaining flat for the duration of the procedure. In the event the patient has a large pannus or body habitus that makes accessing the femoral artery challenging, obtain additional assistance before proceeding with the sterile portion of the procedure.
4. Cleanse the area with 2% chlorhexidine or appropriate alternative. Allow the solution to dry on the surface of the skin completely.
5. Create a sterile field on a stable surface and put on sterile cap, mask, gown, and gloves.
6. Apply eye drape to intended insertion site.
7. Apply sterile probe cover to ultrasound vascular probe, if available.
8. If using ultrasound, perform a brief ultrasonic inspection of the radial artery noting patency of the vessel and where the artery is largest and most superficial. If using palpation only, note the location on the wrist where the pulse feels strongest (Figures 1.1 and 1.2).
9. Using a 21g (or similar size) needle and a sterile 3 to 5 mL syringe, create a wheal at the surface of the skin by instilling 1 to 2 mL of 1% lidocaine at the intended insertion site. If the pulse is difficult to palpate or the target appears very small on ultrasound,

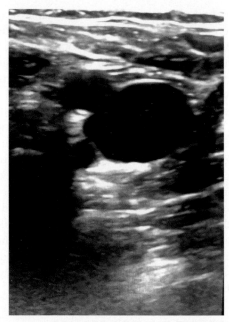

FIGURE 1.1. Sample ultrasound imaging of normal femoral vascular anatomy, noting the smaller femoral artery adjacent to the larger, nonpulsatile femoral vein.

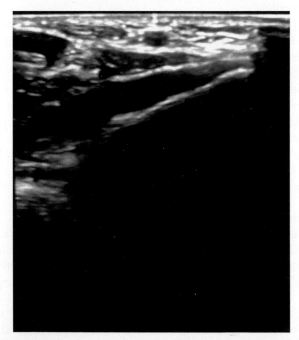

FIGURE 1.2. Sample ultrasound imaging of a normal, patent radial artery.

the instillation of lidocaine may make arterial cannulation more challenging. In lieu of subcutaneous lidocaine, topical anesthetics (e.g., lidocaine-prilocaine cream) may be a suitable alternative.

10. Holding the finder needle, the IV catheter, or the integrated catheter device at a 30° to 45° angle, puncture the skin slightly distal to the palpated artery site, bevel up. If using ultrasound, note the location of the needle tip in the soft tissue and advance the needle slowly until brisk, spontaneous blood appears (Figure 1.3).

11. Once blood appears, advance the catheter slightly to ensure the entirety of the catheter is within the vessel lumen.

12. Lower the angle of the needle by 10° to 15°, then pass the wire through the catheter. If unable to pass the wire, try again to lower the angle of the needle and then attempt to pass the wire again. If the flow of blood is lost, it may be the result of inadvertent advancement of the needle through the vessel. Consider withdrawing slightly until the flow of blood is restored.

13. If using a needle and J-wire, remove the needle, leaving only the wire in place. If using an integrated catheter device, deploy the wire and advance the catheter.

14. If placing a femoral arterial line, it may be necessary to make a small nick in the skin using a scalpel to advance the catheter over the wire. If placing a radial arterial line, the catheter should thread over the wire without difficulty.

15. Remove the wire in its entirety.

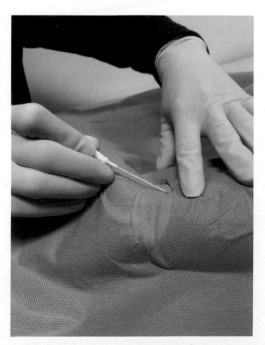

FIGURE 1.3. Visual depiction of the proper angle of approach when inserting a radial arterial catheter using an integrated catheter device.

16. Ensure there is still brisk blood flow through the catheter before attaching the transducer to the catheter. The transducer system is flushed with saline and the pressure bag is inflated to 300 mmHg prior to connecting to the arterial line. Familiarize yourself with transducing equipment, system zeroing, and monitoring prior to arterial line insertion. Note the presence of an arterial waveform on the monitor at the time of attachment.

17. Suture the catheter in place in accordance with institutional guidelines and apply a sterile dressing.

COMPLICATIONS OF THE PROCEDURE

Nuttall et al. conducted a large retrospective study of 52,787 patients who underwent arterial line insertion over a 6-year period. Rates of complication were noted to be very low, estimated at 3.4/10,000. Following are the most common complications of arterial line insertion:

1. **Temporary radial artery occlusion:** A common phenomenon that occurs as a result of arterial vasospasm during arterial line insertion, particularly if multiple attempts are required. While not necessarily a true complication, vasospasm may require the proceduralist to attempt a different insertion site. Perfusion distal to any failed insertion site should be monitored for both hematoma (see following) as well as impaired perfusion.

2. **Arterial thrombus/vessel thrombosis:** Likely related to multiple factors, such as the size of the catheter and the length of time the catheter has remained in place. If there is any concern for malperfusion distal to the catheter, the catheter should be removed and the patient should be evaluated by a vascular surgeon.

3. **Hematoma/bleeding:** In the event of failed cannulation or accidental removal, continuous direct pressure should be held until hemostasis is achieved.

4. **Infection:** While the rates of infection for arterial catheters are low, the catheter site should be monitored regularly for erythema or other signs/symptoms of infection. A meta-analysis by estimates the rate of arterial line–associated bloodstream infections to be similar to that of central venous catheters. The catheter should be removed if infection is suspected.

POSTPROCEDURE CARE

Postprocedure care of the arterial line, aside from managing the potential complications described earlier, is fairly straightforward. As noted, the catheter should be promptly removed if there is concern for impaired circulation or if the catheter ceases to function. The sterile dressing should be maintained in accordance with institutional policy and the site monitored for signs/symptoms of infection. Arterial lines should remain connected to transducer tubing with BP alarms on and audible at all times. Failure to do so may result in life-threatening arterial hemorrhage.

BIBLIOGRAPHY

Evidence-Based Medicine Consult. (2020). *Allen's test: Physical exam*. ebmconsult.com/articles/physica-exam-allens-test

Joly, L., Spaulding, C., Monchi, M., Ali, O. S., Weber, S., & Benhamou, D. (1998). Topical lidocaine-prilocaine cream (EMLA) versus local infiltration anesthesia for radial artery cannulation. *Anesthesia & Analgesia, 87*(2), 403–406. https://doi.org/10.1213/00000539-199808000-00032

Kaur, A. (2006). Caring for a patient with an arterial line. *Nursing, 36*(4), 64cc1–64cc2. https://doi.org/10.1097/00152193-200604000-00047

Nuttall, G., Burckhardt, J., Hadley, A., Kane, S., Kor, D., Marienau, M.S., Schroeder, D.R., Handlogten, K., Wilson, G., & Oliver, W.C. (2016). Surgical and patient risk factors for severe arterial line complications in adults. *Anesthesiology, 124*(3), 590-597. https://doi.org/10.1097/ALN.0000000000000967

O'Horo, J. C., Maki, D. G., Krupp, A. E., & Safdar, N. (2014). Arterial catheters as a source of bloodstream infection. *Critical Care Medicine, 42*(6), 1334–1339. https://doi.org/10.1097/ccm.0000000000000166

Pullen, R. L. (2005). Performing a modified Allen test. *Nursing, 35*(10), 26. https://doi.org/10.1097/00152193-200510000-00020

Scheer, B. V., Perel, A., & Pfeiffer, U. (2002). Clinical review: Complications and risk factors of peripheral arterial catheters used for haemodynamic monitoring in anaesthesia and intensive care medicine. *Critical Care, 6*(3). https://doi.org/10.1186/cc1489

Tegtmeyer, K., Brady, G., Lai, S., Hodo, R., & Braner, D. (2006). Placement of an arterial line. *New England Journal of Medicine, 354*(15), e13. https://doi.org/10.1056/nejmvcm044149

Tiru, B., Bloomstone, J. A., & McGee, W. T. (2012). Radial artery cannulation: A review article. *Journal of Anesthesia & Clinical Research, 3*, 5. https://doi.org/10.4172/2155-6148.1000209

World Health Organization. (2010). *World Health Organization (WHO) guidelines on drawing blood: Best practices in phlebotomy* [WHO Phlebotomy Guideline]. Author.

CHAPTER 2

Central Venous Catheter Placement

Audrey Snyder

INDICATIONS FOR THE PROCEDURE

The purpose of this procedure is to place an indwelling central venous catheter (CVC) to provide venous access for hemodynamic lines, medication administration, or total parenteral nutrition (TPN). Central catheters may be placed in the external jugular, internal jugular, subclavian, or femoral vein to access the central circulation. It is important that the catheter is inserted using maximum barrier precautions to decrease the risk of infection.

Indications for the procedure are:

1. Lack of peripheral veins
2. Inability to cannulate peripheral veins
3. Medication administration (high volume, prolonged delivery, potentially caustic, toxic or irritating solutions, or vasoactive medications)
4. Avoidance of medication interruptions
5. Delivery of incompatible medications with a multilumen catheter
6. Deliver of TPN
7. Central venous access for hemodynamic monitoring of central venous pressure (CVP)
8. Central venous access for pulmonary artery (Swan-Ganz) catheter placement
9. Central venous access for temporary transvenous cardiac pacing

CONTRAINDICATIONS FOR THE PROCEDURE

Relative Contraindications

1. Severe coagulopathy or thrombocytopenia—check platelets and clotting factors before procedure and correct prior to placement. Femoral or external jugular approach is favored in this setting. The subclavian approach is least desirable.
2. Avoid sites of sepsis, trauma, or venous thrombosis.
3. Apical emphysema or bullae contraindicate infraclavicular or supraclavicular approaches to the subclavian vein.
4. Carotid artery aneurysm precludes the use of the jugular vein on the same site.

Absolute Contraindications

None, as an alternative site can usually be accessed.

EQUIPMENT NEEDED

1. Sterile gown, gloves, mask, and goggles
2. Chlorhexidine prep
3. Local anesthetic 1% to 2% lidocaine, 26 gauge needle, and 2 mL syringe
4. Sterile drapes
5. CVC insertion kit, including 16 to 18 gauge needle, 10 mL syringe, guidewire, scalpel, dilator, and catheter (triple lumen if monitoring CVP, cordis for massive infusion or pulmonary artery catheterization)
6. Sterile saline for injection to flush catheter
7. Catheter-securing device
8. Sterile transparent dressing and antimicrobial disk
9. CVP transducer/monitoring equipment if placed for hemodynamic monitoring
10. Ultrasound machine with high-frequency linear probe, sterile ultrasound gel, and sterile sheath cover
11. 14 to 16 gauge needle over catheter available in the event a tension pneumothorax occurs

APPROACHES, LANDMARKS, AND TECHNIQUES

The most common sites used are the internal jugular and subclavian. When selecting a site, take into consideration that insertion on the right side of the patient's body may allow for easier positioning of the catheter tip. If the patient already has a chest tube in place for prior pneumothorax, attempt insertion on the same side as the pneumothorax. There are a few considerations for each approach.

External Jugular Approach

The external jugular approach requires minimal skill. There is decreased success with obesity or short neck. It is best when only fluids and medication infusion are needed. A catheter-over-needle device may be used for this approach versus using the Seldinger technique (described in procedure steps that follow). See Figure 2.1.

Internal Jugular

With the internal jugular approach, there is decreased success with obesity or a flaccid neck. Insertion carries no risk of thoracic duct injury and less risk of pneumothorax because the right pleural dome is lower than the left. There is increased risk of carotid artery puncture.

There are three approaches to the internal jugular vein: the anterior, central (or middle), and posterior approach. The jugular vein lies posterior and lateral to the carotid artery (Figure 2.2). With the patient's head turned to the opposite shoulder, it is easier to access. The vein lies medially to the sternocleidomastoid (SCM) muscle at the top of the neck and passes under the SCM to join the subclavian vein behind the medial aspect

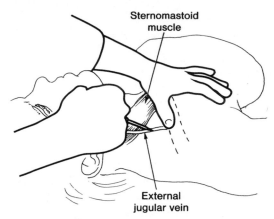

FIGURE 2.1. Entry into the external jugular vein: Distend the vein by applying slight pressure over the vein with thumb placed just above the clavicle. Reprinted with permission from Simon, R. R., Ross, C. P., Bowman, S. H., & Wakim, P. E. (2012). *Cook county manual of emergency procedures.* Wolters Kluwer.

of the clavicle. The two heads of the SCM muscle (sternal and clavicular head) form an anatomic triangle with the medial clavicle as the base (Figure 2.3).

Anterior Approach

With the anterior approach, the needle is inserted at a 45° angle at the medical border of the sternal head of the SCM muscle toward the ipsilateral nipple at a depth of 3 to 5 cm (Figure 2.4).

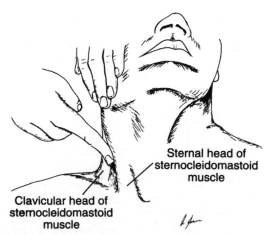

FIGURE 2.2. Anatomic triangle. Reprinted with permission from Simon, R. R., Ross, C. P., Bowman, S. H., & Wakim, P. E. (2012). *Cook county manual of emergency procedures.* Wolters Kluwer.

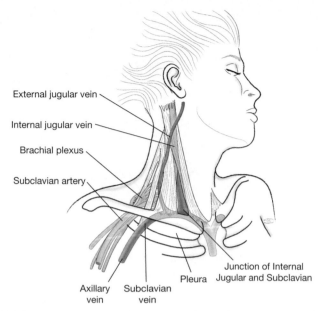

FIGURE 2.3. Anatomy and surface relationships of the internal jugular vein. Reprinted with permission from Simon, R. R., Ross, C. P., Bowman, S. H., & Wakim, P. E. (2012). *Cook county manual of emergency procedures.* Wolters Kluwer.

Central (Medial) Approach

For the central approach, the needle is inserted at a 30 to 40° angle at the apex of the anatomic triangle toward the ipsilateral nipple at a depth of 1 to 3 cm (Figure 2.5).

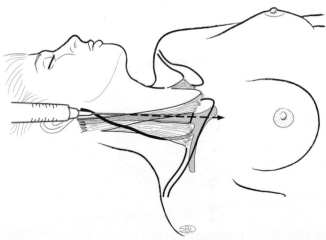

FIGURE 2.4. Anterior approach to the internal jugular vein cannulation. Reprinted with permission from Simon, R. R., Ross, C. P., Bowman, S. H., & Wakim, P. E. (2012). *Cook county manual of emergency procedures.* Wolters Kluwer.

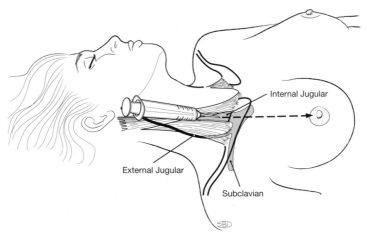

FIGURE 2.5. Central approach to internal jugular vein cannulation. Reprinted with permission from Simon, R. R., Ross, C. P., Bowman, S. H., & Wakim, P. E. (2012). *Cook county manual of emergency procedures.* Wolters Kluwer.

Posterior Approach

With the posterior approach, insert the needle at a 30 to 45° angle at the lateral border of the clavicular head of the SCM muscle toward the suprasternal notch at a depth of approximately 5 cm (Figure 2.6).

Subclavian Approach

One advantage of the subclavian approach is that the anatomy is constant in this region (Figure 2.7). There is increased risk of pneumothorax during subclavian line placement and bleeding potential from the subclavian artery if punctured. There are two approaches to the subclavian vein: infraclavicular and supraclavicular.

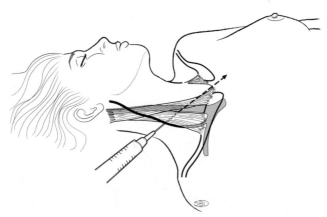

FIGURE 2.6. Posterior approach to cannulation of the internal jugular vein. Reprinted with permission from Simon, R. R., Ross, C. P., Bowman, S. H., & Wakim, P. E. (2012). *Cook county manual of emergency procedures.* Wolters Kluwer.

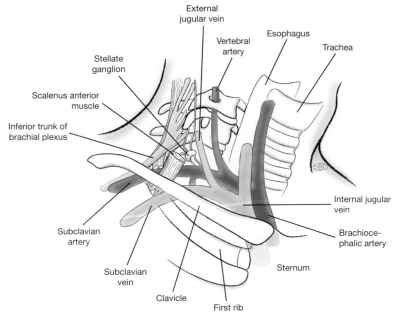

FIGURE 2.7. Anatomy of the subclavian vein. Reprinted with permission from Simon, R. R., Ross, C. P., Bowman, S. H., & Wakim, P. E. (2012). *Cook county manual of emergency procedures.* Wolters Kluwer.

Infraclavicular Approach

Insert the needle at a 20 to 30° angle beneath the clavicle at the middle to medial third of the clavicle parallel to the frontal plane, directing the needle superiorly and medially toward the suprasternal notch advancing to a depth of 3 to 4 cm. Placing a finger of the opposition hand in the notch over the drape will help to define this landmark. Slowly march the needle down the bone to find the space beneath the clavicle while aspirating with the plunger of the syringe with each advancement until blood is returned, indicating the presence of the needle in the vessel (Figure 2.8).

Supraclavicular Approach

The subclavian approach is less commonly used. The needle is inserted above the clavicle at the clavisternomastoid angle (1 cm lateral to clavicular head of SCM and 1 cm superior to clavicle) at a 15° angle, aiming upward toward the contralateral nipple (Figure 2.9).

Femoral Approach

Femoral line placement does not require interruption of cardiopulmonary resuscitation (CPR) for the procedure, but sterility is more difficult to maintain. There is increased risk of femoral artery puncture and hematoma. Anatomically lateral to medial are nerve, artery, vein, empty space, and lymphatics. Landmarks are the anterior superior iliac crest and pubic symphysis; the inguinal ligament lies between the two. Palpate the femoral artery at the midpoint between the anterior superior iliac crest and

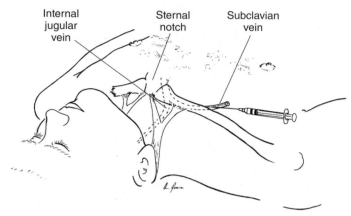

FIGURE 2.8. Infraclavicular approach to the subclavian vein. Reprinted with permission from Simon, R. R., Ross, C. P., Bowman, S. H., & Wakim, P. E. (2012). *Cook county manual of emergency procedures*. Wolters Kluwer.

pubic symphysis, and insert the needle 1 to 2 cm medially and parallel to the femoral artery and 1 to 2 cm below the inguinal ligament, directing the needle at a 45° angle toward the head (Figure 2.10).

GENERAL GUIDANCE FOR THE PROCEDURE

1. Ultrasound guidance for CVC placement should be used by those fully trained in the technique.
2. Do not use a site distal to an injury.
3. Avoid pushing or pulling a guidewire or dilator against resistance.

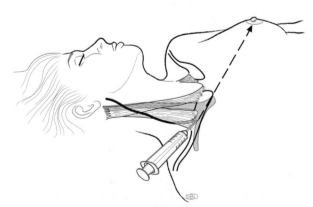

FIGURE 2.9. Supraclavicular subclavian vein approach—direct needle upward toward the ipsilateral nipple. Reprinted with permission from Simon, R. R., Ross, C. P., Bowman, S. H., & Wakim, P. E. (2012). *Cook county manual of emergency procedures*. Wolters Kluwer.

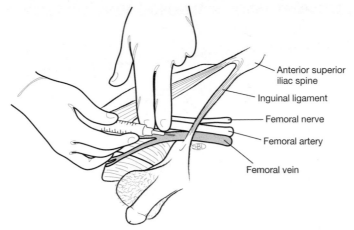

Anterior superior
iliac spine

Inguinal ligament

Femoral nerve

Femoral artery

Femoral vein

FIGURE 2.10. Femoral vein cannulation. Reprinted with permission from Simon, R. R., Ross, C. P., Bowman, S. H., & Wakim, P. E. (2012). *Cook county manual of emergency procedures*. Wolters Kluwer.

STEPS TO PERFORMING THE PROCEDURE

1. Perform standard steps (see Preface).
2. Explain procedure.
3. Ensure patient is on cardiac and pulse oximetry monitoring for procedure.
4. Select vessel site (subclavian, internal jugular, external jugular, or femoral) and mark skin.
5. Perform time-out for procedure.
6. Premedicate with sedation as needed.
7. Position patient supine. For the subclavian or internal jugular approach, place the patient in a 15° angle Trendelenburg position to increase filling of veins with head turned to side opposite of insertion site. For subclavian approach, place a rolled towel between shoulder blades.
8. Wear hair cover, mask, gown, gloves, and eye protection for procedure. In an emergency, wear gloves at minimum. Infection rates are high in emergently placed lines.
9. Using sterile technique clean site with chlorhexidine skin antisepsis. If using the subclavian or internal jugular approach, prep both sites so the other can be used if unsuccessful in the first site.
10. Provide sterile draping of site.
11. Anesthetize insertion site skin with 1% to 2% lidocaine. Aspirate before injecting to ensure you are not in a vessel.
12. If using the subclavian approach, infiltrate toward the clavicle and march down the bone infiltrating the periosteum.
13. Estimate the catheter length required to reach the superior vena cava by placing the catheter over the sterile field in the anatomic position (Table 2.1). The goal is for the catheter to sit in the lower two-thirds of the superior vena cava; aim for 2 to 3 cm inferior to the manubrial–sternal junction.

TABLE 2.1 Guidelines for Insertion Length

Vessel	Right	Left
Internal jugular	12 cm	14 cm
Subclavian	12–14 cm	14–16 cm
Femoral	No limit	No limit

14. Remove port cap from shortest port on catheter.
15. Confirm adequate anesthesia.
16. If ultrasound is available, use ultrasound guidance for placement (Figure 2.11). Apply ultrasound gel to probe prior to placement of sterile probe sleeve over probe. Apply additional sterile ultrasound gel sheath over probe end. Using the probe in the transverse axis to the vessel, watch the needle enter the vessel. Once blood is returned, place the probe along the longitudinal axis (LAX) of the vessel to confirm placement in vessel.
17. If ultrasound is not available, use a 22-gauge finder needle to aspirate venous blood before using larger needle to aspirate venous blood (Figure 2.12). Confirm venous blood by determining oxygen tension via venous blood gas or transduce pressure

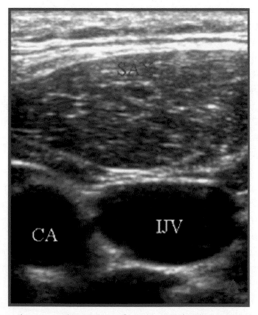

FIGURE 2.11. Ultrasound imaging of neck vessels: the carotid artery (CA) and the internal jugular vein (IJV) can be seen simultaneously in the transverse axis. Reprinted with permission from Savage, R. M., Solomon A., Thomas, J. D., Shanewise, J. S., & Shernan, S. K. (2010). *Comprehensive textbook of intraoperative transesophageal echocardiography* (2nd ed.). Wolters Kluwer.

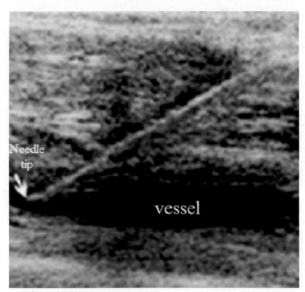

FIGURE 2.12. LAX ultrasound image of the vessel. 2D LAX view of the vessel means that the needle will be "in plane" with the ultrasound beam. From Savage, R. M., Solomon, A., Thomas, J. D., Shanewise, J. S., & Shernan, S. K. (2010). *Comprehensive textbook of intraoperative transesophageal echocardiography* (2nd ed.). Wolters Kluwer. Originally from French, J. L., Raine-Fenning, N. J., Hardman, J. G., & Bedforth, N. M. (2008). Pitfalls of ultrasound guided vascular access: The use of three/four-dimensional ultrasound. *Anaesthesia, 63*(8), 806–813, with permission from John Wiley & Sons. © 2008 The Authors. Journal compilation © 2008 The Association of Anaesthetists of Great Britain and Ireland.

at hub site. After confirming needle is in a vein, you can proceed with guidewire placement, dilation of tract and vessel, and insertion of catheter or introducer. For emergent venous access, proceed with dilation after aspirated blood is sent for oxygen tension, but do not wait for results prior to dilation of tract and insertion of catheter or introducer. Do not infuse fluids until placement in vein is confirmed.

18. Using a needle and 10 mL syringe insert the needle bevel up at the site and angle identified for the vessel approach above, while aspirating with the plunger of the syringe with each advancement until blood is returned, indicating presence in the vessel.

19. When blood return flows freely, remove the syringe and place a finger over the hub of the needle to prevent air entry and possible air embolus.

20. Seldinger technique: passage of guidewire through the needle, removal of needle and passage of catheter over the guidewire (Figure 2.13). See detailed steps below in steps 19 to 23.

21. Place the guidewire through the needle. The wire should pass freely without resistance.

22. Nick the skin at the entry site with the scalpel. It is easier to do this step with the needle still in the skin prior to removing it. If you nick the skin with the wire only in place, you risk nicking and fraying the wire.

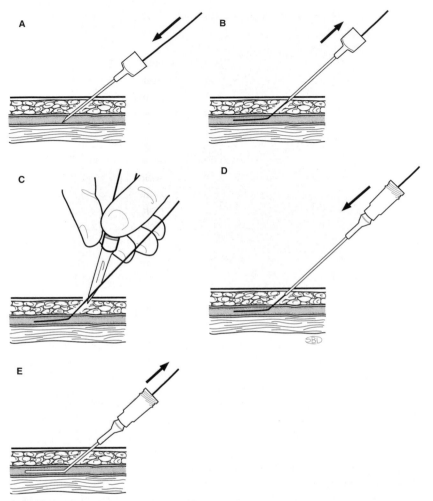

FIGURE 2.13. Seldinger technique for introducing a catheter into a vein. Reprinted with permission from Simon, R. R., Ross, C. P., Bowman, S. H., & Wakim, P. E. (2012). *Cook county manual of emergency procedures.* Wolters Kluwer.

23. Remove the needle over the wire, keeping control of the wire so it does not touch a nonsterile surface.
24. Place the dilator over the guidewire until the guidewire protrudes. Hold on to guidewire and insert dilator several cm through the skin to the estimated depth of the vessel. Remove the dilator. Place the catheter over the wire into the vessel. The guidewire will protrude from a port on the catheter. In the case of a multilumen catheter, it will be the shorted port. Insert catheter to estimated depth.
25. Remove the wire from the catheter while holding the catheter in position.
26. Aspirate blood from each catheter lumen to ensure placement. Obtain blood samples if needed. Flush each lumen with saline and apply cap to the port.
27. Secure the catheter to the skin with an approved catheter-securing device to prevent accidental withdrawal, movement, or kinking of the catheter.

28. Apply antimicrobial disk, such as BIOPATCH*, at entry site and sterile plastic, transparent dressing to help stabilize catheter and maintain skin contact with the antimicrobial disk.
29. Obtain chest x-ray prior to infusion of fluids to evaluate placement of catheter tip and assess for complications. The catheter tip should be at the cavoatrial junction. The catheter is malpositioned if it directs upward into the internal jugular vein in the neck or if the tip is too far into the atria on chest x-ray.

COMPLICATIONS OF THE PROCEDURE

1. **Air embolism:** To help prevent an air embolism, occlude the needle hub after removing the syringe as you advance the wire to prevent air entry. Observe for complaints of shortness of breath during or after central line placement. If suspected, place the patient in the left lateral decubitus position in Trendelenburg and administer 100% oxygen. Consult cardiology and consider aspirating air from the catheter if the catheter is located in the heart. Transesophageal echocardiography, precordial ultrasonography, and end tidal capnography showing a drop in the level can help detect air embolism. Consider immediate hyperbaric oxygen therapy.
2. **Pneumothorax:** Administer 100% oxygen. Obtain chest x-ray to confirm diagnosis. If tension pneumothorax is suspected by assessment, perform immediate needle decompression. (See Chapter 10.) If pneumothorax is present, place tube thoracostomy. (See Chapter 9.)
3. **Arterial puncture:** Remove needle if bright blood is identified in syringe, sit patient upright, obtain chest x-ray, and apply pressure at the site for 10 minutes. If subclavian site, direct pressure will not tamponade bleeding. Obtain hematocrit and monitor patient for blood loss and respiratory distress. Repeat chest x-ray at 12 to 24 hours.
4. **Hemothorax:** Evaluate with chest x-ray. Obtain hematocrit and monitor.
5. **Guidewire embolism:** Consult vascular surgery or interventional radiology for removal of guidewire.
6. **Catheter shear and embolus:** Consult vascular surgery or interventional radiology for removal of catheter.
7. **Inability to place line:** After three attempts at same site, obtain chest x-ray to evaluate for potential pneumothorax before attempting insertion at a different site. Try to stay on the same side of the body for next site insertion.
8. **Dysrhythmias:** Place patient on cardiac monitor during procedure and monitor for dysrhythmias. Stop advancement of line if dysrhythmia occurs.
9. **Cardiac tamponade:** Assess for Beck triad: hypotension, distended neck veins, and muffled heart sounds. Treatment is pericardiocentesis.
10. **Vessel thrombosis:** Identification of vessel thrombosis will require removal of line.
11. **Pulmonary embolus:** Observe for complaints of shortness of breath during or after central line placement. If suspected, place the patient in the left lateral decubitus position and administer 100% oxygen. Obtain a computed tomography (CT) or pulmonary angiography (PA) to diagnose. Treatment is thrombolysis and anticoagulation.
12. **Venous thrombosis:** Treatment is anticoagulation after removal of catheter.
13. **Thoracic duct injury with resultant chyle fistula or chylothorax:** Conservative treatment includes bowel rest, TPN, and somatostatin. Consult thoracic surgeon for operative repair or biologic glue infusion onto leaking area.

14. **Pleural effusion:** Evaluate for and monitor pleural effusion with chest x-ray.
15. **Nerve injury:** Document assessment of nerve injury; will require further evaluation with nerve conduction studies and electromyogram.
16. **Infection at entry site:** Will require removal of line, culture of tip, and treatment with antibiotics.
17. **Hemorrhage at site with hematoma development or bleeding into the mediastinum:** Evaluate and monitor with chest x-ray. May require surgical intervention.
18. **Tracheal puncture:** Assess for respiratory distress. May require intubation and airway management.
19. **Catheter malfunction:** If troubleshooting efforts do not result in a functioning line, this may necessitate removal of the line and placement in a different site.
20. **Catheter malposition:** Obtain a chest x-ray after placement. If malposition is identified, reposition the catheter.
21. **Cardiac tamponade:** Assess for Beck triad to diagnose hypotension, distended neck veins, and muffled heart sounds. The treatment is pericardiocentesis.
22. **Local anesthetic reaction due to allergy:** Confirm patient allergies prior to procedure. Treat allergic reaction.

POSTPROCEDURE CARE

After insertion, check bilateral breath sounds and obtain a chest x-ray prior to infusion of fluids or medications. Reposition catheter if needed. Attach to manometer if continuous CVP reading is required. Document a thorough procedure note in the chart, including date, time, indication(s), staff in attendance, sedation, anesthesia, monitoring, procedure note, if cultures are obtained, estimated blood loss, chest x-ray reading, complications, follow-up required, and number to reach provider. The need for the CVC should be reassessed daily and unnecessary lines removed. Inspect the site daily and evaluate for potential infection. If the patient develops a fever, cultures should be obtained from this site. Nursing instructions should include dressing change every 7 days or sooner if soiled, damp, or loose. Intravenous administration set is replaced no more frequently than every 96 hours. Blood product administration sets are replaced immediately after infusion, and TPN administration sets are replaced every 24 hours.

BIBLIOGRAPHY

Anestis, N., Christos, F.-C., Ioannis, P., Christos, I., Lampros, P., & Stephanos, P. (2012). Thoracic duct injury due to left subclavicular vein catheterization: A new conservative approach to a chyle fistula using biological glue. *International Journal of Surgery Case Reports, 3*(7), 330–332. https://doi.org/10.1016/j.ijscr.2012.03.021

Omar, G. S., Chawala, S., Ganguly, S., Cherian, G., & Tiwari, A. (2013). Supraclavicular approach of central venous catheter insertion in critical patients in emergency settings: Re-visited. *Indian Journal of Critical Care Medicine, 17*(1), 10–15. https://doi.org/10.4103/0972-5229.112145

Saugel, B., Scheeren, T. W. L., & Teboul, J.-L. (2017). Ultrasound-guided central line placement: A structured review and recommendations for clinical practice. *Critical Care, 21*, 225. https://doi.org/10.1186/s13054-017-1814-y

Shaikh, N., & Ummunisa, F. (2009). Acute management of vascular air embolism. *Journal of Emergencies, Trauma, and Shock, 2*(3), 180–185. https://doi.org/10.4103/0974-2700.55330

CHAPTER 3

Transvenous Pacing

Elizabeth Tomaszewski

INDICATIONS FOR THE PROCEDURE

Transvenous pacing (TVP) is used to temporarily stimulate the myocardium to restore heart rate in symptomatic bradycardia. A temporary pacing wire is threaded through an introducer placed in either the internal jugular, subclavian, or femoral vein, with the distal end of the pacing catheter terminating in the right ventricle (RV). Femoral approaches are generally reserved for those being performed under fluoroscopy. Favored sites for bedside blind placement are the right internal jugular and left subclavian, as the trajectory is more direct during insertion. There are also Swan Ganz (SG) catheters that have a pacing component that are located in the RV, provided the SG catheter is located in the proper position. Please refer to Chapter 7 for instructions on placing a SG catheter. In some applications, the need for the pacer may be temporary; however, in others TVP may be used as a bridge to permanent pacemaker placement.

Indications for the procedure are:

1. Hemodynamic instability related to sinus bradycardia, sick sinus syndrome, atrial fibrillation with slow ventricular response, or other losses of sinoatrial (SA) nodal function (asystole)
2. Medication-induced or toxic ingestions of beta- or calcium channel blockers for chronotropic support during medical treatment
3. Failure of transcutaneous pacing (TCP) to achieve capture or prolonged dependence on TCP in a conscious patient
4. Injury to the SA node, as may occur with open heart surgery
5. Overdrive pacing of symptomatic tachyarrhythmias

CONTRAINDICATIONS FOR THE PROCEDURE

Relative Contraindications

1. Asymptomatic bradycardia. If pacing is performed in the presence of a stable rhythm, such as first- or second-degree heart block, or escape rhythms, the patient may become dependent on the pacer.
2. When risk outweighs benefit. As with all procedures, risk/benefit must be evaluated. Risky conditions may include, but are not limited to, dilated cardiomyopathy and coagulopathy.

3. Severe hypothermia. Bradycardia may be normal in this state. May lead to ventricular fibrillation if pacing is attempted. Rewarm patient first.
4. Medical futility or comfort measures only status.

Absolute Contraindications

1. Prosthetic tricuspid valve. Advancing the wire may lead to damage to the prosthetic.

EQUIPMENT NEEDED

1. Code/emergency cart (in event of deterioration)
2. Continuous cardiac monitoring, TCP pads and defibrillator
3. Analgesia/sedation as required
4. Sterile full body length drapes, sterile personal protective equipment (PPE), including caps/masks and eye shield
5. Introducer kit (6Fr cordis)
6. Temporary pacing wire, with pacing wire adapters (should be included)
7. Pacing generator
8. Ultrasound unit
9. Nonsterile assistant

See Figure 3.1 (A) and (B) for examples of temporary pacemakers.

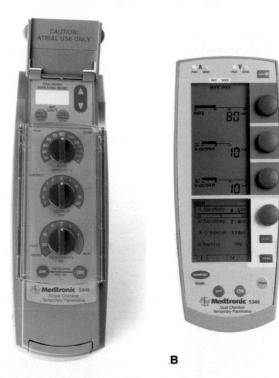

A   **B**

FIGURE 3.1. Pacemakers. (A) Single-chamber temporary pacemaker. (B) Dual-chamber temporary pacemaker. Reproduced with permission from Medtronic.

STEPS TO PERFORMING THE PROCEDURE

1. Perform Standard Steps (see Preface).
2. Explain procedure. If necessary, perform under emergent cover. Patient should be located in a critical care setting (e.g., intensive or cardiac care unit, catheterization laboratory, emergency room), with staff trained in advanced cardiac life support.
3. Patient should be placed on continuous cardiac monitoring. Ideally, TCP pads should be placed on patient, with capacity for TCP/defibrillation should the need arise during the procedure.
4. Perform hand hygiene.
5. Prepare and drape in sterile fashion for the selected insertion site. (Right internal jugular and left subclavian favored for bedside insertions.)
6. Insert introducer. Please refer to Chapter 2 on central venous access. Ultrasound guidance is preferred. Maintain sterile field. Note the length of the introducer prior to insertion.
7. Place the sheath provided with the introducer over the wire *prior to insertion.*
8. Test the pacer balloon to ensure proper inflation. Connect the pacer wire adapters for insertion into the pacer generator (Figure 3.2).
9. Insert the pacer wire through the diaphragm of the introducer. Advance the catheter to a point beyond the tip of the introducer (having noted the length of the introducer prior to insertion). Failure to do so will prohibit the balloon from inflating.
10. At this point, have the nonsterile assistant connect the wires and turn on the pacer generator. There are three settings of concern: rate, sensitivity, and output current (in mAs). Ensure a rate set above the patient's intrinsic rate (or the pacer will not trigger). The sensitivity should be reduced to minimum settings, so the pacer will pace asynchronously (regardless of the patient's intrinsic rhythm). The output current should be started at 20 mAs initially.
11. Inflate the balloon, and begin to advance the catheter until an increase in heart rate is noted with positive capture. Deflate the balloon. If qualified, nonsterile assistant can utilize ultrasound to localize the wire via subcostal view beneath the sterile drape. Otherwise, visualization of the bedside electrocardiogram (ECG) to verify capture is indicative of proper placement (Figure 3.3). Note the depth of the pacer wire once placement is confirmed, and lock the sheath over the wire onto the introducer.

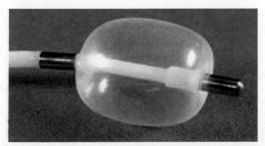

FIGURE 3.2. Test the pacer balloon to ensure proper inflation. Reprinted with permission from Herzog, E. (2017). *Herzog's CCU book.* Wolters Kluwer.

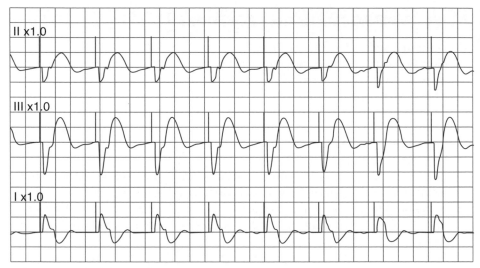

FIGURE 3.3. Rhythm strip for capture determination.

12. Apply sterile dressing and secure pacer wire to prevent migration of the device.
13. Perform chest x-ray to confirm placement and exclude complications from central venous access (such as pneumothorax). Note cardiac size and contour.
14. If capture is intermittent and placement is confirmed, the current may be increased. Ensure that the set rate is above the patient's intrinsic rate for pacing to occur. The sensitivity may be increased to allow for demand pacing in concert with the patient's intrinsic rhythm (however, if sensitivity is set too high, pacing may not occur).
15. Perform a 12-lead ECG.

COMPLICATIONS OF THE PROCEDURE

1. **Misplaced pacer wire**: If failure to capture is observed, the catheter tip may not be in the RV as expected. If unable to place catheter tip in the RV blindly, perform a chest x-ray to ensure proper placement, and reposition as necessary.
2. **Dysrhythmias**: Despite proper placement, an irritable or ischemic heart may begin to experience dysrhythmias. Ventricular dysrhythmias may occur owing to the electrical source floating within the chamber. Supraventricular dysrhythmias can also occur owing to irritability of the right atrium. Antiarrhythmics may be used in conjunction with TVP, but with vigilant monitoring for loss of capture.
3. **Any risk associated with central line placement**: Examples are infection, bleeding, hematoma, pneumothorax. Please refer to Chapter 2.

4. **Ventricular perforation**: Although rare, ventricular perforation is a life-threatening condition. Signs of pericardial tamponade should lead to a high index of suspicion. Treatment may require emergent pericardiocentesis and intervention of cardiac surgery for myocardial repair.
5. **Loss of capture**: Source could be the device but also a change in the patient's condition.

POSTPROCEDURE CARE

A chest x-ray should be ordered to confirm proper placement of the wire and to exclude complications related to the central venous access and pacer wire insertion, such as pneumothorax. Documentation should include a description of the introducer placement, patency of the balloon, depth of the wire, and patient's tolerance of the procedure. Additionally, document the initial settings of the pacer generator and lack or presence of complications. Providers should reassess the pacer function periodically, monitoring for nonsensing or noncapture of the TVP. Settings may require adjustment, or the wire may float out of proper position. In cases where capture is lost or sensing impaired, reassessment of the patient is paramount to exclude a change in his or her condition that is causing the change. Acidemia, electrolyte abnormalities, and hypoxia are leading physiologic reasons for loss of capture. ECGs should be performed after insertions, with any noted change in the patient's cardiac rhythm or condition.

In some cases where the wire is being used for longer than 24 hours, or the patient is completely dependent on the pacer, the wires may lose function. This could require replacement of the wire or battery source or consideration of the placement of a permanent pacemaker.

BIBLIOGRAPHY

Sovari, A. A. (2018a). *Transvenous cardiac pacing technique.* Retrieved January 2, 2019, from https://emedicine.medscape.com/article/80659-technique
Sovari, A. A. (2018b). *Transvenous cardiac pacing.* Retrieved January 2, 2019 from https://emedicine.medscape.com/article/80659-overview

Transcutaneous Pacemakers

Dawn M. Specht

INDICATIONS FOR THE PROCEDURE

Transcutaneous pacemaker use is indicated in symptomatic adults with bradycardia and poor perfusion. Bradycardia may fail to respond to pharmacologic agents such as atropine or present very suddenly when an IV access is not present. The advanced practice provider must first recognize the presence of bradycardia as a heart rate of less than 60 bpm in an adult and determine that the bradycardia is the cause of poor perfusion and serious symptomatology. Serious signs of bradycardia are hypotension, shock, pulmonary congestion, altered mental status, shortness of breath, and chest pain. The purpose of transcutaneous pacemaker application is to deliver externally an electrical current and increase heart rate, heart contraction, and perfusion.

Indications for the procedure are:

1. Symptomatic bradycardia related to heart block
2. Symptomatic bradycardia related to beta-blocker overdose
3. Symptomatic bradycardia related to calcium channel blocker poisoning
4. Symptomatic bradycardia related to dysrhythmia

CONTRAINDICATIONS FOR THE PROCEDURE

Relative Contraindications

1. Severe hypothermia, because the heart will not respond
2. Asystole, because pacing is ineffective with no survival benefit
3. Pulseless electrical activity, because pacing is ineffective with no survival benefit

Absolute Contraindications

1. Bradycardia is not the cause of poor perfusion.
2. Bradycardia is present without serious signs.

EQUIPMENT NEEDED

1. Cardiac monitor with pacing capabilities (pulse generator unit)
2. Cardiac electrodes for chest leads and chest lead cables
3. Cardiac pacing pads and cables
4. Sedation
5. Stethoscope and BP cuff

STEPS TO PERFORMING THE PROCEDURE

The provider will apply transcutaneous pads to the anterior and posterior left chest to encompass the heart or to the right anterior and left lateral chest if unable to turn the patient. Additionally, electrocardiogram chest leads will be applied to allow the rhythm monitoring and coordination of the electrical current with the *r* wave on the electrocardiogram. The electrical current will begin at 10 mA and be increased in increments of 10 mA until electrical and mechanical capture occurs. Capture usually requires at least 50 mA and is increasingly uncomfortable, so consider sedation for the patient.

1. Perform standard steps (see Preface).
2. Apply the cardiac monitor chest leads, examine rhythm. Electrocardiogram chest leads will be applied to allow the rhythm monitoring and coordination of the electrical current with the *r* wave on the electrocardiogram (Figure 4.1).
3. Assess patient for signs of poor perfusion (hypotension, chest pain, etc.).

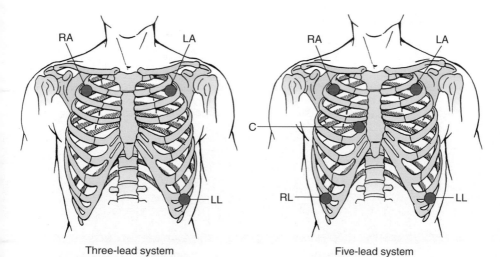

Three-lead system   Five-lead system

FIGURE 4.1. Chest leads. Reprinted with permission from Lynn, P. (2018). *Taylor's clinical nursing skills* (5th ed.). Wolters Kluwer.

4. Apply multifunction pads (for defibrillation and pacing). The provider will apply transcutaneous pads to the anterior and posterior left chest to encompass the heart or the right anterior and left lateral chest if unable to turn the patient (Figures 4.2 and 4.3).
   - May need to shave chest if area is excessively hairy.
   - Remove medication patches.
   - Make sure patient is on dry surface.
5. Turn on pacemaker function.
6. Set heart rate between 60 and 80 bpm; many devices default to a rate in this range.
7. Consider administering sedative, because transcutaneous pacing is uncomfortable.
8. Increase milliamps until capture occurs. The electrical current will begin at 10 mA and be increased in increments of 10 mA until electrical and mechanical capture occurs. Capture usually requires about 50 mA and is increasingly uncomfortable, so consider sedation.
9. Once electrical capture has occurred, assess pulse for mechanical capture (Figure 4.4).
10. Reassess patient for improvement in signs and BP.

COMPLICATIONS OF THE PROCEDURE

1. **Skin irritation at pacing pad site**: Make sure skin is clean and dry before application, and limit pacing time to tie until underlying cause is resolved or a transvenous pacemaker is inserted.
2. **Skin burn at pacing pad site**: Skin should be dry with no medication patches present; limit transcutaneous pacing time.
3. **Failure to capture**: Proceed to transvenous pacemaker insertion.

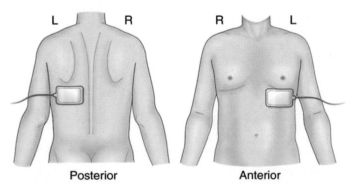

FIGURE 4.2. Anterior–posterior multifunction pad placement options. Reprinted with permission from Lynn, P. (2018). *Taylor's clinical nursing skills* (5th ed.). Wolters Kluwer.

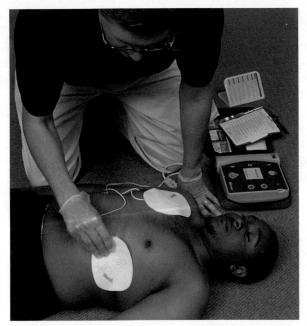

FIGURE 4.3. Anterior multifunction pad placement options. Reprinted with permission from Timby, B. K. (2017). *Fundamental nursing skills and concepts* (11th ed.). Wolters Kluwer.

All patients who are being noninvasively paced should be continually monitored by ECG, under constant direct observation, and be frequently assessed for mechanical and electrical capture.

Electrical capture occurs when a pacing stimulus leads to depolarization of the ventricles. It is confirmed by ECG changes typical of ventricular complexes—a widening of the QRS complex and a tall, broad T wave—displayed on the monitor *(See [A] and [B])*. The deflection of the captured complex may be positive or negative. Capture accompanying noninvasive pacing resembles that seen in permanent or temporary invasive pacing.

Mechanical capture is the contraction of the myocardium and is evidenced by presence of a pulse and signs of improved cardiac output. Both electrical and mechanical capture must occur to benefit the patient.

Many patients achieve capture at 50 to 90 mA, although individual thresholds vary markedly.[1,2,3] Capture thresholds are not related to body surface area or weight,[2,4] but recent thoracic surgery, pericardial effusion, pericardial tamponade, hypoxia, acidosis, and other physiologic variables may lead to higher capture thresholds.[2]

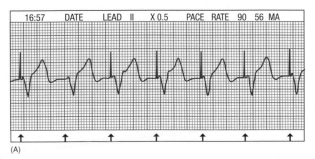

(A)

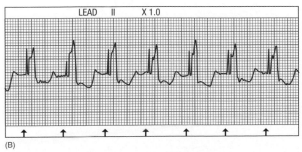

(B)

FIGURE 4.4. Electrical capture. Reproduced with permission from Medtronic.

POSTPROCEDURE CARE

After transcutaneous pacing has occurred, the advanced practice provider will want to monitor the effectiveness. Is electrical capture (a spike followed by a QRS) Figure 4.4(A) and (B) followed by mechanical capture (a pulse)? Reassess serious signs and BP. Search for an underlying cause such as overdose, myocardial infarction, and cardiomyopathy. Check electrolyte levels, especially calcium, magnesium, and potassium. Check the medication history for medications that prolong QT interval. Obtain an electrocardiogram, baseline laboratory studies, and troponins. Consult critical care and/or cardiology because the patient may require cardiac catheterization, critical care admission, and a specialist's care.

BIBLIOGRAPHY

American Heart Association. (2015). American Heart Association guidelines update for cardiopulmonary resuscitation and emergency cardiovascular care. *Circulation*, 132(18.2, Suppl.). www.ahajournals.org

Open Anesthesia. (2019). *Transcutaneous pacing*. https://www.openanesthesia.org/transcutaneous_pacing/

Cardioversion

Jennifer Coates

INDICATIONS FOR THE PROCEDURE

Electrical cardioversion is an important procedure for the management of cardiac dysrhythmias. During cardioversion, an electrical charge is delivered to the myocardium in an attempt to alter the patient's cardiac rhythm. Cardioversion is categorized as either synchronized cardioversion or unsynchronized cardioversion.

Synchronized Cardioversion

Synchronized cardioversion delivers a low-energy electrical charge to the myocardium that is timed with the QRS cycle. This can be done either urgently or nonurgently (electively). The intention of the charge is to cause immediate depolarization and interruption of the current rhythm and allows the sinoatrial node to resume control. Synchronizing the timing of the shock prevents delivery during the relative refractory period of repolarization (R on T), which could put the patient into ventricular fibrillation.

Urgent indications for synchronized cardioversion are:

1. Any persistent atrial tachyarrhythmia causing the patient to become unstable, as evidenced by hypotension, acutely altered mental status, signs of shock, ischemic chest discomfort, or acute heart failure can be considered for cardioversion.
   - Examples are atrial fibrillation, atrial flutter, atrial tachycardia, and supraventricular tachycardia.
2. Monomorphic ventricular tachycardia may also be treated with synchronized cardioversion when serious symptoms exist, such as chest pain, dyspnea, hypotension, change in level of consciousness. If the presence of distinct QRS and T wave is noted, then synchronized cardioversion is likely to be successful.

Nonurgent (elective) indications for synchronized cardioversion are:

1. Patients who have cardiac dysrhythmias but are clinically and hemodynamically stable. Cardioversion would be attempted in this population in an effort to restore normal sinus rhythm and usually occurs in an electrophysiology laboratory.

Unsynchronized Cardioversion (Defibrillation)

Unsynchronized cardioversion (also called defibrillation) delivers a high-energy electrical charge that is not synchronized with the QRS cycle. Defibrillation is used in situations when there is no coordinated intrinsic electrical activity in the heart. Defibrillation may be achieved using monophasic or biphasic energy, depending on the manufacturer of the equipment. In monophasic defibrillation, the energy travels unidirectionally, and a higher amount of energy is required to achieve results. In biphasic defibrillation, the electrical current first travels in a positive direction, then reverses in a negative direction. By delivering two currents of electricity, defibrillation can be achieved using smaller amounts of energy. It is helpful for providers to familiarize themselves with the type of equipment available at their medical institutions.

Indications for unsynchronized cardioversion are:

1. Pulseless ventricular tachycardia
2. Ventricular fibrillation

Anyone performing synchronized or unsynchronized cardioversion should refer to the American Heart Association Guidelines for CPR and ECC (2015).

SPECIAL CONSIDERATIONS AND CONTRAINDICATIONS FOR THE PROCEDURE

Since cardioversion is often an urgent/emergent procedure done on clinically unstable patients, true contraindications are rare. Patients are often at high risk for significant hemodynamic compromise without provider intervention. Primarily, there are special considerations of which the provider must be aware.

Special Considerations

1. Before performing this procedure, the provider must determine whether the patient is stable or unstable and whether the cardiac rhythm is appropriate for cardioversion.
2. Anticoagulation status must be evaluated. Atrial dysrhythmias may put the patient at an increased risk for clot development, which could become dislodged when normal sinus rhythm is restored.
3. In a stable patient, nothing by mouth (NPO) status prior to performing the procedure is preferred.
4. If the patient has an implanted pacemaker or defibrillator, do not place the adhesive pads directly over the device.
5. If the patient has any transdermal medication patch, do not place adhesive pads directly on the patch.
6. In elective cardioversion, consider evaluation of the left atrium/left atrial appendage by ultrasound to assess for presence or absence of a clot.

CONTRAINDICATIONS FOR THE PROCEDURE

Relative Contraindications

None.

Absolute Contraindications

1. Ensure that the provider and patient are in a safe environment prior to performing any electrical intervention on the patient. If environmental hazards exist, do not perform the procedure until safety is established, for example, move from water, dry, and then perform the intervention.

EQUIPMENT NEEDED

1. Cardioverter/defibrillator
2. Self-adhesive electrode defibrillator pads or paddles with conductive electrode gel or conductive gel pads
3. Cardiac monitor with electrodes
4. 12-lead ECG machine
5. Oxygen administration equipment
6. Suction equipment
7. Artificial airway and intubation supplies
8. Handheld resuscitation bag and mask
9. Emergency cardiac medications

STEPS TO PERFORMING THE PROCEDURE

Synchronized Cardioversion

1. Perform standard steps (see Preface).
2. Consider sedation if the patient is awake, alert, and hemodynamically able to tolerate.
3. Establish intravenous (IV) access before cardioversion if possible. Note: do not delay cardioversion if patient is extremely unstable.
4. Turn on the defibrillator and ensure that the device is placed in synchronized or "sync" mode (Figure 5.1).
5. Place cardiac leads on the patient and be sure you can visualize the rhythm on the cardiac monitor. Confirm that you have rhythm appropriate for cardioversion.
6. Place adhesive cardioversion pads on the patient according to instructions on the equipment. There are two typical placements of self-adhesive pads (Figure 5.2).
   a. *Anterolateral placement:* attach one pad to the upper right of the sternum, just below the clavicle. Place the second pad over the fifth or sixth intercostal space at the left anterior axillary line.

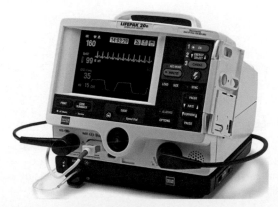

FIGURE 5.1. Portable monitor defibrillator.

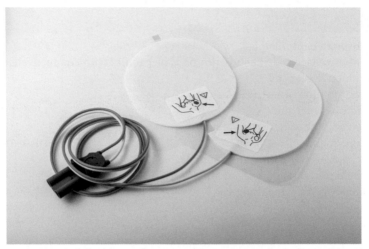

FIGURE 5.2. Multifunction adhesive cardioversion pads. Dario Lo Presti/ Shutterstock.

   b. *Anteroposterior placement*: attach the anterior pad directly over the heart at the precordium to the left of the lower sternal border. Place the posterior pad under the patient's body beneath the heart (Figure 5.3).

7. Observe the monitor; look for the dots or markers on the R waves.
8. Adjust the monitor gain if necessary until sync markers occur with each R wave.
9. Program the energy at the recommended doses for your cardioverter. Initial recommended doses by the American Heart Association Guidelines for CPR and ECC (2015) are as follows:
   a. Narrow regular rhythm: 50 to 100 J
   b. Narrow irregular rhythm: 120 to 200 J biphasic or 200 J monophasic
   c. Wide regular rhythm: 100 J

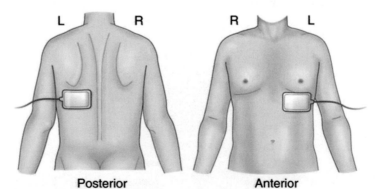

Posterior   Anterior

FIGURE 5.3. Anteroposterior placement of cardioversion pad. Reprinted with permission from Lynn, P. (2018). *Taylor's clinical nursing skills* (5th ed.). Wolters Kluwer.

10. Press the charge button.
11. Announce to the team members, "Charging defibrillator—stand clear." While the defibrillator is charging, ensure that no team members are touching the patient.
12. Press and hold the shock button. Note: there may be a delay between pressing the shock button and the shock delivery. This delay is caused by synchronization with the cardiac cycle.
13. After shock is delivered, assess the patient's heart rhythm to evaluate effectiveness:
    a. If narrow complex tachycardia persists, increase the energy level as per the manufacturer's specifications and American Heart Association guidelines, and repeat the shock.
    b. If the rhythm is terminated, obtain a 12-lead ECG and initiate supportive care.
    c. If the rhythm transitioned into ventricular fibrillation, proceed to defibrillation (unsynchronized cardioversion) and cardiopulmonary resuscitation (CPR).

Unsynchronized Cardioversion (Defibrillation)

It is important to note that defibrillation is only one part of the cardiac resuscitation process. It must be done in conjunction with high-quality CPR, airway management, and pharmacologic management. Please refer to the American Heart Association guidelines for more information.

1. Perform standard steps (see Preface).
2. Turn on the defibrillator.
3. Place cardiac leads on the patient and be sure you can visualize the rhythm on the cardiac monitor. Confirm that you have rhythm appropriate for defibrillation.
4. Place adhesive cardioversion pads on the patient according to instructions on the equipment. There are two typical placements of self-adhesive pads.
    a. *Anterolateral placement*: Attach one pad to the upper right of the sternum, just below the clavicle. Place the second pad over the fifth or sixth intercostal space at the left anterior axillary line.
    b. *Anteroposterior placement*: Attach the anterior pad directly over the heart at the precordium to the left of the lower sternal border. Place the posterior pad under the patient's body beneath the heart.
5. Program the energy at the recommended doses for your defibrillator. Initial recommended doses by the American Heart Association Guidelines for CPR and ECC (2015) are as follows:
    a. Monophasic device: 360 J
    b. Biphasic device: 200 J
6. Press the charge button.
7. Announce to the team members, "Charging defibrillator—stand clear." While the defibrillator is charging, ensure that no team members are touching the patient.
8. Press the shock button.
9. Resume chest compressions according to Advanced Cardiac Life Support (ACLS) guidelines.

COMPLICATIONS OF THE PROCEDURE

1. There is the risk that performing synchronized cardioversion will cause the rhythm to change into a lethal rhythm such as ventricular fibrillation or asystole.
2. There is the risk that the patient may suffer electrical burns on the skin from the cardioversion.
3. There is a risk of accidental electric shock to the team members during shock delivery. This can be minimized by ensuring that no team member is touching the patient prior to shock delivery.

POSTPROCEDURE CARE

Postprocedure care should focus on the patient's clinical condition and indication for cardioversion. In the case of an elective cardioversion, monitor the patient's heart rhythm, oxygenation status, and blood pressure (BP) post procedure. Most patients who are clinically stable after an elective cardioversion can be discharged home the same day. Ensure that the patient is provided with follow-up instructions, including any antidysrhythmic medication or anticoagulants that may be prescribed.

If the patient had an urgent synchronized cardioversion heart rhythm, oxygenation status and BP should be monitored post procedure. Differential diagnoses should be explored to determine the cause of the dysrhythmia, so appropriate treatment can be initiated. Pharmacologic agents should be considered to help promote heart rate and rhythm stabilization. If the patient had unsynchronized cardioversion as a component of a resuscitation attempt, postprocedure care would depend on the clinical outcome of the resuscitation. Postresuscitation care with the return of spontaneous circulation (ROSC) should include maintaining oxygen saturation greater than 94%, SBP greater than 90, assessing 12-lead ECGs, laboratory studies, and the need for targeted temperature management or coronary reperfusion.

BIBLIOGRAPHY

American Heart Association (2015). 2015 American Heart Association Guidelines update for cardiopulmonary resuscitation and emergency cardiovascular care. *Circulation, 132*(18), S313-S314. https://doi .org/10.1161/CIR.0000000000000307

American Heart Association (2016). *Advanced cardiac life support: Provider manual.* American Heart Association: Dallas, Texas.

Kirchhoh, P., Eckardt, L., & Loh, P. (2003). Anterior-posterior vs. anterior-lateral electrode positions for external cardioversion of atrial fibrillation: A randomized trial. *ACC Current Journal Review, 12*(2), 87. https://doi.org/10.1016/s1062-1458(03)00089-8

Knight, B. (2019). *Cardioversion for specific arrhythmias. UpToDate*, Topic 983, Version 38.0. https://www .uptodate.org

Starting an Intraosseous Infusion

Elizabeth Tomaszeweski

INDICATIONS FOR THE PROCEDURE

Intraosseous (IO) access provides a quick alternative when peripheral intravenous (IV) access is not possible or is difficult. Accomplished quickly with an intraosseous needle or commercially available devices, a large-bore needle is placed into the medullary cavity of a large bone mass. This provides a conduit for the infusion of fluids, medications, and blood products. Favored sites for insertion in adults include proximal tibia, proximal humerus, and sternum.

Indications for the procedure are:

1. Trauma
2. Cardiac arrest
3. Rapid deterioration in patient condition requiring vascular access

CONTRAINDICATIONS FOR THE PROCEDURE

Relative Contraindications

1. Ability to rapidly establish intravascular access

Absolute Contraindications

1. Fracture involving the bone of the intended site of insertion. This would permit the fluids to leak out of the cavity into the surrounding tissue.
2. Proximal ipsilateral vascular injury. This would allow the fluids/medications to leak out of the vessel.
3. Osteogenesis imperfecta.

EQUIPMENT NEEDED

1. Chlorhexidine or facility-approved skin preparation agent
2. Gloves
3. Commercial IO drill with needle, or bone marrow aspiration needle (such as Jamshidi), or IO infusion needle
4. Sterile stabilization dressing.

STEPS TO PERFORMING THE PROCEDURE

1. Perform standard steps (see Preface).
2. Choose infusion site.
   a. In adults, proximal humerus is favored for patient tolerance and easy accessibility. The arm should be placed in mild adduction, with the hand on the abdomen. This allows for better identification of the humeral head. The insertion point is 1 cm above the surgical neck, pointing into the greater tuberosity.
   b. Medial malleolus is also acceptable, inserting the IO needle along the medial surface of the distal tibia at the junction of the medial malleolus directed cephalad.
   c. Tibial placement in adults is often difficult due to hardened bone and is better accessed with a commercial device. The IO should be inserted 1 to 3 cm distal of the tibial tuberosity, over the medial tibia, and pointed away from the joint space on insertion.
   d. The sternum may also be used, because it is a large, flat bone with rapid transit.
3. Prepare the skin in sterile fashion.
4. Stabilize the site with the nondominant hand.
5. If using a commercial drill device, puncture the skin and use gentle pressure while squeezing the trigger on the drill. Proceed until resistance is relieved, indicating that the needle has entered the marrow cavity (Figure 6.1).

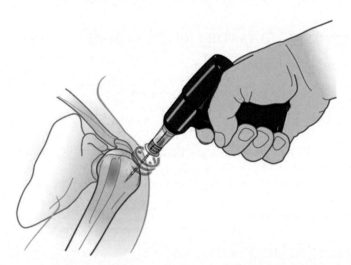

FIGURE 6.1. Proximal humerus intraosseous (IO) insertion site. IO insertion is the greater tubercle approximately 1 cm above the surgical neck and directed at a 45° angle to the anterior plane to avoid the epiphyseal plate. The patient's hand should rest on the abdomen, with the elbow adducted to internally rotate the humerus and protect the intertubercular groove. Image courtesy of Teleflex Incorporated. © 2021 Teleflex Incorporated. All rights reserved.

6. If using a manual needle, hold perpendicular to the bone and use constant pressure with a twisting motion until resistance is relieved. Remove the stylet (Figure 6.2).
7. Confirm placement by aspiration of marrow, or flow of fluids without extravasation.
8. Secure the IO needle with gauze and bulky dressing or commercial stabilization dressing.
9. X-ray to confirm placement and exclude iatrogenic fracture.

COMPLICATIONS OF THE PROCEDURE

1. **Dislodgement:** The IO should be immediately discontinued and another site accessed.
2. **Infiltration:** The IO should be immediately discontinued and another site accessed.
3. **Osteomyelitis/site infection:** The IO should be immediately discontinued and another site accessed. Antibiotics should be administered.

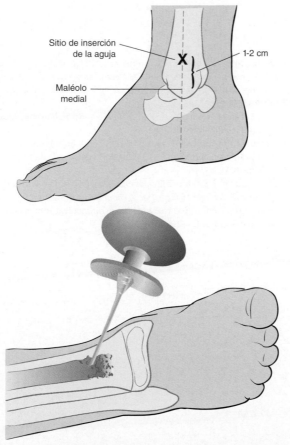

FIGURE 6.2. Intraosseous infusion. Reprinted with permission from Hodge, D. III. (2007). Intraosseous infusion. In C. King, & F. Henretig (eds.), *Textbook of pediatric emergency procedures* (2nd ed.). Williams & Wilkins.

4. **Fracture or epiphyseal plate injury:** The IO should be immediately discontinued and another site accessed.
5. **Fat embolus:** Supportive care should be provided.

POSTPROCEDURE CARE

After insertion, an x-ray should be performed to determine proper placement and exclude fracture of the bone. If fracture or misplacement is noted, the IO should be removed and another site chosen. All fluids and medications should be discontinued from a site with fracture or extravasation, because tissue necrosis or sloughing could occur.

If the patient is responsive to pain, providers may consider the use of lidocaine instillation prior to infusion. Slowly infuse 2 to 5 mL of 2% preservative-free lidocaine followed by 10 mL of normal saline over 1 minute. Analgesic effect is approximately 1 hour. The patient may require further pain control, such as opiates, owing to the pain of infusion.

BIBLIOGRAPHY

Deitch, K. (2019). Intraoseous infusion. In A. S. Chanmugam, C. R. Chudnofsky, P. M. DeBlieux, A. Mattu, S. P. Swadron, & M. E. Winters (Eds.), *Roberts and Hedges' clinical procedures in emergency medicine and acute care* (Chapter 25, pp. 461–475.e3). Elsevier. https://www-clinicalkey-com.ezproxy2.library.drexel .edu/#!/content/book/3-s2.0-B9780323354783000257

Marcucci, C., Gierl, B. T., & Kirsch, J. R. (2020). *Avoiding common anesthesia errors* (2nd ed.). Wolters Kluwer. Originally © 2017 Teleflex Incorporated.

Shah, K. H., & Mason, C. (2015). *Essential emergency procedures* (2nd ed.). Wolters Kluwer. Originally from Hodge, D. III. (2008). Intraosseous infusion. In C. King & F. Henretig (Eds.), *Textbook of pediatric emergency procedures*. Williams & Wilkins.

Wyatt, C. (2019). Vascular access. In J. E. Tintinalli, J. Stapczynski, O. Ma, D. M. Yealy, G. D. Meckler, & D. M. Cline (Eds.), *Tintinalli's emergency medicine: A comprehensive study guide (8th ed.)*. McGraw-Hill. Retrieved December 16, 2019, from http://accessmedicine.mhmedical.com.ezproxy2.library.drexel.edu/ content.aspx?bookid=1658&sectionid=109427625

CHAPTER 7

Pulmonary Catheter Insertion

Steven Bocchese

The first known cardiac catheterization was in 1929. The rudimentary catheterization occurred when a Dr. Werner Forssmann inserted a urinary catheter into his basilic vein and into the right side of his heart. This groundbreaking technique led to further cardiac catheterizations as well as development of the pulmonary artery catheter (PAC).

In 1970, Dr. Jeremy Swan developed a balloon-tipped catheter with the purpose of floating it into the pulmonary artery. The idea was developed while he was on vacation with his family, watching sailboats sailing with ease with even the lightest of breezes. Simultaneously, Dr. William Ganz was developing thermodilution technology to calculate cardiac output as well as other cardiac pressures. The combination of the two became known as the Swan–Ganz catheter.

The Swan–Ganz catheter measures:

- Right pulmonary systolic and diastolic pressures (PAP)
- Pulmonary artery wedge pressure (PAWP)
- Cardiac index (CI)
- Systemic and pulmonary vascular resistance (SVR, PVR)
- Core body temperature
- Mixed venous oxygen saturation

The use of the Swan–Ganz catheter or PAC has revolutionized the treatment of the critically ill. The use of a PAC has decreased in recent years owing to noninvasive technology for cardiac monitoring but is still used in critically ill patients that fit the criteria.

INDICATIONS FOR THE PROCEDURE

The use of a PAC can yield important information about the critically ill patient. It can provide real-time data that will influence management. The indications for pulmonary artery insertion are:

1. Severe cardiogenic shock
2. Pulmonary artery hypertension—suspected or known
3. Unknown volume status in shock state
4. Unexplained dyspnea

5. Evaluation of left-to-right intracardiac shunt
6. Evaluation for pericardial tamponade
7. Severe underlying cardiopulmonary disease status post cardiothoracic surgery
8. Multiorgan failure

CONTRAINDICATIONS FOR THE PROCEDURE

The PAC is a useful tool when used correctly in the previously mentioned indications. However, insertion is not always an acceptable or safe option.

Absolute Contraindications
1. Infection at the insertion site
2. Lack of consent
3. Right ventricular assist device (RVAD) in place
4. Insertion during cardiopulmonary bypass

Relative Contraindications
1. Coagulopathy: international normalized ratio (INR) greater than 1.5
2. Thrombocytopenia: platelet count less than 50,000/μL
3. Electrolyte disturbances (hypo- or hyperkalemia, -calcemia, -magnesium)
4. Severe acidosis or alkalosis

EQUIPMENT NEEDED

The advanced practice provider should bring into the room all the necessary equipment and place it in an orderly fashion. Assistance from another healthcare professional is also important. Equipment needed includes

1. Sterile gown, drapes, gloves
2. Sterile central line dressing kit
3. PAC
    a. Sheath
    b. Lumens
4. Thermodilution catheter introducer set
5. 500 mL 5% dextrose
6. Cardiac output module and cable
7. Electrocardiogram (ECG) and two pressure modules and cables
8. Pressure bag
9. Two pressure transducers
10. Two pressure line extension tubing
11. 500 mL 0.9% sodium chloride
12. 5 and 10 mL syringes
13. Scalpel
14. 4×4 gauze
15. 2-0 silk suture

16. Two 3-way stopcocks
17. 21G, 23G, and 25G needles

STEPS TO PERFORMING PULMONARY ARTERY INSERTION

It is important for the advanced practice provider to develop a strategy when inserting a PAC. Performing the steps for PAC insertion the same way every time ensures that no step is missed and safety is maintained.

Insertion of sheath

1. Put on sterile personal protective equipment (PPE) (gown, gloves, and mask).
2. Prepare and drape the intended insertion site.
3. Place patient into preferred position. Trendelenburg positioning may help make insertion easier.
4. Prime lines and level transducers.
5. Inject 1% lidocaine to surgical site.
6. Attach the introducer needle to the 10 mL syringe.
7. With the use of the ultrasound, find the desired vein and insert introducer needle using the Seldinger technique.
8. Once the introducer needle is in the desired vessel, check for dark nonpulsatile blood when aspirating.
9. Remove the introducer needle and use the ultrasound to confirm that the guide-wire is in the vein and not in the artery or soft tissue.
10. Make a small skin incision with the scalpel and dilate the soft tissue with the dilator.
11. Thread the sheath over the guidewire while simultaneously pulling the wire out through the port. Once the wire is removed and the line in place, suture the line to the skin.

Insertion of PAC

1. Flush the PAC through all the ports and inflate the balloon to ensure patency. Hook the transducer to the PAC and the monitor.
2. Insert the PAC through the hemostasis valve on the sheath. Generally, the balloon on the catheter is clear of the sheath after it has been inserted about 18 cm.
3. Next, inflate the balloon and close the red port to ensure the balloon remains inflated.
4. Continued to advance the catheter into the right atrium and look to the monitor for a central venous pressure (CVP)/right atrial (RA) waveform.
5. Advance the catheter with the balloon inflated through the right atrium into the right ventricle and into the pulmonary artery. Monitor for the appropriate waveform on the module with the associated region of the heart (RA–RA–PA) (Figure 7.1).
6. Deflate the balloon and confirm the PAP tracing on the module. The catheter insertion length is between 50 and 60 cm when inserting from the internal jugular or subclavian vein. Mark the exact insertion length in the documentation.

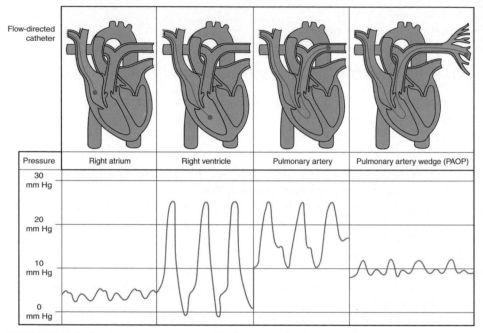

FIGURE 7.1. Pulmonary artery catheter (PAC) waveforms as the catheter progresses through the cardiac chambers. Reprinted with permission from Shaffner, D. H., & Nichols, D. G. (2015). *Rogers's textbook of pediatric intensive care* (5th ed.). Wolters Kluwer.

7. Transduce the CVP or the proximal port and assess the waveform. The practitioner may now hook up medications or intravenous fluids to the extra ports on the catheter. Connect the thermodilution cable and temperature cable to the red port.
8. The insertion site should be cleaned and a dressing should be placed.
9. Order a chest x-ray to confirm placement and to assess for any lung damage caused during the sheath insertion (Figure 7.2). The catheter should be 2 cm left of the mediastinal border.
10. Check the cardiac monitoring numbers.
11. Document the procedure.

COMPLICATIONS OF THE PROCEDURE

When inserting a PAC, the advanced practice provider must consider all possible complications that may occur with insertion and attempt to minimize the risk. Unfortunately, complications do occur, especially in a critically ill population. These complications are broken down into three categories: insertion, maintenance and use, and misinterpretation.

Insertion
1. **Dysrhythmias:** Ventricular dysrhythmias, right bundle branch block (in about 5% of insertions), left bundle branch block (which places patient at risk for complete heart block)

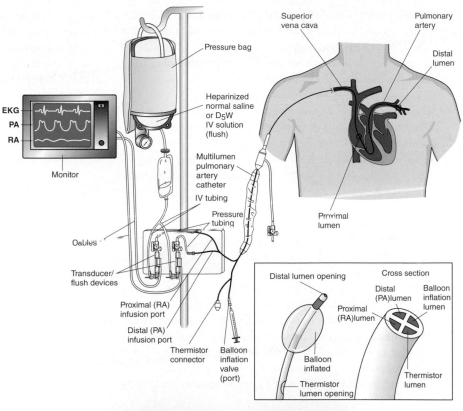

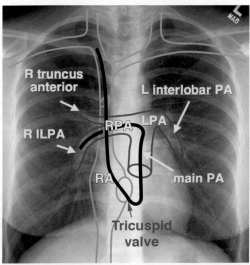

FIGURE 7.2. Correct placement of a PAC evidenced on a chest x-ray. EKG, electrocardiogram; ILPA, interlobar pulmonary artery; LPA, left pulmonary artery; PA, pulmonary artery; IV, intravenous; RA, right atrial; RPA, right pulmonary artery. Reprinted with permission from Smeltzer, S. C., & Bare, B. G. (2000). *Textbook of medical-surgical nursing* (9th ed.). Lippincott Williams & Wilkins.

2. **Misplacement:** Tip of the of catheter loops in the right atrium or right ventricle
3. **Knotting:** Suspect when the PAC does not reach the pulmonary artery or the advanced practice provider meets resistance with withdrawal. If knotting is suspected, the provider should order a chest x-ray or computed tomography of the chest to assess for knotting. The knot may be released by injecting 10 to 20 mL of cold sterile saline, placement of a guidewire to unknot, or even a surgical intervention
4. **Myocardial, vessel, or valve rupture:** Suspect if the patient develops an acute onset of shortness of breath or respiratory failure and shock
5. **Pneumothorax:** Upon sheath introduction
6. **Arterial cannulation:** Remove and hold pressure; hold for 5 minutes per French sheath (i.e., for an 8 Fr sheath, hold pressure for 40 minutes.)

Maintenance and Use
1. **Pulmonary artery perforation:** Occurs when the balloon is overinflated. This commonly occurs when the distal end is positioned in the distal pulmonary artery. This complication results in a range of 30% to 70% mortality rates
2. **Pulmonary infarction:** May occur when the catheter migrates and blocks the smaller pulmonary artery branches, leading to infarction
3. **Thromboembolism:** Catheter-induced thrombus
4. **Infection:** Endocarditis or central line-related bacteremia; perform proper sterile central line care during insertion and during maintenance to prevent infection
5. **Valvular vegetations:** Generally develop when the PAC is left in place for a prolonged period
6. **Venous air embolism:** Caused by open infusion ports on the catheter

Misinterpretation
1. Owing to miscalibration of the monitoring system or if the pressure monitors are unleveled. Remember that data interpretation should take place when the patient is lying flat and supine and the pressure monitors should be leveled at the phlebostatic axis
2. Variability among providers of waveform interpretation
3. Improper estimation of the PAWP caused by improper inflation of the balloon, possibly because of migration of the catheter

POSTPROCEDURE CARE

Once the sheath and PAC are in place, a sterile dressing should be maintained to avoid a central line infection or potential bacteremia. The insertion site should be checked daily to monitor for any signs of infection at the skin insertion site. A sheath sleeve can be used to cover the entire PAC outside of the body to allow for sterility if manipulation of the PAC is required. The advanced practice provider should assess the need and utility of the PAC catheter daily. Once it is decided that the PAC is no longer needed, it should be removed promptly.

BIBLIOGRAPHY

Gerald, W. (2019a). Pulmonary artery catheterizations: Indications, contraindications, and complications in adults. *UptoDate.*

Gerald, W. (2019b). Pulmonary artery catheterizations: Insertion technique in adults. *UptoDate.*

Nekic, P. (2016). *Pulmonary artery catheter learning package. Intensive Care: Learning Packages.* https://www.aci.health.nsw.gov.au/__data/assets/pdf_file/0004/306589/Pulmonary_Catheter_Learning_Package.pdf

CHAPTER

8 Endotracheal Intubation

Steven Bocchese

Endotracheal intubation is commonplace for the emergency department, intensive care units, and the emergency room. It is a procedure that can be accomplished when all correct steps are taken and the patient has a normal anatomy. Unfortunately, this is not always the case. When the proper steps are not taken, the operator is unskilled at endotracheal intubation or inefficient, or the patient has a difficult airway, life-threatening outcomes occur.

The procedure of endotracheal intubation requires planning and, at times, quick decision making. Difficulty during the procedure can lead to hypoxemia, hypotension, and even cardiac arrest.

INDICATIONS FOR THE PROCEDURE

Indications for endotracheal intubation fit into a few categories. However, it is for the operator to assess a patient's indication for endotracheal intubation and act on this. The timing for intubation is a learned skill. Using clinical judgment and knowing the indications for intubation will help the practitioner acquire that skill. Indications are:

1. Poor oxygenation and/or ventilation
2. Airway protection
   a. Decreased level of consciousness
   b. Status epilepticus
   c. Confusion with vomiting
3. Prolonged course
   a. Worsening respiratory failure
   b. Sepsis: bacterial or viral causes
   c. Acute respiratory distress syndrome (ARDS)
   d. Recurrent operations needed
   e. Profuse hemoptysis

CONTRAINDICATIONS FOR THE PROCEDURE

Few absolute contraindications exist for endotracheal intubation. However, endotracheal intubation may not be indicated in certain patients because of difficulty performing the procedure. In that case, other airway securement procedures must be performed.

Absolute Contraindications
1. **Severe airway trauma:** Consider surgical airway procedure
2. **Airway obstruction:** Consider surgical airway procedure

Relative Contraindications
1. **Severe laryngeal or supralaryngeal edema:** Caused by infection, burn or anaphylaxis
2. **Anatomy:** Abnormal anatomical features
3. **Operator:** Experience or skill of the operator
4. **Reported as difficult intubation:**
   a. Prior difficult intubation
   b. Thyromental distance
   c. Sternomental distance
   d. Decreased head and neck extension
   e. Mallampati score of 3 or 4
   f. Mandibular protrusion
   g. Neck circumference of greater than 40 cm
   h. Submental compliance
   i. Poor dentition

If a patient meets the criteria for contraindications but requires a mechanical airway, a surgical airway (i.e., cricothyrotomy, emergency tracheostomy), fiberoptic, or awake intubation must be considered.

EQUIPMENT NEEDED

Preparation and having equipment available can make the difference between a safe and quick intubation versus multiple attempts with potential decompensation of the patient. Developing a checklist of equipment and personnel needed before intubating is crucial.

1. Suction and yankauer available
2. Oral airway
3. Nasopharyngeal airway
4. Oxygen-nasal cannula, bag-valve mask, noninvasive ventilation machine, nonrebreather mask, Venti-mask
5. Bag-valve mask with positive end-expiratory pressure (PEEP) valve
6. Cardiac monitoring and continuous pulse oximetry monitoring
7. Multiple-sized endotracheal tubes
8. Stylet

9. Lubricant jelly
10. Macintosh #3 or #4 blade, Miller blade, or video laryngoscopy (Figure 8.1)
11. Light source
12. Bougie
13. Good intravenous (IV) access
14. IV fluids, isotonic fluids
15. Medications
    a. Analgesia: fentanyl, dilaudid
    b. Paralytic/muscle relaxant: vecuronium, succinylcholine, rocuronium
    c. Anesthetic agent: etomidate
    d. Vasopressor: phenylephrine, norepinephrine
    e. Ketamine or benzodiazepine for delayed sequence intubation
    f. Sedation after endotracheal tube is placed (i.e., propofol, versed, fentanyl)
16. Qualified personnel: Nurses, nursing technicians, respiratory therapist, other advanced practice providers, and anesthesiologist if a difficult airway is reported
17. Ventilator
18. Capnography
19. Arterial blood gas (ABG) kit for postintubation ABG sample
20. Surgical airway setup close by

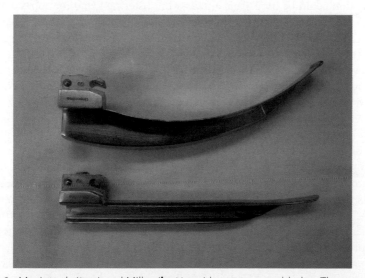

FIGURE 8.1. Macintosh (**top**) and Miller (**bottom**) laryngoscope blades. The curved blade is a size 4 German Macintosh, which is a good blade for routine use in adults, unlike the American design, which has a taller flange height. The straight blade is a size 3 Miller, for normal-sized adults. Most Miller blades have the light on the left side (as shown here), which can embed in the tongue, but better designs place the light on the right side of the blade. From Brown, C. A. III, Sakles, J. C., & Mick, N. W. (2017). *Walls manual of emergency airway management* (5th ed.). Wolters Kluwer and The Difficult Airway Course (www.theairwaysite.com). Used with permission.

STEPS TO PERFORMING THE PROCEDURE

An advanced practice provider that follows the proper steps for intubation will provide a safe and effective intubation. Depending on the clinical condition, some of the steps will be changed or canceled. It is important during those times to have anesthesia available if needed.

Oral intubation
1. Have all the appropriate staff and equipment available and ready.
2. Begin preoxygenating the patient, using a nasal cannula, nonrebreather mask, bag-valve mask (BVM) or noninvasive ventilation machine (BiPap, CPAP).
3. Positioning of the patient is key. If there is no cervical injury suspected, place the patient in the "sniffing" position. The "sniffing" position is when the patient performs an atlanto-occipital extension with head elevation (Figure 8.2).
4. Have a bag of IV fluids hooked to the patient's IV access and slowly infusing.
5. In a firm voice, tell the healthcare professional who is drawing up medications which medications you would like to be given and the exact dosage you will use.
6. The gold standard for medication selection is a rapid sequence intubation (RSI). This includes the administration of an anesthetic agent followed immediately by the administration of a muscle relaxant. If RSI is not an option, a delayed sequence intubation could be used. This entails administering ketamine to relax the patient without compromising the respiratory status prior to RSI.
7. Select your blade and size (direct laryngoscopy would include a light source to attach the blade to, and the blade to a video laryngoscopy is usually attachable and disposable) as well as endotracheal tube size. Place the stylet into the endotracheal tube and lubricate the tip with the lubricant jelly.
8. Begin the RSI as you slowly ventilate the patient.
9. Once the patient is properly anesthetized, open the jaw with your nondominant hand in a scissors motion. For a Macintosh blade, next insert the blade into the side of the mouth and move the tongue out of the way with the blade. Next, take the blade and elevate the tongue and soft tissue in an upward motion, being careful not to rock the blade against the teeth. At this point, you should see the vocal cords and epiglottis. Gently push the tip of the blade superior to the epiglottis to the vallecula to provide a better view of the vocal cords. At this time cricoid pressure may be applied if the advanced practice provider chooses to ask for it (Figure 8.3).
10. Once the vocal cords are in view and any suctioning of oral secretions is completed, take the endotracheal tube with the stylet in place and insert into the vocal cords.
11. Once the endotracheal tube is in place, inflate the balloon cuff.
12. Monitoring with a pulse oximetry and telemetry should be taking place during the entire procedure. The use of end-tidal carbon dioxide measuring should be used as real-time data measurement for proper placement.
13. Ordering a confirmatory chest x-ray may be policy at your institution (Figure 8.4).

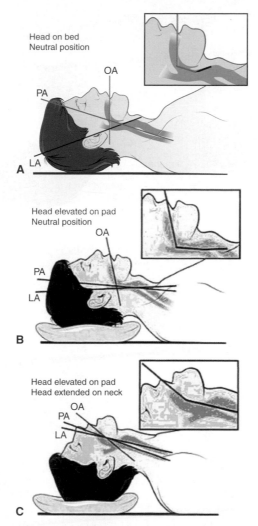

FIGURE 8.2. Understanding aligning the oral axis (OA), pharyngeal axis (PA), and laryngeal axis (LA). (A) Anatomical neutral position. The OA, PA, and LA are at greater angles to one another. (B) Head, still in neutral position, has been lifted by a pillow flexing the lower cervical spine and aligning the PA and the LA. (C) The head has been extended on the cervical spine, aligning OA with the PA and the LA, creating the optimum sniffing position for intubation. Reprinted with permission from Brown, C. A., Sakles, J. C. & Mick, N. W. (2017). *The Walls Manual of Emergency Airway Management* (5th ed.). Lippincott Williams & Wilkins.

Nasal intubation
1. Perform the same setup as for an oral intubation.
2. After the patient is preoxygenated and anesthetized, insert the endotracheal tube through the selected nostril.

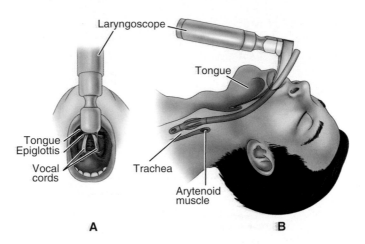

FIGURE 8.3. Endotracheal intubation in a patient without a cervical spine injury. (A) The primary glottis landmarks for tracheal intubation as visualized with proper placement of the laryngoscope. (B) Positioning the endotracheal tube. Reprinted with permission from Honan, L. (2018). *Focus on adult health* (2nd ed.). Wolters Kluwer.

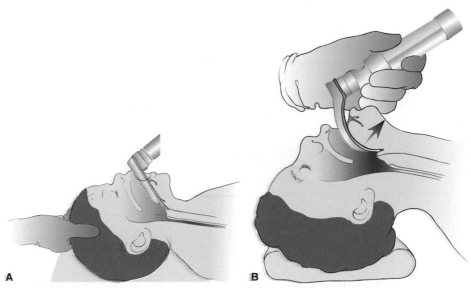

FIGURE 8.4. (A) Direct laryngoscopy using a straight blade. The tip of the blade is used to directly retract the epiglottis, revealing the vocal cords and glottic opening. (B) Direct laryngoscopy using a curved blade. The blade is inserted under direct vision until the tip is positioned in the vallecula. Pulling upward on the laryngoscope handle at 45° angle retracts the tongue while elevating the epiglottis, revealing the vocal cords and glottis. Reprinted with permission from King, C., & Stayer, S. A. (2007). Emergent endotracheal intubation. In C. King, & F. Henretig (eds.), *Textbook of pediatric emergency procedures* (2nd ed.). Williams & Wilkins.

3. Use a Macintosh blade to perform direct laryngoscopy.
4. When the tube is visualized, use a Magill forceps to pull the tube proximal to the cuff toward the glottic opening.
5. Continue to guide the tube with the Magill forceps while inserting the tube through the nostril until it is past the vocal cords.
6. Confirm placement with an end-tidal carbon dioxide measurement and/or a chest x-ray.

COMPLICATIONS OF THE PROCEDURE

Patients can undergo endotracheal intubation in a controlled environment such as prior to surgery for general anesthesia or in emergent situations as in respiratory failure. Complications are more likely to occur in the acute situations but can still happen in the elective intubation. A difficult airway or a challenging intubation can cause complications that may be life threatening. Complications include:

1. Sore throat
2. Hemodynamic changes
3. Aspiration
4. Hypoxia
5. Airway trauma
6. Bronchospasm
7. Damage to vocal cords
8. Damage to teeth
9. Esophageal intubation
10. Airway edema
11. Bleeding
12. Right main stem intubation
13. Pneumothorax
14. Cardiac arrest and death

POSTPROCEDURE CARE

Once the endotracheal tube is securely attached, a trained professional should assess bilateral lung sounds. If lung sounds are not heard or are softly auscultated on the left side, there is a chance the endotracheal tube is in the right main stem bronchial. If this is the case, the endotracheal tube must be withdrawn. IV fluids should be ordered if there is no contraindication for them, and a sedation infusion should be started if deemed necessary. A chest x-ray is to be ordered to assess placement of the endotracheal tube and the surrounding structures. The tip of the endotracheal tube should be 2 to 3 cm above the carina. Once the endotracheal tube placement is checked, the ventilator should be set up with the settings you have chosen. After an hour of the ventilator setup, an ABG should be drawn to assess for hypercapnia and for hypoxemia. After receiving the results of the ABG, make proper changes to the ventilator. Document your procedure and any important information not covered by the electronic note writer. Document the patient's dentition and at what measurement the endotracheal tube is located. For nasal intubations, the steps are similar, but a surgical airway kit should be placed at the bedside.

Placing an endotracheal tube can make the difference between saving a person's life or not. Improperly placing the endotracheal tube or being unprepared for the intubation can result in patient harm and poor outcomes. It is the advanced practice provider's job to be prepared with all the equipment needed and to surround the patient with important members of the multidisciplinary team.

BIBLIOGRAPHY

Avva, U. (2021, January 15). *Airway management*. StatPearls [Internet]. https://www.ncbi.nlm.nih.gov/books/NBK470403/

Orebaugh, S., & Snyder, J. (2020). Direct laryngoscopy and endotracheal intubation in adults. *UpToDate*.

Waltz, C. F., Strickland, O. L., & Lenz, E. R. (2017). *Measurement in nursing and health research*. Springer Publishing Company.

Tube Thoracostomy (Chest Tube) Placement

Dana McCloskey
Salina Wydo

INDICATIONS FOR THE PROCEDURE

Tube thoracostomy (chest tube) insertion is one of the most common procedures performed in cases of thoracic trauma or in the critical care patient. The goal of chest tube placement is to evacuate the pleural space of blood, air, or fluid; allow reexpansion of lung parenchyma; and permit adequate oxygenation and ventilation. The decision to place a chest tube should be dictated by the clinical status of the patient but is supplemented by imaging such as conventional chest radiograph, computed tomography (CT), or ultrasound scan.

The most common indications for chest tube placement are:

1. Hemothorax
2. Pneumothorax with or without tension (Figure 9.1)
   a. It is recommended that a chest tube be placed in any patient with traumatic pneumothorax who requires positive pressure ventilation to prevent the development of a tension pneumothorax. In all other cases, a chest tube should be placed in cases of pneumothorax greater than or equal to 20% of the pleural space.
3. Symptomatic pleural effusion
4. Empyema

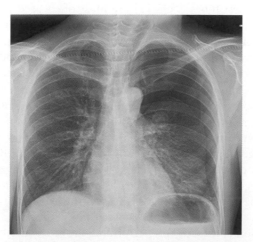

FIGURE 9.1. Expiratory radiograph shows enlargement of the pneumothorax. Reprinted with permission from Daffner, R. H., & Hartman, M. (2013). *Clinical radiology* (4th ed.). Wolters Kluwer.

CONTRAINDICATIONS FOR THE PROCEDURE

Ultimately, the decision to pursue chest tube placement should be made after careful consideration of the risks versus benefits to the individual patient.

Relative Contraindications

1. Blebs or severe bullous disease, as injury to blebs or bullous segments increases the risk of persistent air leak
2. Dense adhesions, as seen in patients who have previously undergone thoracic surgery or pleurodesis, as adhesive disease increases the risk for iatrogenic lung injury
3. Coagulopathy or systemic anticoagulation

Absolute Contraindications

There are no absolute contraindications to chest tube placement.

EQUIPMENT NEEDED

1. Antiseptic for skin preparation (the authors use chlorhexidine)
2. Personal protective equipment, including sterile drape for surgical field
3. Local anesthetic, such as 1% lidocaine with or without epinephrine (the authors also administer intravenous analgesia and occasionally sedation if the patient's clinical status permits)
4. Scalpel
5. Two hemostats or two Kelly clamps
6. Chest tube (the authors most commonly use 28 Fr)
   a. There is no consensus recommendation for chest tube size. In trauma, large-bore chest tubes (>32 Fr) are most often used because the increased diameter is believed to allow for faster evacuation of hemothorax and reduce the risk of chest tube clotting and obstruction; however, this is not currently supported by published data. In a large prospective study comparing small-bore (28–32 Fr) with large-bore (36–40 Fr) chest tubes in the management of hemothorax and pneumothorax, no statistically significant difference in the rate of complications was found. In the hemothorax group, there was no statistically significant difference in initial chest tube output or the incidence of retained hemothorax between small-bore and large-bore groups. In the pneumothorax group, there was no statistically significant difference in the rate of unresolved pneumothorax or need for chest tube reinsertion in small- and large-bore groups. For patients with uncomplicated pneumothorax, a 14 Fr pigtail catheter is associated with less pain without any clinically significant advantages compared with tube thoracostomy. The size of chest tube used is at the discretion of the surgeon performing the procedure.
7. Nonabsorbable suture such as 0 silk
8. Sterile dressings: split 4×4 gauze, ABD pad, silk tape

9. Drainage and collecting system, such as a Pleur-evac®, assembled per manufacturer instructions

STEPS TO PERFORMING THE PROCEDURE

The location of chest tube placement may vary according to indications. Small-bore (e.g., 14 Fr) chest tubes may be placed via the Seldinger technique at the second or third inter-costal space anteriorly for pneumothorax or posteriorly at the sixth intercostal space for pleural effusions. In this section, we describe the classic placement of a large-bore tube thoracostomy in the midaxillary line at the level of the fifth intercostal space (Figure 9.2). If chest tube placement is not emergent, the procedure should be described to the patient and informed consent obtained. During the procedure, the patient should be observed on a cardiac monitor with supplemental oxygen available

1. Perform Standard Steps (see Preface).
2. The patient should be supine, head of bed elevated to approximately 30° with ipsi-lateral arm abducted to at least 90° and flexed. This permits exposure of the planned insertion site and expansion of intercostal spaces to facilitate chest tube placement.
3. Identify anatomical landmarks, including the lateral edge of the pectoralis major (anteriorly), base of the axilla (superiorly), anterior border of the latissimus dorsi

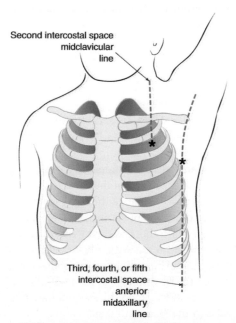

Second intercostal space midclavicular line

Third, fourth, or fifth intercostal space anterior midaxillary line

FIGURE 9.2. Possible sites for chest tube placement. Reprinted with permission from Connors, K. M., & Terndrup, T. E. (1997). Tube thoracostomy and needle decompression of the chest. In F. M. Henretig, & C. King (eds.), *Textbook of pediatric emergency procedures.* Lippincott Williams & Wilkins.

(posteriorly), and the nipple (inferiorly). In males, the fifth intercostal space is traditionally identified at the level of the nipple. In females, the inframammary fold should be used as a landmark to identify the fifth intercostal space.

4. If indicated by clinical status, administer systemic sedation and analgesics.
5. Prior to putting on sterile gown and gloves, the Pleur-evac® drainage system should be connected to suction and set up according to manufacturer instructions to create a water seal.
6. Set up a sterile field, including equipment and chest tube. A Kelly clamp (or hemostat) should be placed on the distal end of the chest tube to avoid leakage of fluid once the chest tube is inserted into the pleural space. A Kelly clamp should also be placed on the proximal end of the chest tube to guide insertion into the pleural cavity. The tip of the Kelly clamp should be in line with (i.e., parallel to) the end of the chest tube to avoid trauma to surrounding tissues on insertion.
7. Widely prepare the area of insertion with chlorhexidine or betadine solution.
8. Place sterile drapes over the procedure area (the authors use a full-body drape).
9. Inject local anesthetic at the previously determined insertion site, including the skin, subcutaneous tissues, and periosteum of the underlying ribs.
10. Create a 2 cm transverse skin incision over the fifth intercostal space.
11. Using a Kelly clamp, bluntly dissect the subcutaneous tissue until reaching the periosteum of the sixth rib/intercostal muscles of the fifth intercostal space (Figure 9.3(A)).
12. Using steady pressure, guide the tip of the Kelly clamp over the superior border of the sixth rib to enter into the pleural space. One finger should be placed approximately 2 cm away from the tip of the Kelly clamp prior to insertion to limit the risk of parenchymal injury on entry into the pleural space (see Figure 9.3(A)).
13. Once in the pleural space, open the Kelly clamp widely in the direction of the intercostal space to dissect the intercostal muscles, and develop a tract for chest tube insertion. Remove the Kelly clamp.
14. Using an index finger, explore the pleural cavity for adhesions. If able, gently dissect any adhesions. If adhesions are dense and prominent, an alternative chest tube site must be identified (Figure 9.3(B)).
15. Insert the chest tube alongside your index finger within the dissected tract using the Kelly clamp on the proximal end of the chest tube as a guide (Figure 9.3(C)).
16. Once within the pleural space, remove the Kelly clamp from the proximal end of the tube and direct the chest tube posteriorly and apically.
17. Insert the chest tube to a depth that ensures all drainage holes are within the pleural cavity. Any resistance encountered with advancing the chest tube should indicate the need for the chest tube to be redirected or an alternative site to be chosen.
18. Connect the chest tube to the drainage system with suction set at negative 20 cm H_2O. An assistant may be asked to do this, so you may maintain sterility.
19. Secure the chest tube to the skin with 0 silk suture. The securing stitch should be placed to reapproximate the edges of the incision around the chest tube to limit the risk of air leak.
20. Place sterile dressings over the chest tube site; usually, split gauze and ABD trauma pads with silk tape will suffice.
21. Follow-up chest x-ray must be obtained to confirm intrathoracic placement, satisfactory depth of placement, and resolution of underlying pathology.

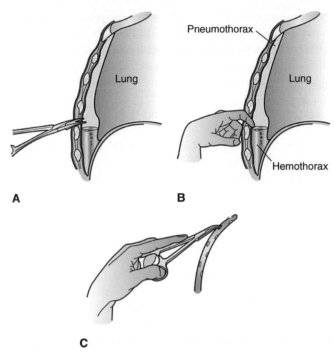

FIGURE 9.3. Tube thoracostomy placement. (A) Pleural space entered by blunt spreading of the clamp over the top of the adjacent rib. (B) A finger is introduced to ensure position within the pleural space and to lyse adhesions. (C) The thoracostomy tube is placed into the tunnel and directed with the help of a Kelly clamp. The tube is directed posteriorly and caudally for an effusion or hemothorax and cephalad for a pneumothorax. Reprinted with permission from Klingensmith, M. E. (2016). *The Washington manual of surgery* (7th ed.). Wolters-Kluwer.

COMPLICATIONS OF THE PROCEDURE

Detailed information is beyond the scope of this chapter; however, generally:

1. **Retained hemothorax (or failure to resolve hemothorax):** Retained hemothorax may lead to empyema (see later) or fibrothorax, restricting pulmonary expansion and ventilation. If, on initial chest tube insertion, postprocedure chest x-ray does not show improvement, a second chest tube should be placed. Cross-sectional imaging should be obtained on postprocedure day 3 to evaluate the degree of retained hemothorax. A retained hemothorax with estimated volume less than 300 mL may successfully resolve without further intervention. A retained hemothorax larger than 300 mL warrants operative evacuation. In the modern era, video-assisted thoracic surgery (VATS) is now the procedure of choice for management of post-traumatic retained hemothorax. Although early VATS is an effective and efficient approach to retained hemothorax evacuation, there is no well-established timeline

for intervention. Intrapleural tissue plasminogen activator (tPA) has also proven to be an effective option for treatment of posttraumatic retained hemothorax, particularly in patients with delayed presentation.

2. **Empyema:** Empyema is a feared complication of retained hemothorax estimated to occur in up to 30% of patients with retained hemothorax. Risk factors for empyema after retained hemothorax or thoracic trauma include the presence of rib fractures, greater injury severity score, ISS of greater than or equal to 25, and any invasive prior intervention for evacuation of retained hemothorax. Empyema often will not improve with only antibiotic administration and often requires decortication surgical intervention via thoracotomy or VATS.

3. **Persistent pneumothorax:** A new or persistent air leak may be a sign of parenchymal injury or injury to the tracheobronchial tree. A significant or continuous air leak present at the time of chest tube placement warrants cross-sectional imaging (CT) and bronchoscopy to evaluate for an airway injury. An air leak lasting more than 3 days may be caused by parenchymal injury. In such cases, VATS for posttraumatic air leak is a safe option for identifying the source of air leak and management. In patients otherwise stable for discharge, VATS decreases the number of chest tube days and length of stay compared to nonoperative management.

4. **Ectopic chest tube:** Iatrogenic compilations of chest tube placement are estimated to occur in 10% to 30% of cases. The stomach, diaphragm, and pulmonary parenchyma are the most commonly injured organs in cases of misplaced chest tubes. Although rare, there are cases of fatal injuries resulting from chest tube perforation of atria, ventricles, and hilar vessels. Careful identification of landmarks and digital exploration of the pleural cavity prior to chest tube insertion may reduce the risk of ectopic chest tube placement.

5. **Reexpansion pulmonary edema:** Rapid reexpansion of pulmonary parenchyma after chest tube placement may lead to pulmonary edema, which can be fatal in up to 20% of cases. This rare sequela of chest tube insertion is more commonly seen in cases of prolonged pulmonary collapse. Overall incidence is approximately 10%, most commonly occurring in patients aged 20 to 39 years. Onset of persistent cough during evacuation of air or fluid from the pleural space, unilateral pulmonary edema on follow-up chest x-ray, and hypoxia should raise suspicion for reexpansion pulmonary edema. Management involves oxygenation, diuretics, hemodynamic support, and positive pressure mechanical ventilation if clinically indicated.

POSTPROCEDURE CARE

Chest Tube Output

Chest tube output should be quantified immediately after placement and for as long as the chest tube is in place. In cases of traumatic hemothorax, thoracotomy is indicated if the initial chest tube output is greater than 1,500 mL, greater than 200 mL/h over 4 hours, or if the patient is hemodynamically unstable. To decrease the risk of reexpansion pulmonary edema in cases of pleural effusion, it is recommended that no more than 1,500 mL be drained initially and no more than 500 mL/h.

Follow-Up X-Ray

A postprocedure chest x-ray should be ordered on all patients to demonstrate correct chest tube placement and to confirm evacuation of the pleural space and lung reexpansion. Failure of the lung to reexpand after chest tube placement for pneumothorax or evacuation of the pleural space in cases of hemothorax may warrant additional chest tube placement or more invasive intervention. For as long as the chest tube is in place, a daily chest x-ray should be obtained to monitor resolution of hemothorax or pneumothorax and monitor position. It is recommended that cross-sectional imaging be obtained on postprocedure day 3 in cases of hemothorax to evaluate for retained hemothorax and assess the need for further intervention.

Draining the Pleural Space

Chest tubes should be placed to negative pleural suction no greater than 20 cm H_2O for approximately 24 hours to aid in the evacuation of the pleural space and facilitate pleural apposition. After this time, if the patient remains stable, the team may consider placing chest tubes to water seal to allow for passive drainage of the pleural space. Chest tubes may be removed once there is resolution of hemothorax or pneumothorax on chest x-ray, air leak has sealed, and chest tube output is less than 200 mL/day or 2 mL/kg/day.

Use of Antibiotic Therapy

There is no established standard of care for presumptive antibiotic administration while chest tubes are in place. Several reports show no difference in infectious complications from tube thoracostomy in patients receiving antibiotics. One randomized trial published by Maxwell et al. found that neither a short course of antibiotics nor a continuous course reduced the incidence of empyema or pneumonia. Further, the authors argued against the use of presumptive antibiotics as a pattern of resistance was identified in patients receiving antibiotics. The EAST Practice Management Guidelines Work Group found insufficient data to support the use of antibiotics as standard of care in cases of thoracostomy tube placement in isolated chest trauma. Current guidelines suggest that the risk of pneumonia in patients with tube thoracostomy may be reduced with the use of a first-generation cephalosporin; however, administration should be limited to 24 hours.

BIBLIOGRAPHY

Carrillo, E., Schmacht, D., Gable, D., Spain, D. A., & Richardson, J. D. (1998). Thoracoscopy in the management of posttraumatic persistent pneumothorax. *Journal of the American College of Surgeons, 186*(6), 636–639.

DuBose, J., Inaba, K., Demetriades, D., Scalea, T. M., O'Connor, J., Menaker, J., Morales, C., Konstantinidis, A., Shiflett, A., Copwood, B., & AAST Retained Hemothorax Study Group. (2012). Management of post-traumatic retained hemothorax: A prospective, observational, multicenter AAST study. *Journal of Trauma and Acute Care Surgery, 72*(1), 11–22; discussion 22-24; quiz 316.

DuBose, J., Inaba, K., Okoye, O., Demetriades, D., Scalea, T. M., O'Connor, J., Menaker, J., Morales, C., Shiflett, A., Brown, C., Copwood, B., & AAST Retained Hemothorax Study Group. (2012). Development of posttraumatic empyema in patients with retained hemothorax: Results of a prospective, observational AAST study. *Journal of Trauma and Acute Care Surgery, 73*(3), 752–757.

Enderson, B., Abdalla, R., Frame, S., Casey, M. T., Gould, H., & Maull, K. I. (1993). Tube thoracostomy for occult pneumothorax: A prospective randomized study of its use. *The Journal of Trauma: Injury, Infection, and Critical Care, 35*(5), 726–730.

Inaba, K., Lustenberger, T., Recinos, G., Georgiou, C., Velmahos, G. C., Brown, C., Salim, A., Demetriades, D., & Rhee, P. (2012). Does size matter? A prospective analysis of 28-32 versus 36-40 French chest tube size in trauma. *Journal of Trauma and Acute Care Surgery, 72*(2), 422–427.

Kong, V. Y., & Clarke, D. L. (2014). The spectrum of visceral injuries secondary to misplaced intercostal chest drains: Experience from a high volume trauma service in South Africa. *Injury, 45*(9), 1435–1439.

Kulvatunyou, N., Erickson, L., Vijayasekaran, A., Gries, L., Joseph, B., Friese, R. F., O'Keeffe, T., Tang, A. L., Wynne, J. L., & Rhee, P. (2014). Randomized clinical trial of pigtail catheter versus chest tube in injured patients with uncomplicated traumatic pneumothorax. *The British Journal of Surgery, 101*(2), 17–22.

Laws, D., Neville, E., & Duffy, J. (2003). Pleural Diseases Group, Standards of Care Committee, British Thoracic Society: BTS guidelines for the insertion of a chest drain. *Thorax, 58*, 53–59.

Luchette, F. A., Barrie, P. S., Oswanski, M. F., Spain, D. A., Mullins, C. D., Palumbo, F., & Pasquale, M. D. (2000). Practice Management Guidelines for prophylactic antibiotic use in tube thoracostomy for traumatic hemopneumothorax: The EAST Practice Management Guidelines Work Group. Eastern Association for Trauma. *The Journal of Trauma: Injury, Infection, and Critical Care, 49*(4), 753–757.

Mahajan, V. K., Simon, M., & Huber, G. L. (1979). Reexpansion pulmonary edema. *Chest, 75*(2), 192–194.

Matsuura, Y., Nomimura, T., Murakami, H., Matsushima, T., Kakehashi, M., & Kajihara, H. (1991). Clinical analysis of reexpansion pulmonary edema. *Chest, 100*(6), 1562–1566.

Maxwell, R. A., Campbell, D. J., Fabian, T. C., Croce, M. A., Luchette, F. A., Kerwin, A. J., Davis, K. A., Nagy, K., & Tisherman, S. (2004). Use of presumptive antibiotics following tube thoracostomy for traumatic hemopneumothorax in the prevention of empyema and pneumonia—a multi-center trial. *The Journal of Trauma: Injury, Infection, and Critical Care, 57*(4), 742–749.

Meyer, D. M., Jessen, M. E., Wait, M. A., & Estrera, A. S. (1997). Early evacuation of traumatic retained hemothoraces using thoracoscopy: A prospective, randomized trial. *The Annals of Thoracic Surgery, 64*(5), 1396–1401.

Schermer, C., Matteson, B., Demarest, G., Albrecht, R. M., & Davis, V. H. (1999). A prospective evaluation of video assisted thoracic surgery for persistent air-leak due to trauma. *The American Journal of Surgery, 177*, 480–484.

Stiles, P. J., Drake, R. M., Helmer, S. D., Bjordahl, P. M., & Haan, J. M. (2014). Evaluation of chest tube administration of tissue plasminogen activator to treat retained hemothorax. *American Journal of Surgery, 207*(6), 960–963.

Utter, G.H. (2013). The rate of pleural fluid drainage as a criterion for the timing of chest tube removal: Theoretical and practical considerations. *Annals of Thoracic Surgery, 96*(6), 2262–2267.

Weissberg, D., & Refaely, Y. (2000). Pneumothorax. *Chest, 117*(5), 1279–1285.

Younes, R., Gross, J., Aguiar, S., Haddad, F. J., & Deheinzelin, D. (2002). When to remove a chest tube? A randomized study with subsequent prospective consecutive validation. *Journal of the American College of Surgeons, 195*(5), 658–662.

Audrey Snyder

INDICATIONS FOR THE PROCEDURE

A tension pneumothorax occurs when air accumulates in the pleural space without a means of escape, causing complete lung collapse, compression of the heart, and tracheal and mediastinal shift, resulting in decreased cardiac output. The purpose of this procedure is to relieve the life-threatening tension pneumothorax by releasing the air trapped in the pleural cavity, which is causing compression of the structures in the mediastinum. Needle decompression, therefore, is a temporizing measure for the treatment of a tension pneumothorax. After release of the tension, the patient will need a chest thoracostomy (Figure 10.1).

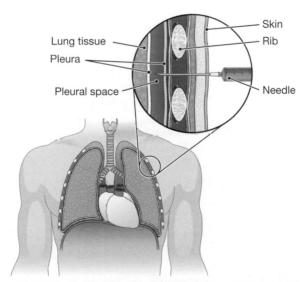

FIGURE 10.1. Technique for needle decompression. Reprinted with permission from Hawkins, S. C. (2017). *Wilderness EMS*. Wolters-Kluwer.

CONTRAINDICATIONS FOR THE PROCEDURE

There are no relative or absolute contraindications. A needle decompression is performed when a life-threatening tension pneumothorax emergency exists.

EQUIPMENT NEEDED

1. A 14 to 16 gauge catheter-over-needle device or 14 to 16 gauge needles with 10 cc syringe with 1 cc normal saline in syringe attached
2. Skin disinfectant: alcohol prep or chlorhexidine prep
3. Gloves
4. Tape to secure catheter

STEPS TO PERFORMING THE PROCEDURE

1. Identify site for catheter insertion on affected side (Figure 10.2):
   a. Midclavicular line second or third intercostal space
2. Disinfect the skin at the identified site (Figure 10.3).

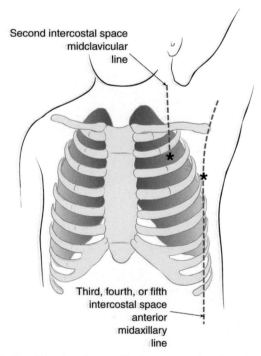

Second intercostal space midclavicular line

Third, fourth, or fifth intercostal space anterior midaxillary line

FIGURE 10.2. Possible sites for needle decompression. Reprinted with permission from Connors, K. M., & Terndrup, T. E. (1997). Tube thoracostomy and needle decompression of the chest. In F. M. Henretig, & C. King (eds.), *Textbook of pediatric emergency procedures*. Lippincott Williams & Wilkins.

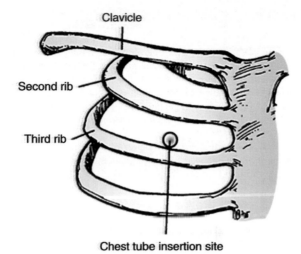

Clavicle

Second rib

Third rib

Chest tube insertion site

FIGURE 10.3. Needle insertion sites. Reprinted with permission from Jaffe, R. A. (2014). *Anesthesiologist's manual of surgical procedures* (5th ed.). Wolters Kluwer.

3. Advance catheter-over-needle device over the rib in the identified intercostal space while aspirating. Once air is returned (confirms tension pneumothorax), advance catheter and withdraw the needle and syringe.
4. Tape catheter in place, being careful not to occlude the catheter.
5. Once the chest tube is placed, the catheter is removed.

COMPLICATIONS OF THE PROCEDURE

1. **Puncture or injury to lung or pleura:** Once the catheter-over-needle device is inserted and air is returned in the needle, stop advancing the device and push the catheter in over the needle.
2. **Risk for injury to intercostal nerve, artery, or vein:** This can be prevented by going directly over the superior aspect of the rib and by going two to three finger breadths below the clavicle to avoid the subclavian vein.

POSTPROCEDURE CARE

Following needle decompression, the provider should observe for chest expansion and assess for bilateral breath sounds. Monitor for reoccurrence of tension pneumothorax. A second needle decompression may be needed on the same side. The patient should be placed on supplemental oxygen and placed on a cardiac and pulse oximetry monitor. The provider should prepare for tube thoracostomy (see Chapter 9) or call a provider who can complete this procedure. Following tube thoracostomy a chest x-ray should be ordered. Once the chest tube is placed, the catheter can be removed. After removing the catheter, apply topical antibiotic ointment and dressing.

BIBLIOGRAPHY

Ball, C. G., Wyrzykowski, A. D., Kirkpatrick, A. W., Dente, C. J., Nicholas, J. M., Salamone, J. P., Rozycki, G. S., Kortbeek, J. B., & Feliciano, D. V. (2010). Thoracic needle decompression for tension pneumothorax: Clinical correlation with catheter length. *Canadian Journal of Surgery, 53*(3), 184–188. http://canjsurg.ca/

Dezube, R. (2019). *How to do needle thoracostomy.* https://www.merckmanuals.com/professional/pulmonary-disorders/how-to-do-pulmonary-procedures/how-to-do-needle-thoracostomy

Hammond, B., & Zimmerman, P. (2012). *Sheehy's manual of emergency care* (7th ed.). Mosby/Elsevier.

Henretig, F. M., & King, C. (Eds.). (1997). *Textbook of pediatric emergency procedures* (p. 399). Lippincott Williams & Wilkins.

Tintinalli, J. E., Ma, O. J., Yealy, D. M., Meckler, G. D., Stapczynski, J. S., Cline, D. M., & Thomas, S. H. (2016). *Tintinalli's emergency medicine: A comprehensive study guide.* McGraw-Hill Medical.

11   Removing Chest Tubes

William Pezotti

INDICATIONS FOR THE PROCEDURE

The purpose of this procedure is to allow the practitioner to safely discontinue a chest tube (see Figure 11.1 for an image of a chest-drainage system). This procedure will take place when an indwelling chest tube needs to be removed. This may be because the chest tube is no longer needed or because it is no longer functioning.

Indications for the procedure are:

1. Complete resolution of the initial indication for placement, and the lungs have re-expanded based on chest x-ray findings (Figure 11.2).

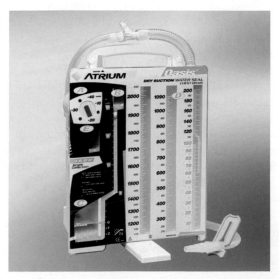

FIGURE 11.1. The Atrium Oasis is an example of a dry suction water seal chest drainage system that uses a mechanical regulator for vacuum control, a water seal chamber, and a drainage chamber. (A) Dry suction regulator; (B) water seal chamber; (C) air leak monitor; (D) collection chamber; (E) suction monitor bellows. Reprinted with permission from Hinkle, J. L., & Cheever, K. H. (2013). *Brunner & Suddarth's textbook of medical-surgical nursing* (13th ed.). Wolters Kluwer. Photos from Atrium Medical Corporation, Hudson, NH.

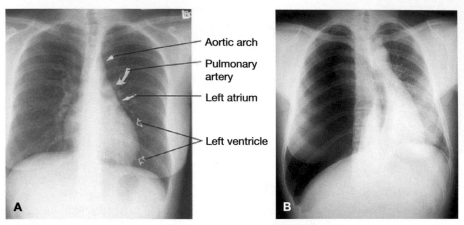

FIGURE 11.2. (A) Normal chest x-ray. (B) X-ray of right tension pneumothorax. (A) Reprinted with permission from Lippincott, Williams, & Wilkins. (2018). *Cardiovascular care made incredibly visual!* Wolters Kluwer. *Cardiovascular care made incredibly visual!* Wolters Kluwer; (B) Reprinted with permission from LoCicero, J. (2018). *Shields' general thoracic surgery* (8th ed.). Wolters Kluwer.

2. Amount of drainage has decreased significantly to 50-200 mL in the prior 24 hours if the tube was placed for hemothorax, empyema, or pleural effusion.
3. If the tube was placed for cardiac surgery, the tube may be considered for discontinuation if the drainage has changed from bloody to serosanguineous, no air leak is present, and the amount of fluid in the collection device is less than 100 mL in the past 8 hours.
4. Mediastinal chest tubes are typically removed 24 to 36 hours after cardiac surgery.
5. The drainage system is no longer holding suction, as indicated by the absence of air leaks in the drainage system.
6. The chest tube is clogged and unable to be cleared.
7. Stable respiratory status: respiratory rate less than 24/min; no acute respiratory distress noted; equal breath sounds bilaterally; symmetrical respiratory excursion.
8. Fluctuations are minimal or absent in the water-seal chamber of the collection device, and the level of solution rises in the chamber.
9. All coagulation parameters are within normal limits.

CONTRAINDICATIONS FOR THE PROCEDURE

Relative Contraindications

The provider should consider the following relative contraindications before removing the chest tube:

1. 24-hour output is greater than 300 mL.
2. Coagulation parameters are not within normal limits.
3. Arterial blood gases are not yet resolved.

Absolute Contraindications

The provider should consider the following absolute contraindications before removing the chest tube:

1. Air leak.
2. Lungs are not reexpanded on chest x-ray.
3. Unstable respiratory status: RR greater than 25, acute respiratory distress.

EQUIPMENT NEEDED

1. Suture-removal set
2. Antiseptic swabs (chlorhexidine gluconate with alcohol, etc.)
3. Clean gloves and sterile gloves
4. Prepared sterile dressing: petrolatum-impregnated gauze or Xeroform gauze, 4 × 4-inch gauze dressings, and large dressings (two to four)
5. 2- to 4-inch adhesive tape or elastic bandage (Elastoplast) cut into strips
6. Steri-strips
7. Stethoscope, sphygmomanometer, pulse oximeter
8. Mask with face shield
9. Local analgesic, if needed
10. Linen-saver pads
11. Hazard trash bags

STEPS TO PERFORMING THE PROCEDURE

1. Ensure proper patient identification by obtaining two patient identifiers.
2. Provide privacy.
3. Evaluate most recent chest x-ray to examine if lung reexpansion has occurred (Figure 11.2).
4. Confirm that bubbling in water-seal chamber has stopped and that any drainage has decreased to less than 100 to 200 mL in the last 24 hours.
5. Have someone available to assist to apply the dressing and maintain an occlusive seal at the time of tube removal.
6. Explain the procedure to the patient.
7. Position the patient comfortably with adequate access to the surgical site. Semi-Fowler's position is best, if the patient can tolerate it.
8. Perform a timeout and document all appropriate steps, if nonemergent.
9. Wash your hands and maintain aseptic technique.
10. Administer an analgesic medication (such as fentanyl 25–50 mg IV) 15 minutes before the procedure.
11. Put on clean gloves, mask with face shield, to comply with standard precautions.
12. Discontinue suction, if needed from the chest-drainage system, and assess for air leaks when the patient coughs. If bubbling in the air leak detector is present, then an air leak may be present. Removal of the chest tube with an air leak present may

cause a pneumothorax to develop, and removal of the chest tube should not take place.

13. Cover the patient's bed and lower body with linen-saver pads to protect them from drainage and to provide a place to put the chest tube after removal.
14. With clean gloves, remove the dressing covering the chest tube insertion site. Discard the soiled drainage.
15. Clean the area around the chest tube with chlorohexidine or antiseptic swabs.
16. Remove suture(s) holding the chest tube in place. If a purse-string suture was used, leave the long ends intact.
17. Take the 4 × 4's with Xeroform gauze, petroleum gauze, or other dressing based on institution protocol and place over chest tube removal site; hold dressing firmly in place (Figure 11.3).
18. Instruct the patient to take a deep breath and hold it while bearing down (Valsalva maneuver). The provider may decide to encourage a few practice breaths first, if possible. If the patient is ventilated, cycle with ventilator and remove the chest tube during peak inspiration. The primary goal of chest tube removal is removal of the tubes without introducing air into the pleural space. A complication associated with removal of chest tubes is a recurrent pneumothorax, which can occur when patients inhale during tube removal.

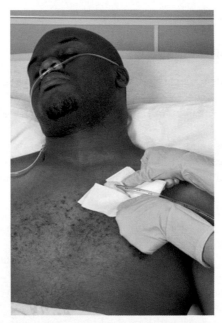

FIGURE 11.3. Applying the dressing for a chest tube wound. Reprinted with permission from Lippincott, Williams, & Wilkins. (2008). *Lippincott's nursing procedures and skills*. Wolters Kluwer.

19. In one smooth and rapid motion, remove the chest tube completely during exhalation, applying direct and immediate pressure with the dressing.
20. Have a second person apply the adhesive tape while maintaining occlusive pressure.
21. Inspect the end of the chest tube before disposal to ensure entire removal. On rare occasions, tubing can become damaged by instruments or manipulation that can cause it to break during removal.
22. Tape dressing firmly in place.
23. Instruct the patient to breathe normally.
24. Obtain a chest x-ray within 4 to 6 hours of removal (based on institution protocol, or STAT, if signs of respiratory distress, subcutaneous emphysema, or bleeding from site should occur).
25. Review the chest x-ray for a new pneumothorax or hemothorax that may have resulted from the procedure.
26. Have the patient's vital signs monitored. Assess the patient's postprocedure respiratory status and oxygen saturation levels.
27. Be sure to dispose of all contaminated supplies in appropriate receptacle, remove and dispose of your gloves, and perform hand hygiene.
28. Be sure to identify any abnormalities.
29. Document per your institution's policy.

COMPLICATIONS OF THE PROCEDURE

1. **Recurrent pneumothorax:** If it is small (under 10%–15%), it may resolve with no treatment. If it is larger or causes respiratory distress, the patient may need another chest tube inserted. The patient should be ordered daily chest x-rays to assess the progress of reabsorption and to rule out progression of the pneumothorax. A large pneumothorax may cause a change in vital signs, tachypnea, decreased oxygen saturation, or clinical instability. Intubation may be needed.
2. **Subcutaneous emphysema:** Although this issue may not be significant alone, the provider should continue to assess the patient for expansion of subcutaneous emphysema up to the neck and face or throughout the thorax. If this occurs, the asymptomatic patient may require serial chest x-rays. The development of rapid, symptomatic, or persistent subcutaneous emphysema may indicate an air leak from the thoracic cavity and, if serious, may require intubation and placement of a new chest tube.
3. **Sudden respiratory distress:** In this event, immediate attention is warranted. Consider intubation while you assess the cause of the respiratory distress and assess the need for insertion of another chest tube.
4. **Infection:** If fever, purulent or foul-smelling drainage, and erythema at the removal site develop, then obtain a culture specimen from the removal site or wound. Consider starting broad-spectrum antibiotics until the laboratory can identify the pathogen and sensitivities. Any chest tube left in place for more than 7 days increases the risk of infection along the chest tube tract.

5. **Hemorrhage:** Consult a surgeon immediately to assist in identifying and correcting the cause of bleeding, and assess the patient's vital signs, hemoglobin, and hematocrit. If appropriate, consider drawing a type-and-cross test for the transfusion of packed red blood cells, should the need arise. Infuse blood and intravenous fluids to replace lost volume. Obtain a chest x-ray to assess for a hemothorax; if one is present, then a new chest tube should be inserted to collect related drainage from the thorax.

6. **Lung damage:** Consult a thoracic surgeon to further assess the lung.

7. **Injury of the heart or mediastinal structures:** Immediately consult the cardiothoracic surgeon to further assess the injury. Assess the patient's vital signs and assess for signs of dysrhythmia, bleeding, and ischemia.

POSTPROCEDURE CARE

Once the chest tube has been removed and the steps for performing the procedure have been followed, the practitioner should document their note within the electronic medical record. Documentation should consist of the pretreatment evaluation and any abnormal physical findings. Further documentation should include indication for the procedure, type and size of the chest tube removed, estimated blood loss, the outcome, how the patient tolerated the procedure, medications used, complications, and the care plan, as well as any teaching and discharge instructions. Documentation should also include that the x-ray was obtained and results noted. It is important to note that all abnormal findings should be reviewed with the collaborating physician. Nursing staff should be instructed to call you if signs or symptoms of complications develop, particularly fever, erythema, or new drainage from the wound site, which could indicate infection.

If the patient will be discharged home, then they should be instructed to leave the chest tube dressing in place for 48 hours and reposition frequently, as well as to perform coughing and deep-breathing exercises. Once the chest tube dressing is removed, the patient may shower or wash the incisions daily with mild soap and water. It is important to educate the patient that they should not soak in a bathtub or hot tub or go swimming until the incisions have healed. The patient should be instructed not to apply lotions or powders to the site and should always pat the incisions dry. Patients should also be instructed to call the physician if any signs or symptoms of infection develop, which include increased redness, purulent drainage, excess swelling, sudden onset of sharp chest pain with shortness of breath, or fever.

BIBLIOGRAPHY

Huggins, J., Carr, S. R., & Woodward, G. A. (2019). Placement and management of thoracostomy tubes and catheters in adults and children. In A. B. Wolfson, A. M. Stack, E. M. Bulger, V. C. Broaddus, & E. Vallières (Eds.), *UpToDate*. https://www.uptodate.com/contents/placement-and-management-of-thoracostomy-tubes-and-catheters-in-adults-and-children

Kirkwood, P. (2017). Chest tube removal (perform). In D. Weigand (Ed.), *AACN procedure manual for critical care* (7th ed.). Elsevier.

Novoa, N., Jiménez, M. F., & Varela, G. (2017). When to remove a chest tube. *Thoracic Surgery Clinics, 27*(1), 41–46.

Oncology Nurses Society (ONS). (2018). *Toolkit for safe handling of hazardous drugs for nurses in oncology.* https://www.ons.org/clinical-practice-resources/toolkit-safe-handling-hazardous-drugs-nurses-oncology

The Joint Commission (TJC). (2020). *National patient safety goals, Oakbrook Terrace, IL*. Retrieved June 30, 2019, from http://www.jointcommision.org/standards_information/npsgs.aspx

Weigand, D. L. (2017). *AACN procedure manual for high acuity, progressive, and critical care* (7th ed.). Elsevier.

Ella Hawk

INDICATIONS FOR THE PROCEDURE

A thoracentesis is a percutaneous procedure whereby a needle or catheter is inserted into the pleural space between the lungs and the chest wall in order to aspirate an excessive amount of fluid that has accumulated within that space; this is known as a pleural effusion. A small amount of fluid is normally found in this space as part of healthy lymphatic drainage, providing lubrication between the lung parenchyma and musculoskeletal structures of the rib cage during expansion (inhalation) and recoil (exhalation). Thoracentesis can be performed during an inpatient stay or as an outpatient procedure with a trained provider.

The indications for a thoracentesis are relatively broad, including diagnostic and/ or therapeutic intent.

Indications for the procedure are:

1. **Diagnostic:** Patients with a new finding of a pleural effusion can undergo a diagnostic thoracentesis to ascertain the nature of the effusion (i.e., transudate, exudate) to determine its underlying cause. The exceptions to the aforementioned are a small amount of pleural fluid, which can be caused by atelectasis, viral pleurisy, or clinical diagnosis of the patient with uncomplicated congestive heart failure. In this case, observation, in lieu of diagnostic thoracentesis, may be warranted in uncomplicated heart failure.
2. **Therapeutic:** Thoracentesis for therapeutic intent is done primarily for dyspnea related to pleural effusion(s). Thoracentesis will alleviate the large volume of fluid in the pleural space, making it easier for the lungs to fully expand. Therapeutic thoracentesis is also indicated for patients with pleural conditions that risk pleural thickening and restrictive functional impairment, such as effusions caused by postprimary or reactivation tuberculosis and hemothorax.

CONTRAINDICATIONS FOR THE PROCEDURE

Relative Contraindications

1. Insufficient amount of pleural fluid, deeming thoracentesis procedure unsafe.
2. Skin infection or wound at the needle insertion site.

3. Bleeding disorder or anticoagulation. The decisions to reverse the coagulopathy and/or correct the thrombocytopenia should be individualized and based on perceived benefits versus risks, urgency of thoracentesis, and the probability of bleeding into the pleural space. The ability of a patient to tolerate a hemothorax and a procedure to drain intrapleural blood should also be considered.

4. Uncertain fluid location. Very small, free-flowing pleural effusions less than 30 mL, less than 1 cm distance from the pleural fluid line to the chest wall on a decubitus chest radiograph, have been considered too small to justify thoracentesis because of the low diagnostic yield and high risk of pneumothorax. With the advent of ultrasound-guided thoracentesis, the safe window for thoracentesis has been estimated as a point where maximum pleural fluid depth is greater than 1 cm adjacent to the parietal pleura.

5. Uncontrolled cough or hiccups.

6. Defer thoracentesis in patients with severe hemodynamic or respiratory compromise until the underlying condition is stabilized.

7. Caution must be exercised when performing thoracentesis in mechanically ventilated patients. The positive pressure of the ventilator may expand the lung to greater than normal volumes, increasing the potential risk of pneumothorax. Ultrasound-guided thoracentesis is recommended in this situation.

Absolute Contraindications

No absolute contraindications.

EQUIPMENT NEEDED

Diagnostic testing inclusive of chest radiographic posteroanterior and lateral chest radiography is the most commonly used initial diagnostic workup for patients with suspected pleural effusions. There is extensive, well-established data to support the utilization of ultrasound, which allows the operator to identify the most accessible area of the pleural fluid, measure the exact distance a needle must travel to enter the pleural effusion, avoid important surrounding structures, and localize intercostal vessels, reducing the rate of complications from thoracentesis.

Ultrasound machine with two-dimensional brightness, motion mode capability, and Doppler to identify vascular structures and free fluid movement, with an appropriate transducer.

Sterile gloves, gowns, and sterile drapes; skin sterilizing fluid 0.05% chlorhexidine or 10% povidone–iodine solution; and sterile occlusive wound dressing.

Local anesthetic agent 1% to 2% lidocaine with the appropriate needles—25-gauge for skin infiltration and 21- or 22-gauge for deeper tissue infiltration—through the ribs and syringe for injection.

Thoracentesis needle, an 8-French over-the-needle catheter, an 18-gauge needle, a stopcock, hemostats, 35 to 60 mL syringe, and thoracentesis drainage bag/system and vacuum bottle.

- If the thoracentesis is performed for diagnostic purposes with only a small volume withdrawal (i.e., 30 mL), an 18-gauge needle without catheter may be used.
- If the thoracentesis is performed for therapeutic intent, use of a needle alone for drainage is contraindicated owing to risk of lacerating the visceral pleural surface. The needle is used transiently to introduce the drainage catheter using an over-the-needle catheter system utilizing a technique called Seldinger, which entails utilizing a wire/dilator/catheter system. For drainage of a large volume pleural effusion, typical catheter size is 8 French, while Seldinger technique catheters range in size from 6 to 14 French.

Emergency equipment would include:

- Thoracotomy tray with chest tubes for emergency chest tube placement in the event of a pneumothorax
- Emergency Code Cart

STEPS TO PERFORMING THE PROCEDURE

1. Perform Standard Steps (see Preface).
2. Position the patient in the sitting position, leaning forward with arms and head resting supported on a bedside adjustable table (Figure 12.1).
   If the patient is unable to sit upright, the patient should lie at the edge of the bed on the affected side with the ipsilateral arm over the head and the midaxillary line accessible for the insertion of the needle. Ensure the head of the bed is elevated to 30° (Figure 12.2).
3. Utilize real-time ultrasound guidance to identify a safe access site. Choose an access site in the triangle of safety, an anatomic triangle bordered by the lateral pectoralis major anteriorly, lateral latissimus dorsi laterally, fifth intercostal place inferiorly, and the base of the axilla superiorly (Figure 12.3).
4. Select and mark the site in an interspace below the point of dullness to percussion in the midposterior line for posterior insertion or midaxillary line for lateral insertion.
5. Sterile technique is used to gown, glove, and prep the skin with antiseptic solution 0.05% chlorhexidine or 10% povidone–iodine solution and apply a sterile drape.

Anesthetize the skin over the insertion site with 1% to 2% lidocaine using a 5- or 10-mL syringe with the 25- to 27-gauge needle, utilize a 21- to 22-guage needle for deep tissue infiltration through the ribs for injection. Next, anesthetize the superior surface of the rib and the pleura. The needle is inserted over the top of the rib (superior margin) to avoid the intercostal nerves and blood vessels that run along the underside of the rib. The needle should be "walked" along the superior edge of the rib, alternately injecting anesthetic and pulling back on the plunger every few millimeters to rule out intravascular placement and to check for proper intrapleural placement (Figure 12.4).

Once pleural fluid is aspirated, additional lidocaine should be injected to anesthetize the highly sensitive parietal pleura, and the needle should no longer be advanced.

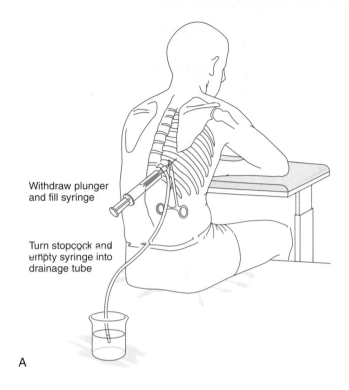

A

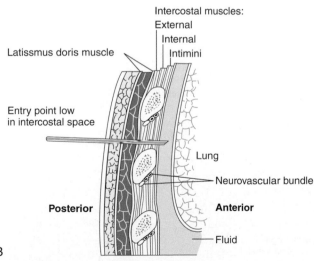

B

FIGURE 12.1. Patient positioning for thoracentesis. (A) Posterior thoracentesis to drain a pleural effusion is performed through an intracostal space above the ninth rib with the patient in the upright position. (B) Posterior thoracentesis is performed at the inferior aspect of the interspace because there is only one neurovascular bundle at the inferior aspect of each rib. Reprinted with permission from Benumof, J. (1991). *Clinical procedures in anesthesia and intensive care*. Lippincott.

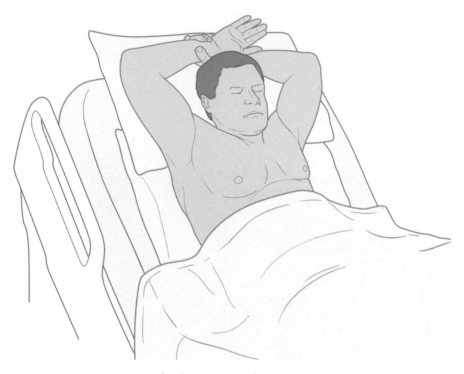

FIGURE 12.2. Patient position for thoracentesis if unable to assume seated position.

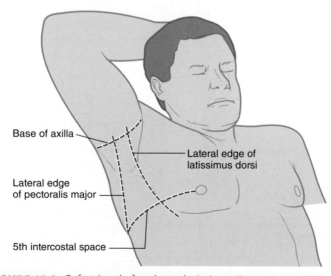

Base of axilla

Lateral edge of
latissimus dorsi

Lateral edge
of pectoralis major

5th intercostal space

FIGURE 12.3. Safe triangle for chest drain insertion.

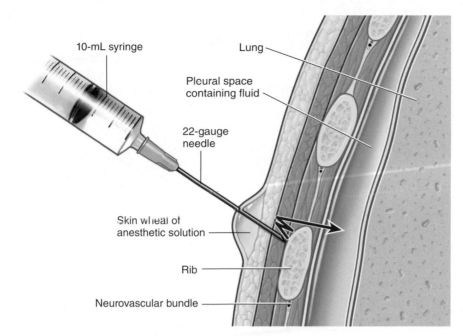

10-mL syringe

Lung

Pleural space
containing fluid

22-gauge
needle

Skin wheal of
anesthetic solution

Rib

Neurovascular bundle

FIGURE 12.4. Anesthetize on an angle, then insert needle over the top of the rib (see red arrow).

Note the depth of the needle and mark it with a hemostat; this gives the approximate depth for insertion of the angiocatheter or thoracentesis needle. Remove the anesthetizing needle. Place a gloved finger over the open hub of the catheter to prevent the entry of air into the pleural cavity, attach the three-way stopcock and tubing to the catheter hub, and aspirate the amount of pleural fluid needed (Figure 12.5).

Turn the stopcock and evacuate the fluid through the tubing—usually 30 to 100 mL for diagnostic intent and generally no more than 1,500 mL at one time for therapeutic intent secondary to increased risk of pleural edema or hypotension (Figure 12.6).

When the fluid draining is complete, have the patient take a deep breath and "hum" as you gently remove the catheter/needle. Always remove the needle when the patient is at end expiration. This maneuver increases intrathoracic pressure and decreases the chance of a pneumothorax. Cover the insertion site with a sterile occlusive dressing.

COMPLICATIONS OF THE PROCEDURE

1. **Pneumothorax:** Pneumothorax is the most common complication of thoracentesis, with incidental rates as high as 19%, according to Cantey et al. (2016). Pneumothorax caused by thoracentesis is usually small and resolves spontaneously,

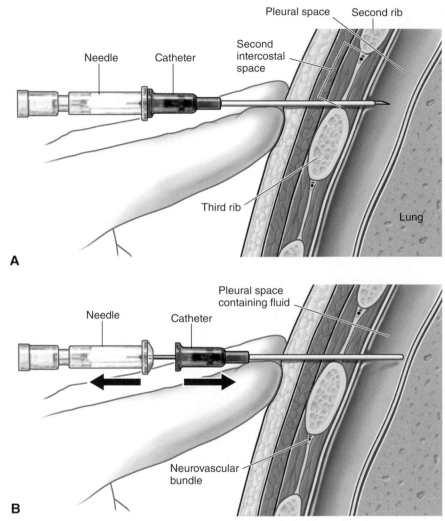

FIGURE 12.5. (A) Insertion of a catheter over needle into the pleural space. (B) The catheter remains, and the needle is withdrawn.

although up to one-third of patients require a chest tube for drainage. A chest tube should be considered if the pneumothorax is large and progressive and the patient is symptomatic or on mechanical ventilation.

2. **Hemothorax (bleeding):** Bleeding diathesis, anticoagulation, and abnormal hemostasis, including elevated international ratio (INR) or partial thromboplastin time (PTT) and low platelet count, are felt to be the best predictors of bleeding complications. However, based on research done by Ault et al. (2015), only 0.18% bleeding complication was noted post thoracentesis. Any bleeding diathesis must

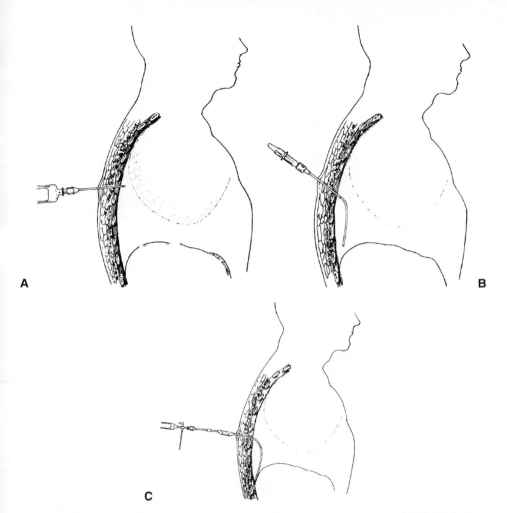

FIGURE 12.6. (A–D) Therapeutic thoracentesis. (A) A standard 14-gauge needle attached to a syringe is introduced into the pleural space. (B) A 14-gauge catheter is threaded through the needle and is directed down toward the costodiaphragmatic recess. (C) The needle is withdrawn from the pleural space, and its end is covered immediately with the guard. Fluid can be withdrawn from the pleural space using the three-way stopcock and the syringe. Reprinted with permission from Light, R. W. (2013). *Pleural diseases* (6th ed.). Wolters Kluwer.

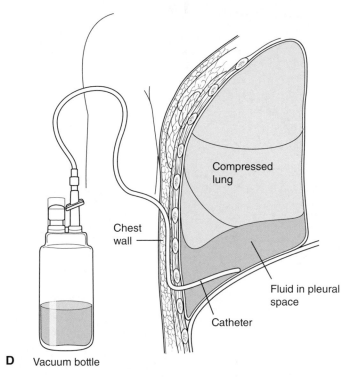

D   Vacuum bottle

FIGURE 12.6. (*continued*) (D) Connection of a pleural drain is possible after removal of the stopcock. Figure D: courtesy of Joseph Pangrace, Artist, 2016.

be corrected prior to start of the procedure, and the risk versus benefit must be assessed by an experienced clinician.

3. **Infection**: Infection at the insertion site is extremely rare. In one observational study, there were no serious infections following more than 2,000 ultrasound-guided thoracenteses; however, it remains a possible complication to the procedure. Utilize proper handwashing and sterile technique while doing the procedure. Clean the area of injection appropriately with chlorhexidine 0.05% and or povidone iodine.

4. **Puncture of the liver or spleen**: This can occur when the patient is not sitting upright; as a patient moves toward recumbency, the abdominal viscera move cephalad. In the event of a puncture to the organs, the patient must be immediately assessed hemodynamically and radiographically with the possibility of surgical intervention.

5. **Reexpansion pulmonary edema**: This is the development of hypoxia and new alveolar infiltrates within 24 hours of pleural fluid drainage of greater than 1,500 mL. Studies indicate that increased hydrostatic forces in the reexpanded lung and direct injury to the alveolar–capillary barrier may contribute to this pathogenesis. Limit the fluid removal to less than 1,500 mL to avoid reexpansion pulmonary edema.

POSTPROCEDURE CARE

Postthoracentesis chest radiographs are not routinely required after an uncomplicated thoracentesis, but should be obtained if:

- Air was aspirated from the pleural space during the procedure.
- The patient develops chest pain, dyspnea, or hypoxemia during or after the procedure.
- Multiple needle insertions were required.
- The patient is critically ill.
- The patient is being mechanically ventilated.

You can also utilize the ultrasound to examine the ipsilateral chest for pneumothorax. Continue to hemodynamically monitor the patient's vital signs, heart rate, and BP for any signs of compromise for approximately 1 to 2 hours post procedure. Provide postprocedural analgesics as needed. Instruct the patient to call the physician or 911 and return to the emergency department if they develop chest pain, increased cough, shortness of breath, respiratory distress, or signs and symptoms of infection. Send specimens collected and properly labeled to the laboratory if thoracentesis is done with diagnostic intent.

BIBLIOGRAPHY

Ault, M. J., Rosen, B. T., Scher, J., Feinglass, J., & Barsuk, J. H. (2015). Thoracentesis outcomes: A 12-year experience. *Thorax Journal, 70,* 127–132. https://doi.org/10.1136/thoraxjnl-2014-206114

Brauner, M. E., & Bailey, R. A. (2018). *Thoracentesis.* https://emedicine.medscape.com/article/80640-overview

Cantey, E. P., Walter, J. M., Corbridge, T., & Barsuk, J. H. (2016). *Complications of thoracentesis: Incidence, risk factors, and strategies for prevention.* www.co-pulmonarymedicine.com

Heffner, J. E., Mayo, P., Broaddus, V. C., & Finlay, G. (2018a). *Diagnostic evaluation of a pleural effusion in adults: Initial testing.* https://www.uptodate.com/contents/diagnostic-evaluation-of-a-pleural-effusion-in-adults-initial-testing

Heffner, J. E., Mayo, P., Broaddus, V. C., & Finlay, G. (2018b). *Ultrasound guided thoracentesis.* Retrieved December 24, 2018, from https://www.uptodate.com/contents/ultrasound-guidedthoracentesis

Juarez, M., & Nemer, J. (2019). "Thoracentesis," Chapter 52. In E. F. Reichman (Ed.), *Reichman's emergency medicine procedures* (3rd ed.). McGraw-Hill.

Krackov, R., & Rizzolo, D. (2017). Real-time ultrasound-guided thoracentesis. *Journal of the American Academy of Physician Assistants, 30,* 32–37. https://doi.org/10.1097/01.JAA.0000508210.40675.09

Lechtzin, N. (2016). *How to do thoracentesis.* In *Merck Manual Professional Version.* https://www.merckmanuals.com/professional/pulmonary-disorders/diagnostic-and-therapeutic-pulmonary-procedures/how-to-do-thoracentesis

Oxford Medical Education, Ltd. (2017). https://www.oxfordmedicaleducation.com/clinical-skills/%20procedures/intercostal-drain/

Queens University School of Medicine. (n.d.). *Indications.* https://meds.queensu.ca/central/assets/modules/ts-thoracentesis/indications.html

Satish, K., & Pastores, S. M. (2017). *Thoracentesis, Chapter 108.* In J. M. Oropello, S. M. Pastores, & V. Kvetan. *Critical care.* McGraw-Hill.

Simel, D. L. (n.d.). *Make the diagnosis: Thoracentesis.* https://jamaevidence.mhmedical.com/content.aspx?sectionid=75186098&bookid=845

Standardized Procedure Thoracentesis (Adult). (n.d.). https://health.ucsd.edu/medinfo/
medical-staff/application/Documents/SP42%20Thoracentesis%20(Adult).pdf

Stevic, R., Colic, N., Bascarevic, S., Kostic, M., Moskovljevic, D., Savic, M., & Ercegovac, M. (2018).
Sonographic indicators for treatment choice and follow-up in patients with pleural effusion. *Canadian Respiratory Journal,* 2018, 1–6. https://doi.org/10.1155/2018/9761583

Thoracentesis [Computer generated image]. (2009). commons.m.wikimedia.org/wiki/File: Thoracentesis.jpg

Wiederhold, B. D., & O'Rourke, M. C. (2018). Thoracentesis. In *StatPearls [Internet].* StatPearls Publishing.
Retrieved December 24, 2018, from https://www.ncbi.nlm.nih.gov/books/NBK441866/

Steven Bocchese

INDICATIONS FOR THE PROCEDURE

With the growing numbers of advanced practice providers in the acute care setting, providers are learning and performing bronchoscopy. The purpose of flexible bronchoscopy is for both diagnostic and therapeutic intentions. Performing bronchoscopy can aid in the diagnosis of bacterial infection, fungal infection, and malignancy. Examples of collections include biopsies of a node to rule out malignancy or even a bronchoalveolar lavage (BAL). The information obtain by bronchoscopy may not be obtainable in any other manner or would require high-risk invasive procedures. The bronchoscope can also be used as a therapeutic intervention such as clearing secretions from the bronchi or placing an endotracheal tube in a difficult airway.

Indications for the procedure are:

Diagnostic Indications:
1. Concern for pulmonary disease
   a. Hemoptysis
   b. Stridor/hoarseness
   c. Unilateral wheezing
   d. Unexplained chronic cough
2. Suspected pulmonary infections
   a. Pneumonia in an immunocompromised host or unresolved pneumonia
   b. Cavitary lesions
   c. Suspected resistant organism
   d. Ventilator-associated infections
3. Diffuse lung disease
   a. Interstitial lung disease
   b. Diffuse alveolar damage or hemorrhage
   c. Drug-induced lung disease (i.e., amiodarone toxicity)
   d. Lung parenchymal nodule or mass
4. Known or suspected malignancy
   a. Endobronchial tumor
   b. Mediastinal or hilar adenopathy or mass
   c. Compressed airway caused by tumor invasion
   d. Detection of central lung cancer; staging or restaging lung cancer

5. Miscellaneous
   a. Airway stent evaluation
   b. Evaluation of benign airway disease and strictures
   c. Lung transplant surveillance
   d. Thermal or chemical airway injury
   e. Confirmation of endotracheal tube position
   f. Bronchopleural fistula

Therapeutic Indications:
6. Malignant central airway obstruction
   a. Endobronchial obstruction
   b. Extrinsic tumors
7. Benign central airway obstruction
   a. Radial cuts
   b. Balloon dilation
   c. Airway stenting
   d. Intrabronchial injections
8. Tracheoesophageal fistula
   a. Stenting
   b. Laser-induced closure
9. Hemoptysis
   a. Hemostasis of centrally located bleeding lesions
10. Bronchopleural fistulas closure
    b. Airway spigots or endobronchial valves
11. Miscellaneous
    a. Aspiration of cyst/abscess drainage
    b. Endoscopic lung volume reduction
    c. Bronchoscopic intubation
    d. Mucous plugging
    e. Foreign body removal

CONTRAINDICATIONS FOR THE PROCEDURE

As with any invasive procedure, there are contraindications for performing bronchoscopy. Most are relative contraindications but there are a few absolute contraindications to be considered prior to bronchoscopy.

Relative Contraindications

1. Severe hypoxemia: The provider must consider what the results of an attempted bronchoscopy on a patient with severe hypoxemia would yield and whether this would change management.
2. Severe pulmonary hypertension.
3. Myocardial ischemia, decompensated heart failure, acute asthma, or chronic obstructive pulmonary disease (COPD) for at least 6 weeks.
4. Coagulopathy: The provider should consider the risk of bleeding in a coagulopathic patient.

5. Renal insufficiency: Uremia can increase the risk of bleeding in this patient population.
6. Superior vena cava syndrome.
7. Increase intracranial pressure: owing to airway stimulation and increased intrathoracic pressure.

Absolute Contraindications

1. Refractory hypoxemia
2. Hemodynamic instability
3. Life-threatening dysrhythmias
4. Lack of informed consent
5. Inadequate equipment or inexperienced operator

EQUIPMENT NEEDED

Prior to performing a bronchoscopy, the equipment should be gathered and placed in order of use.

1. Bronchoscope (Figure 13.1): Flexible bronchoscope has three parts (control handle, flexible shaft, and distal tip with camera and light).
2. Image processor: Used to store videos and pictures taken during the bronchoscopy

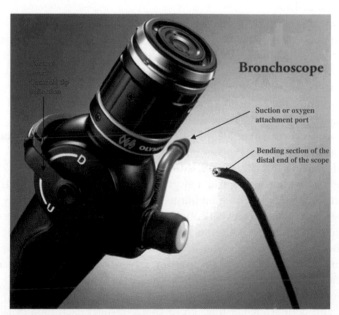

FIGURE 13.1. Bronchoscope. Reprinted with permission from Chu, L. F., & Fuller, A. (2011). *Manual of Clinical Anesthesiology*. Wolters Kluwer.

3. Personal protective equipment (PPE): Mask (N95 mask if needed), gloves, gown, shoe covers
4. Needle aspirator, laser, cryosurgery: If needed for diagnostic indication
5. Topical anesthetic: Lidocaine most commonly used
6. IV access
7. Sedatives: Commonly used sedatives include midazolam and fentanyl
8. Specimen traps and syringes: Traps for airway secretions, BAL, and bronchial washing
9. Sterile normal saline for flushing
10. Suction and suction tubing
11. Equipment for endotracheal intubation (i.e., endotracheal tube, laryngoscope, bag-valve mask, supraglottic devices, oxygen tubing, and medications for rapid sequence intubation)
12. Cardiac monitoring and trained personnel to monitor
13. Resuscitation medications, reversal agents, and code cart

STEPS TO PERFORMING THE PROCEDURE

Performing invasive procedures should be done methodically so as to prevent mistakes. The provider must consider risk versus benefit for any invasive procedure along with the potential complications that can be caused by the procedure.

1. Gather the needed equipment for the procedure. Ensure proper personnel are available and at bedside.
2. Put on the proper PPE for this particular patient.
3. Place the patient flat or with head of bed elevated up to 30°. The patient should have nothing by mouth (NPO) 6 to 8 hours prior to the procedure unless it is an emergency.
4. Administer a sedative (i.e., midazolam) and analgesia (i.e., fentanyl).
5. Place the tip of the bronchoscope into the mouth of the patient and visualize the oral mucosa. Identify the vocal cords and epiglottis.
6. Once the vocal cords are identified, visualize any lesions and movement if conscious sedation is given. Process an image of the vocal cords.
7. After visualizing the vocal cords, administer 1 to 2 mL of 2% to 4% lidocaine. If persistent coughing occurs, you may give additional aliquots of lidocaine. Spraying lidocaine in the subglottic region immediately distal to the vocal cords provides the best anesthetic effect to prevent coughing. To prevent lidocaine toxicity, do not use more than 20 mL of 2% lidocaine. Do not use 4% lidocaine past the vocal cords.
8. After the patient is properly anesthetized, pass the bronchoscope through the vocal cords into the trachea during inspiration. Do not force the bronchoscope through the vocal cords or during expiration.
9. Continue moving the distal tip down to the carina while inspecting the trachea, carina, and endobronchial tree. From there, inspect each lobe of the lungs, the bronchial segments and subsegments, and proceed with the intended indication for bronchoscopy (Figure 13.2).

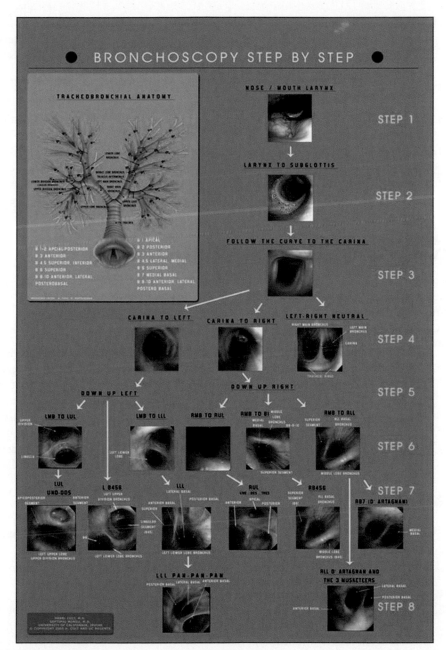

FIGURE 13.2. Bronchoscopy Step-by-Step© is a series of exercises that teaches muscle memory and systematic approach to bronchoscopic inspection so bronchial segments are entered with ease and accuracy. Using a nasal and oral approach from the head and from in front of the patient, images are intentionally intermixed to enhance learning. Bronchoscopy Step-by-Step© is best taught in models. It can be used in patients to help learners master technical skills. Available at: https://bronchoscopy.org/step-by-step. With permission, Henri Colt, Bronchoscopy International.

10. BAL is the most commonly performed procedure during a bronchoscopy.
11. If during inspection mucus is identified, the operator instills 10 to 30 mL of sterile normal saline via a syringe into a port in the bronchoscope. Once the saline is instilled in the lung, suction is than applied to remove the secretion.
12. A specimen trap is connected to the bronchoscope and the suction so that it can collect the BAL specimen to be sent to the laboratory.
13. This step may be repeated as long as needed to remove the secretion and open the collapsed airway.
14. After the operator feels that all the secretions are removed and a specimen is collected, they will do a final check of each segmental bronchus to ensure that each segmental bronchus is open and patent.
15. After this step, the bronchoscope is removed, and the patient is supported while the sedation wears off (Figure 13.3).

COMPLICATIONS OF THE PROCEDURE

Invasive procedures include some level of risk for complications. While generally safe when performed using the proper techniques, flexible bronchoscopy does carry risks for complications depending on a patient's status or an operator's skill, as follows:

Common complications:

1. **Mild hypotension and hypoxia**: Have IV fluids at the bedside ready to be administered for hypotension. Vasopressor medications should be readily available in cases where the patient is critically ill. Oxygen administration devices should be at the bedside (i.e., nasal cannula, nonrebreather mask, bag-valve mask, supraglottic airway device, endotracheal tube and equipment, surgical airway kit in extreme cases).
2. **Iatrogenic pneumothorax**: Rare unless advanced procedure such as biopsy or needle aspiration is being performed. If suspected, order chest x-ray or use bedside ultrasound to confirm. A pigtail catheter chest tube kit should be readily available in such cases.
3. **Bleeding**: If minimal, have ice cold saline or epinephrine available to inject to site of bleeding. If life threatening, treatment would include argon plasma coagulation, embolization, or surgical intervention.

Less common complications:

1. **Nausea/vomiting cause aspiration**: Provide antiemetics as needed.
2. **Airway injury**: bronchospasm, epistaxis, laryngospasm, laryngeal edema—Provide supportive care and nebulizer treatments (i.e., albuterol, racemic epinephrine).
3. Topical agent toxicity (lidocaine).
4. **Pneumonia and bacteremia**: Monitor vitals post procedure. If pneumonia is suspected, check chest x-ray and consider antibiotic administration.
5. **Death**: Extremely rare in flexible bronchoscopy but is often related to patient instability owing to critical illness, severe hypoxemia, tension pneumothorax, or massive bleeding.

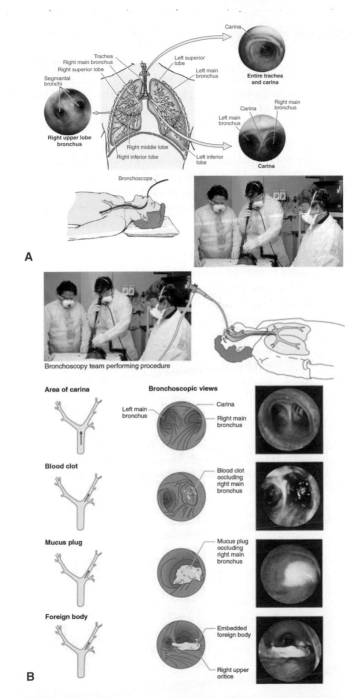

FIGURE 13.3. Bronchoscopy done through a fiberoptic scope. (A) Expected findings; (B) Abnormal findings. (A) Reprinted with permission from Feinsilver, S. H., & Fein, A. (1995). *Textbook of bronchoscopy*. Williams & Wilkins. (B) Reprinted with permission from Willis, M. C. (2005). *Medical terminology: The language of health care* (2nd ed.). Lippincott Williams & Wilkins.

POSTPROCEDURE CARE

The postprocedure care provided to patients following a bronchoscopy varies depending on the clinical indication for the bronchoscopy. If the patient is an inpatient on a ventilator, the patient will return to the intensive care unit for further care. If the patient is not on a ventilator, the patient will, following the procedure, recover in the postanesthesia care unit while the sedation wears off. Monitoring of cardiac and vital signs should be instituted. A chest x-ray may be ordered after the procedure to visualize any therapeutic benefit of the bronchoscopy. If a patient has respiratory distress or bleeding, a chest x-ray or bedside ultrasound should be obtained to assess for pneumothorax. If the pneumothorax is less than 2 cm and the patient is not in distress or hemodynamically unstable, the pneumothorax can be monitored with a repeat chest x-ray in 4 hours. If the patient complains of chest pain, shortness of breath, or respiratory distress and the chest x-ray or ultrasound confirms a pneumothorax, then a small-bore (pigtail catheter) chest tube should be inserted to reexpand the lung. A repeat chest x-ray would be ordered and assessed following placement of the chest tube.

The provider should review the findings of the bronchoscopy with the patient after the patient is no longer sedated. The provider should provide the patient with proper education on postprocedural effects such as sore or scratchy throat, low-grade fever, or mild hemoptysis. Information on more life-threatening effects such as chest pain, sudden onset of shortness of breath, or significant hemoptysis should be provided to the patient. If these were to occur, the patient should be instructed to call 9-1-1 or go to the nearest emergency room.

BIBLIOGRAPHY

Ernst, A., & Herth, F. (2017). *Introduction to bronchoscopy.* Cambridge University Press.
International, B. (2020). *Bronchoscopy step-by-step.* https://bronchoscopy.org/step-by-step
Islam, S. (2021). *Flexible bronchoscopy in adults: Indications and contraindications.* https://www.uptodate.com/contents/flexible-bronchoscopy-in-adults-indications-and-contraindications
Miller, R. I., Casal, R. O., Lazarus, D., Ost, D., & Eapen, G. (2018). *Interventional pulmonology: An update.* Elsevier.

14 Changing Tracheostomy

Troy Derose

INDICATIONS FOR THE PROCEDURE

The purpose of a tracheostomy change is to remove a previously surgically placed tracheostomy tube and exchange it with a new tracheostomy tube of the exact same size as opposed to replacing it with one whose cannula is of different size and length. A tracheostomy tube may also be changed depending on the need for an addition or removal of a balloon cuff depending on the clinical reasoning for the tracheostomy change, e.g., clinical decompensation, that requires positive pressure ventilation.

A tracheostomy can be exchanged for several indications. After a tracheostomy is initially placed, it is best practice to remove the original tracheostomy tube within 5 to 7 days post procedure to establish a formed tracheostomy tract that does not adhere to the tracheostomy's indwelling portion of the cannula.

Indications for tracheostomy change are:

1. After the initial surgical placement of a tracheostomy, best practice is to replace the tracheostomy 5 to 7 days post initial surgical placement to establish a well-healed tract that does not adhere to the surrounding tissue of the tracheostomy tube. This replacement is done to lessen the risk of creating a false passage into the surrounding subcutaneous tissue.
2. To upsize or downsize the cannula portion of the tracheostomy depending on ventilatory requirements needed for maximal ventilatory function.
3. To exchange a nonfunctional, poorly functioning, or poorly fitting tracheostomy tube with a functional or working tracheostomy tube.
4. To add or remove a balloon cuff at the distal end of the cannula, depending on the need for positive pressure ventilation as opposed to no longer needing a ventilator and attempting to establish the means for phonation (speaking) on a patient post tracheostomy placement by removing a tracheostomy with a balloon cuff at the distal end of the cannula.

CONTRAINDICATIONS FOR THE PROCEDURE

Relative Contraindications

1. An early tracheostomy exchange prior to the initial 5 days of the surgical placement of the tracheostomy is a relative contraindication. This increases the likelihood of replacing the tracheostomy tube into a *false passage* or false tract in the anterior subcutaneous tissue of the neck not leading into the airway.

2. A technically difficult surgical placement of a tracheostomy in which the potential loss of the tracheotomy tract is considered high or profound. In this case, a technically difficult tracheostomy may be safest to maintain intact and only cut the stay sutures of the tracheostomy after 7 days of the original placement. Timing of a tracheostomy change may then be decided in the future, when the airway may be considered more stable.
3. Clinician inexperience and unavailability of staff versed in airway management and care.

Absolute Contraindications

1. Extremely high ventilation settings would increase the risk of a tracheostomy decannulation.
2. If a patient is not cooperative with ancillary assistance and support, it is safest to wait until staffing is more readily available and the patient is more cooperative to lessen the risk of poor placement and dislodgment during the tracheostomy change.

EQUIPMENT NEEDED

1. Bag valve mask/manual resuscitator (as emergency equipment)
2. Adequate lighting
3. Neck roll to hyperextend the neck, offering adequate exposure of the anterior neck
4. A 10-to-14-French suction catheter connected to a functioning wall or portable continuous suction canister with compatible suction tubing
5. A replacement tracheostomy with a properly fitting inner cannula and obturator
6. Suture scissors and forceps to remove the initial surgically placed stay sutures at all four corners of the baseplate of the tracheostomy (if present)
7. Tracheostomy ties
8. Saline-soaked sterile gauze to wipe away stomal crust, secretions, and debris underneath the previous baseplate of the tracheostomy
9. Nasopharyngolaryngoscope (if available) to assess adequate placement of the tracheostomy after the exchange for direct visualization of tracheal rings and carina

STEPS TO PERFORMING THE PROCEDURE

A tracheostomy change is generally recommended to be performed by two clinicians, one flanking the patient on each side of the examination chair/table, operating room table, or hospital bed. The reason for this technique is to ensure the tracheostomy tube does not become dislodged when sutures are cut or ties or unfastened. The flanked clinician (on the opposite side of the field) holds the baseplate in place while the opposing clinician is either cutting stay sutures or unfastening tracheostomy ties. A two-clinician technique also allows one person to remove the tracheostomy and cleanse the neck and tracheotomy incision, while the other flanked clinician replaces the tracheostomy in a matter of seconds. This approach optimizes safe clinical practice to lessen the chances of losing an airway because of the need for multiple hands to complete the tasks required during a tracheostomy exchange.

Traditional Technique

1. Have the patient lying flat and supine in bed with siderails down on each side flanked by a clinician on each side of the patient's head of bed, with the bed elevated to a position comfortable to the clinicians.
2. Place a neck roll (i.e., rolled towel, blanket, IV bag wrapped with towel) under the patient's cervical posterior neck to assist with hyperextension of the neck.
3. Ensure that adequate overhead lighting is available and functioning properly. Utilization of a head lamp is appropriate for this acute care procedure (if available).
4. Ensure that a bag valve mask is present and functioning, readily available if needed.
5. Set up a 14-French suction catheter with a working suction canister.
6. Set up a sterile field complete with scissors, forceps, and new tracheostomy tube unpackaged and obturator set in place into the cannula of the prepared tracheostomy tube with tracheostomy ties already fastened to each side of the base plate See Figure 14.1 for tracheostomy change equipment on sterile field.
7. While one flanked clinician/practitioner at the head of the bed holds the sutured baseplate in place, the other clinician/practitioner cuts the stay sutures, then hands off the suture scissor to the partner clinician to snip the remaining sutures while holding the baseplate in place (Figure 14.2).
8. The tracheostomy that will be placed in the stoma after removal of the old tracheostomy is prepared and positioned in line with the stoma (Figure 14.3).

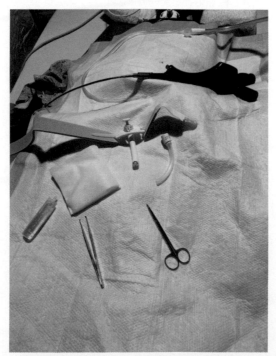

FIGURE 14.1. Equipment for use in changing a tracheostomy.

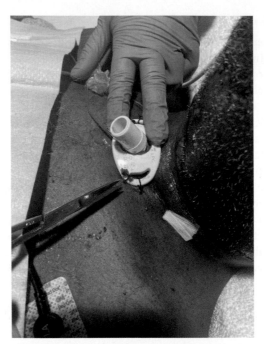

FIGURE 14.2. One clinician holds the sutured baseplate of the tracheostomy as the other cuts and removes sutures.

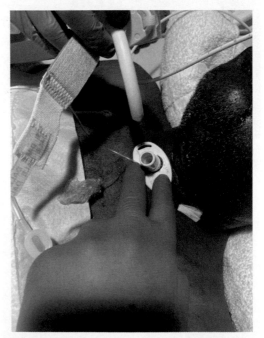

FIGURE 14.3. The preprepared new tracheostomy with Velcro ties is positioned above the old tracheostomy.

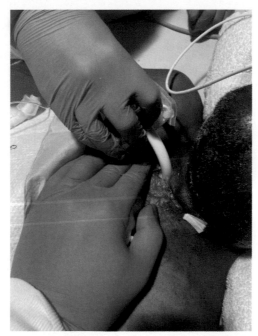

FIGURE 14.4. Note the caudal direction of the replacement tracheostomy through the stoma.

9. While one clinician removes the original tracheostomy while wiping the area clean with sterile saline-soaked gauze, the clinician/practitioner on the other side of the patient replaces the tracheostomy with a one-motion lateral turning caudal motion entering the inspected airway (Figures 14.4 and 14.5).
10. The obturator is removed (Figure 14.6).
11. The new inner cannula is readily replaced (Figure 14.7).
12. If available, a nasopharyngoscope is passed via the inner cannula for inspection of airway, anticipating a visualized clear and patent airway to the patient's carina, which confirms proper placement.
13. Ties are fastened and secured (Figure 14.8).
14. The neck roll is removed.
15. The patient is assisted to a more comfortable sitting position (if able).
16. Bed is lowered and siderails are raised.
17. A documented note in the patient's chart is written documenting ease of tracheostomy versus any significant events, size of tracheostomy previously, and new tracheostomy size and cuff status. It is important to document pulse oxygenation percentage prior to tracheostomy change, during the tracheostomy change, and after completion of tracheostomy change. Confirmation of an adequate airway should be documented along with postprocedure care of the tracheostomy and/or ties.

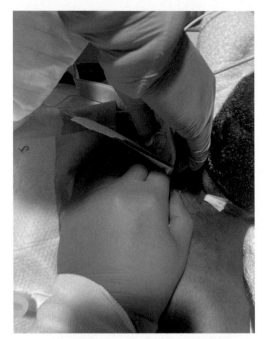

FIGURE 14.5. New tracheostomy has an obturator in place.

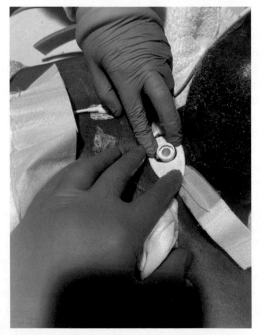

FIGURE 14.6. New tracheostomy after obturator removed.

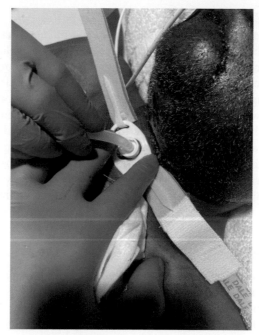

FIGURE 14.7. A disposable inner cannula is placed.

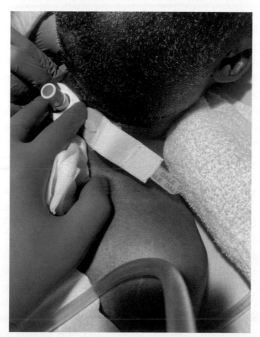

FIGURE 14.8. Notice one provider holds the tracheostomy plate while the other provider secures the Velcro ties.

Modified Seldinger Technique

Referencing *"Tracheostomy Tube Replacement Using a Modified Seldinger Technique,"* a *letter to the editor* in the *Journal of Critical Care*, August 1998, volume 16, issue 8, first describes a common procedure performed in intensive care and nonintensive care units of changing the tracheostomy tube over a catheter or inner cannula (stiff Salem sump, flexible nasopharyngolaryngoscope, Levine tube, Robnel catheter, etc.). First described for use in arteriography, this maneuver is described as replacement of a tracheostomy through a tract without an obturator. The tracheostomy is placed over the top of the curled end of the catheter or nasopharyngolaryngoscope. The appropriate catheter or nasopharyngolaryngoscope is introduced into the airway and a direct visualization of a clear and patent carina should be confirmed. The tracheostomy is then slid down over the catheter or pigtailed flexible end of a scope and reintroduced into the airway. Tracheostomy ties are fastened and secured.

COMPLICATIONS OF THE PROCEDURE

1. **Loss of airway, inability to properly ventilate the airway, or placement of a tracheostomy into a false passage:** Difficulty reestablishing an airway after a tracheostomy tube exchange is a life-threatening emergency. Proper replacement of a tracheostomy into an airway needs the immediate attention of an educated and trained respiratory therapist, experienced nurse, nurse practitioner, physician assistant, or physician. Use of a mouth bag mask ventilation, oral intubation, or introduction of an endotracheal tube into the patient's tracheotomy incision or stoma should be decided and performed quickly, but soundly. A misplaced or ill-positioned tracheostomy as an airway emergency requires an immediate attempt to reintroduce the tracheostomy tube into the airway and at times may require surgical intervention including, but not limited to, a tracheostomy revision or tracheal dilation. In a hospital setting, the initiation of a rapid response alert or of a respiratory "code blue" is recommended to help gather teams of providers to assist in critical airway emergencies and advanced cardiac and respiratory life support. Outpatient clinic replacement or home dislodgement often requires urgent emergency medical service calls and responses from a trained clinician and physicians. The previously described techniques of tracheostomy replacement should be attempted to establish an adequate airway. Cardiopulmonary resuscitation and advanced cardiac life support as recommended by the American Heart Association should always be considered depending on the patient's vital signs and respiratory and mental status.

2. **Bleeding:** Patients at high risk for bleeding or past medical histories of blood dyscrasias should be considered for delay of tracheostomy change until stable from a hematologic standpoint. Local bleeding from surrounding tissue can often be treated with pressure, topical hemostatic agents such as thrombin, local packing such as oxidized cellulose sheets, and possibly bedside electrocautery if refractory to local packing and topical agents. Severe cases may require an urgent or emergent

return to the operating room for hemostatic control in a controlled operating room environment.

3. **Airway obstruction from mucous plugging or crust:** Tracheostomy changes can often dislodge mucous plugs or crust that may have been present in the airway prior to the tracheostomy change but perhaps were not obstructive prior to the change. After a tracheostomy change, clearing the airway with a 14-French suction catheter can be advantageous to the respiratory tract by removing airway mucous, crust, and debris. Saline lavages followed by soft suctioning of the airway on nonventilated patients with a good cough reflex may promote a moistened and humidified airway, loosening any airway secretions for expectoration and/or manual removal by a trained clinician or nurse. If airway crust or mucous plugs collect in the tracheostomy tube after the tracheostomy change, removing and cleansing the tracheostomy inner cannula with half-strength hydrogen and peroxide solution and a wire brush is an appropriate intervention.

POSTPROCEDURE CARE

After a tracheostomy change, the person caring for the tracheostomy, whether it be the patient with the tracheostomy or a designated caregiver, should clean the tracheostomy tube twice daily. Cleansing the baseplate with sterile saline solution, moistened gauze, and sterile tip applicators is typically standard of care in most practice settings. If dried secretions and crusting builds up on the baseplate, half-strength peroxide solution mixed with sterile saline solution in equal parts can be used for débridement and cleansing of the tracheostomy. The inner cannula should be removed twice daily and cleansed with a wire brush in half-strength hydrogen peroxide and half-strength sterile saline solution and then rinsed with sterile saline solution. The tracheostomy ties should be secured around the neck, and two-finger breadths should be able to fit underneath the ties to assess tightness. Future tracheostomy changes should be considered every 3 to 6 months to maintain a clean and patent airway and tracheostomy tube.

BIBLIOGRAPHY

Aronow, J., & Bromley, H. R. (1988). Tracheostomy tube replacement using a modified Seldinger technique. *Critical Care Medicine, 16*(8), 818–819. https://doi.org/10.1097/00003246-198808000-00021

CHAPTER

15 Paracentesis

Kristopher Jackson
Starr Tomlinson

INDICATIONS FOR THE PROCEDURE

Abdominal paracentesis is a procedure in which a catheter or needle is introduced into the peritoneal cavity to sample or drain ascitic fluid for diagnostic and/or therapeutic purposes. Indications for the procedure are:

1. A diagnostic paracentesis is performed in order to determine the etiology of new-onset ascites or to rule out an infection, as in the case of spontaneous bacterial peritonitis.
2. A therapeutic, or large-volume paracentesis, is performed both for patient comfort and to prevent respiratory compromise when tense ascites is present.
3. Serial therapeutic paracenteses may be required if a patient has refractory ascites not responsive to diuretic therapy.
4. Approximately 85% of patients with ascites requiring paracentesis have been diagnosed with cirrhosis.
5. The remaining 15% of patients demonstrate nonhepatic causes of ascites, which include cancer, heart failure, nephrotic syndrome, tuberculosis, or pancreatitis.

Ascites from a patient's initial paracentesis should be sent for cell count, culture, total protein or albumin, and amylase to determine the underlying cause. If malignancy is suspected, cytology should also be obtained.

CONTRAINDICATIONS FOR THE PROCEDURE

Relative Contraindications

1. Disseminated intravascular coagulation and hyper-fibrinolytic states, as these patients require treatment to decrease the risk of bleeding
2. Intra-abdominal adhesions
3. Bowel obstruction or ileus
4. Pregnancy

Although not an absolute contraindication, careful thought is imperative when performing an abdominal paracentesis on a patient with a significant coagulopathy derangement or thrombocytopenia, particularly in a patient with comorbid renal dysfunction.

EQUIPMENT NEEDED

A variety of prepackaged paracentesis kits are commercially available and vary by institution. You should familiarize yourself with the specific device used at your facility prior to starting this or any other procedure.

For sterile preparation:

1. Skin cleansing agent
2. Sterile gauze
3. Sterile gloves and drape
4. Face shield
   For anesthesia administration:
5. Skin marking pen
6. 5 cc 1% to 2% lidocaine
7. 10 mL syringe
8. 22 to 25-gauge needle
   For ascites fluid collection:
9. Over-the-needle catheter device, such as a Yueh Centesis catheter needle
10. 60 mL syringe
11. High-pressure drainage tubing
12. Large evacuated containers
13. Specimen tubes
14. Sterile occlusive dressing

STEPS TO PERFORMING THE PROCEDURE

1. The patient should be in bed and placed in a supine position. The head of the bed should be mildly elevated at about 15°.
2. Identify a suitable site; this is typically performed using an ultrasound and a curvilinear or phased array ultrasound probe. Ultrasound increases procedural success, reduces chances of procedural complication, and may identify patients in whom there is insufficient ascites for paracentesis.
   a. Typical sites for abdominal paracentesis include the left lower quadrant, the right lower quadrant, and the avascular midline 2 cm below the umbilicus.
   b. If the left or right lower quadrants are chosen, be sure to make the puncture lateral to the rectus sheath to avoid puncture of the inferior epigastric artery.
   c. If a midline subumbilical approach is used, complete bladder emptying must be confirmed prior to initiation of the procedure.
   d. Take care to avoid passing the needle or catheter through sites of cutaneous infection, surgical scars, engorged blood vessels, or abdominal wall hematomas.
3. Once an appropriate location is chosen, the site should be marked with a skin marker.
4. Sterile gloves and a face shield must be applied prior to continuing the procedure. A sterile gown is not required but recommended. Once sterile, the site should be cleansed with an antiseptic solution, and a sterile drape should be placed.

5. A 22 to 25-gauge needle should be used to anesthetize the site with 1% or 2% lidocaine. A wheal should be injected superficially on the skin, and then the needle should be advanced to anesthetize the deeper tissues (Figure 15.1).

6. When advancing the catheter, pull back on the syringe intermittently until ascitic fluid is visible in the syringe. Once ascites fluid is seen, inject the remainder of the lidocaine in order to anesthetize the sensitive peritoneal lining.

7. An 18-gauge needle or scalpel should be used to make a small puncture at the site of insertion to ensure that the paracentesis catheter device can advance through the tough cutaneous tissue.

8. Hold the syringe with your dominant hand and the shaft of the catheter device in your nondominant hand close to the skin. Advance the paracentesis catheter device in 2 to 3 mm increments while intermittently pulling back on the plunger of the syringe.

9. The catheter should be advanced via an angular entry approach or a Z-tract technique in order to reduce the risk for postprocedure ascitic fluid leak.

10. When using the angular entry approach, the catheter is inserted at a 45° angle so that the cutaneous puncture site does not overlie the peritoneal puncture site. When using the Z-tract technique, the abdominal tissue is displaced 2 cm upward prior to catheter insertion so that the cutaneous insertion site retracts after removal.

11. You may feel a sudden loss of resistance when you enter the peritoneal cavity. When this occurs, or when ascitic fluid enters the syringe, stop the forward advancement of the needle and catheter immediately.

12. Advance the catheter over the needle and then remove the needle.

13. For a diagnostic paracentesis, attach a syringe to the catheter and remove 30 to 60 mL for ascitic fluid for analysis (Figure 15.2). For a large-volume or therapeutic paracentesis, attach one end of the high-pressure connection tubing to the catheter and the other end to the evacuated vacuum container.

14. Once adequate fluid has been removed, remove the catheter quickly and apply an occlusive sterile dressing.

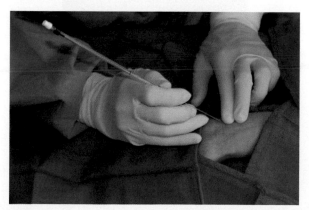

FIGURE 15.1. Optimal insertion angle with either palpation or ultrasound. Reprinted with permission from Freer, J. (2016). *Washington manual of bedside procedures.* Wolters Kluwer Health and Pharma.

COMPLICATIONS OF THE PROCEDURE

1. **Bleeding/hemorrhage:** Abdominal hematoma at the puncture site occurs in up to 1% of patients but is seldom serious. Acute arterial or venous hemorrhage can be life threatening but is very rare, with an incidence of less than 0.2%. The most serious bleeding complication involves puncture of the inferior epigastric artery, which requires emergent repair.
2. **Hemodynamic instability/hypotension:** This can occur owing to intravascular volume depletion and the large fluid shifts that commonly occur following a large-volume paracentesis. The use of colloid replacement is recommended for patients undergoing large-volume paracentesis of greater than 5 L to minimize fluid shifts and prevent hepatorenal syndrome.
3. **Infection:** Infection following paracentesis is very rare and is most often the result of concomitant bowel perforation. Regular monitoring of the paracentesis site for erythema, induration, or other signs of local infection is also important.
4. **Ascitic fluid leak:** This is probably the most common complication of paracentesis, with an occurrence of as high as 5% of cases. Measures to avoid ascitic fluid leak include the Z-track technique or angular entry approach. Utilizing a smaller bore needle and ensuring the smallest skin incision possible will also reduce this risk.
5. **Bowel perforation:** If the bowel is perforated by the paracentesis needle, infection and peritonitis may result and should be promptly treated with antibiotic therapy and surgical consultation.

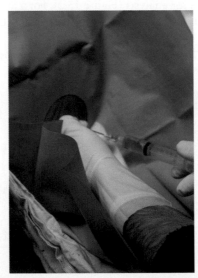

FIGURE 15.2. Insertion of blunt catheter over Caldwell needle. Reprinted with permission from Freer, J. (2016). *Washington manual of bedside procedures*. Wolters Kluwer Health and Pharma.

POSTPROCEDURAL CARE

Postprocedural care after paracentesis is minimal and fairly straightforward, barring any of the aforementioned complications. At the end of the procedure, the paracentesis catheter should be removed promptly in one quick motion and a sterile occlusive dressing placed. Aspirated ascites fluid should be placed in the appropriate tubes, labeled at the bedside, and sent to the laboratory immediately after the procedure. The use of colloid replacement after paracentesis remains controversial and is not usually recommended for paracentesis with fluid removal of less than 5 L. If appropriate, the recommended dose colloid replacement is 6 to 8 g of albumin per liter of ascites given intravenously post procedure.

BIBLIOGRAPHY

American Association for the Study of Liver Diseases (AASLD). (2013). *Management of adult patient with ascites due to cirrhosis: Update 2012.* https://www.aasld.org/publications/practice-guidelines

Aponte, E. M., & O'Rourke, M. C. (2018, October 27). *Paracentesis.* https://www.ncbi.nlm.nih.gov/books/NBK435998

Carpenter, D., Bowen, M., & Subramanian, R. (2016). Paracentesis. In: D. Taylor, S. Sherry, & R. Sing (Eds.), *Interventional critical care: A manual for advanced care practitioners* (pp. 299–310). Springer.

Gines, P., Cardenas, A., Arroyo, V., & Rodes, J. (2004). Management of cirrhosis and ascites. *New England Journal of Medicine, 350,* 1646–1654. https://doi.org/10.1056/nejm200407153510321

Gottardi, A. D., Thévenot, T., Spahr, L., Morard, I., Bresson–Hadni, S., Torres, F., Giostra, E., & Hadengue, A. (2009). Risk of complications after abdominal paracentesis in cirrhotic patients: A prospective study. *Clinical Gastroenterology and Hepatology, 7*(8), 906–909. https://doi.org/10.1016/j.cgh.2009.05.004

Lin, S., Wang, M., Zhu, Y., Dong, J., Weng, Z., Shao, L., Chen, J., & Jiang, J. (2015). Hemorrhagic complications following abdominal paracentesis in acute on chronic liver failure. *Medicine, 94*(49), e2225. https://doi.org/10.1097/md.0000000000002225

Moore, K. P. (2006). Guidelines on the management of ascites in cirrhosis. *Gut, 55*(suppl 6), vi1–vi12. https://doi.org/10.1136/gut.2006.099580

Runyon, B. A. (2009). Management of adult patients with ascites due to cirrhosis: An update. *Hepatology, 49*(6), 2087–2107. https://doi.org/10.1002/hep.22853

Sandhu, B. S., & Sanyal, A. J. (2005). Management of ascites in cirrhosis. *Clinics in Liver Disease, 9*(4), 715–732. https://doi.org/10.1016/j.cld.2005.07.008

Inserting Small-Bore Feeding Tubes (Nasoduodenal and Nasogastric)

Diana Filipek-Oberg

INDICATIONS FOR THE PROCEDURE

Enteral nutrition is the preferred method of feeding the critically ill patient. Enteral feeding can be through a Dobhoff tube or a surgically placed feeding tube (percutaneous endoscopic gastrostomy [PEG] tube, gastrostomy [G] tube, jejunostomy [J] tube) (Figure 16.1). For those who will not need prolonged feedings, a Dobhoff tube (nasoenteric tube) can be placed (Figure 16.2). Please note that a Dobhoff tube is different than a nasogastric tube (NGT) in that Dobhoff tubes are smaller in diameter and only for feeding and medication administration because they do not allow suctioning.

Enteral feeding provides multiple benefits to patients, such as maintaining the gut mucosa, stimulating the return of bowel function, and stimulating the immune barrier function and decreasing infectious complications. Of note, if therapy is needed for

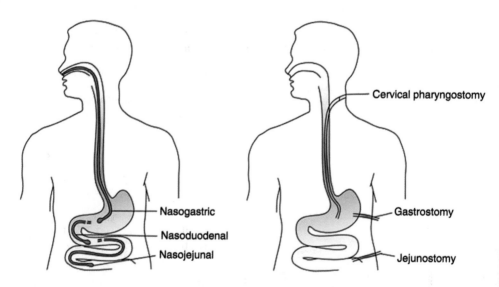

FIGURE 16.1. Nasoenteric and enterostomy feeding sites. Reprinted with permission from Alldredge, B. K., Corelli, R. L., Ernst, M. E., Guglielmo, B. J., & Jacobson, P. A. (2012). *Koda-Kimble & Young's applied therapeutics: The clinical use of drugs* (10th ed.). Wolters Kluwer.

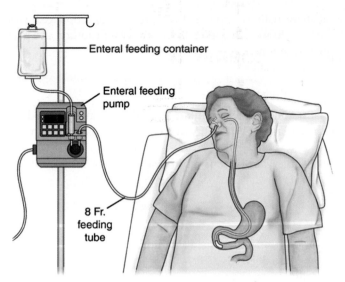

Enteral feeding container

Enteral feeding pump

8 Fr. feeding tube

FIGURE 16.2. Nasoenteric tube feeding by continuous controlled pump. The head of the bed should be elevated to prevent aspiration. Reprinted with permission from Hinkle, J. L., & Cheever, K. H. (2013). *Brunner & Suddarth's textbook of medical-surgical nursing* (13th ed.). Wolters Kluwer.

longer than 1 month, discuss with the family and medical team if a surgical feeding tube (PEG, G, GJ, or J) is warranted for long-term feeding options.

Indications for enteral feeding are:

1. Prolonged anorexia
2. Liver failure
3. Severe protein-energy undernutrition
4. Coma, altered mental status
5. Head or neck trauma, causing an inability to have oral intake
6. Metabolic stress secondary to critical illnesses
7. Malabsorption that could be related to chronic illness such as Crohn disease
8. Closure of enterocutaneous fistulas
9. Other conditions that limit oral intake
10. Postpyloric feedings are indicated for those with increased risk of aspiration, significant esophageal reflux, or gastric outlet obstruction.

CONTRAINDICATIONS FOR THE PROCEDURE

Relative Contraindications

1. Inability to protect the airway

2. Esophageal abnormalities—note that the presence of esophageal varices is not an absolute contraindication; however, there is a risk of rupture, and placement under fluoroscopy is recommended.
3. Coagulation abnormalities

Absolute Contraindications

1. Maxillofacial trauma, especially midface, as there is an increased risk of the tubing entering the cranial vault on placement. High risk if the cribriform plate is disrupted.
2. Recent facial surgery, as there is an increased risk of tubing entering the cranial vault.

EQUIPMENT NEEDED

1. Sterile gloves, gown, and face shield (medical institution requirement)
2. Dobhoff tubing (usually an 8–12 Fr)
3. Lubrication jelly
4. Cup of water with straw
5. Oral tip syringe with feeding tube water
6. Suction setup, oxygen setup at bedside in case of emergency
7. Tape/safety pin to secure the tubing after placement

STEPS TO PERFORMING THE PROCEDURE

1. Perform Standard Steps (see Preface for discussion of consent and patient identity).
2. Gather all supplies as above and set up at patient's bedside. Discuss the plan with the patient if able.
3. Patient should be sitting up (high Fowler). Measure the tubing to estimate insertion. Use the tube to measure the distance from the tip of the patient's nose to their earlobe, and then the earlobe to the xiphoid process for gastric placement. If intestinal placement is warranted, add approximately 10 inches or 25 cm.
4. A stylet can facilitate passage of the tube into the stomach. If a stylet is being inserted, using a syringe to inject 10 mL of water into the tube, because this activates the hydromer coating.
5. Lubricate the tip of the tubing.
6. Using the most patent nares, insert the tubing with the stylet. Keep a hand on the stylet the entire time you are inserting the tubing. Have patient flex their neck to help with guidance on insertion. Allow the patient to take sips of water to facilitate the passage of the tubing once the tubing has entered the oropharynx. Do not manipulate or pull stylet back and forth within the feeding tube. Advance tubing to the measured distance. Do not force tubing if you hit resistance. If the placement is proving difficult, consider fluoroscopic guided tube insertions (Figure 16.3).
7. Placement is to be confirmed from x-ray (Figure 16.4). Make sure tubing and stylet are secured prior to confirmation, because you cannot lose the stylet into the tubing.
8. Once placement is confirmed, flush with another 10 mL of water to help remove the stylet. Secure tubing with tape (Figure 16.5).

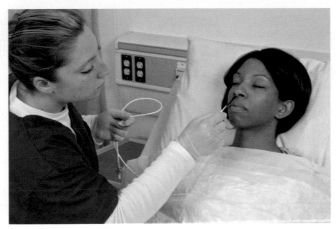

FIGURE 16.3. Feeding tube insertion and removal. Inserting the tube nasally. Insert the curved, lubricated tip into the more patent nostril and direct it along the nasal passage toward the ear on the same side. When it passes the nasopharyngeal junction, turn the tube 180° to aim it downward into the esophagus. Tell the patient to lower their chin to their chest to close the trachea. Then give the patient a small cup of water with a straw or ice chips. Direct the patient to sip the water or suck on the ice and swallow frequently. This will ease the tube's passage. Advance the tube as the patient swallows. Reprinted with permission from Springhouse. (2008). *Lippincott's visual encyclopedia of clinical skills.* Wolters Kluwer Health.

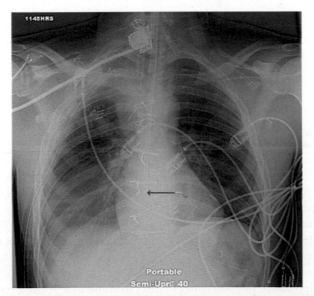

FIGURE 16.4. Radiograph showing initial insertion of the feeding tube into the distal esophagus to confirm midline positioning beyond the carina. Reprinted with permission from Dimick, J. B., Upchurch, G. R., & Sonnenday, C. J. (2012). *Clinical scenarios in surgery: Decision making and operative technique.* Wolters-Kluwer.

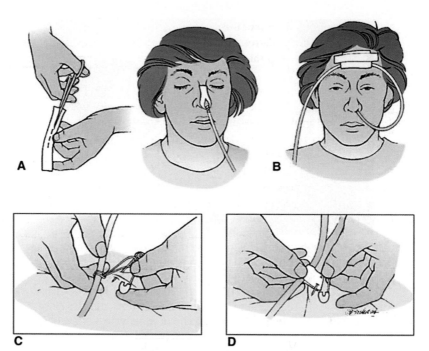

FIGURE 16.5. Securing nasogastric and nasoenteric tubes. (A) The nasogastric tube is secured to the nose with tape to prevent injury to the nasopharyngeal passages; the cheek may also be used. (B) Tape is placed on the forehead, and the nasoenteric tube is taped to it, thereby allowing the tube to be advanced until the desired placement is achieved. (C, D) Secure tubing to the patient's gown with an elastic band or tape attached to a safety pin to prevent tension on the line during movement. Reprinted with permission from Rosdahl, C. B., & Kowalski, M. T. (2012) *Textbook of basic nursing* (10th ed.). Wolters-Kluwer.

COMPLICATIONS OF THE PROCEDURE

1. **Aspiration pneumonia:** Associated with long-term use of nasoenteric feeding. Remember to discuss with the patient/medical team/family the long-term plan for nutrition if this discussion is warranted. Surgical feeding tube will likely be necessary if feeding is to be over 4 to 6 weeks.
2. **Clogged tube:** Flush after feedings with water to keep tube patent. Flush after medication administration with water. Discuss with your clinical pharmacist if you have a clog zapper medication that can be administered to the Dobhoff tube to break up the clogged tubing.
3. **Tube malposition, pneumothorax:** This can result in a pneumothorax if the tube is placed into the trachea or, less commonly, the distal tracheobronchial tree. It can also result in pleural effusions or pneumonia. Monitor for these if tube was not in

the correct location. If placement imaging comes back and shows misplacement or patient shows respiratory distress, remove Dobhoff tube immediately and obtain a stat chest x-ray. Treat respiratory distress appropriately. For radiograph of tube malposition and correction.

4. **Dislodgement/inadvertent removal:** Increased risks are those who are agitated, altered mental status. Assess the need for restraints based on your medical institution's policy. Use appropriate measures to tape the tubing to the patient so it cannot be accidentally caught on something or removed.

5. **Esophageal perforation:** This is a rare but serious complication more likely to occur in patients with previous gastric surgery. A frontal and lateral chest x-ray would be advisable to confirm correct placement.

6. **Epistaxis:** This is a minor complication from Dobhoff tube insertion, and those at risk include those with a history of sinusitis, coagulation disorders, and nasal polyps. If warranted, can consider a consult to an ear, nose, and throat specialist for nasal packing.

7. **Sinusitis:** This is a long-term complication from longer time frame on tube feedings. Increased risk for those who require long-term ventilation support.

POSTPROCEDURE CARE

Once the tube is placed, get the chest x-ray to confirm location of the tube. On x-ray, the tube should pass vertically midline below the level of the carina, with the tip of the tube visible below the level of the diaphragm. The tube should not enter the right or left bronchi. Electromagnetic placement device (EMPD) may offer a method to verify feeding tube placement with a decrease in radiation exposure to the patient; however, studies have mixed results. The radiograph of the lower chest/upper abdomen for "feeding tube placement" is the standard of care. Once placement is verified and the tube is visualized to be centrally present distal to the carina, crossing the diaphragm, into the gastric region with the tip dependent in the stomach, an order for feedings can occur. Consult nutrition and dietary services. Combined, these services will be able to discuss with you and the patient the appropriate tube feeding, goals, and supplements needed for the patient. Assess daily for whether the patient is stable for Dobhoff removal and oral trial. Also assess daily for patency as well as positioning. Document the measurement visible each day. A speech therapist should also be following the patient if there was a risk of aspiration that warranted the feedings.

BIBLIOGRAPHY

Abidali, A., Dzandu, J. K., Mangram, A., Moeser, P., Shirah, G.R., & Wilson, W. (2018). Bilateral pneumothoraces in a trauma patient after Dobhoff tube insertion. *American Journal of Case Reports, 19*, 244–248.

Abrams, K., Bryant, V., & Phang, J. (2015). Verifying placement of small-bore feeding tubes: Electromagnetic device images versus abdominal radiographs. *American Journal of Critical Care, 24*(6), 525–530.

Baskin, W. N. (2006). Acute complications associated with bedside placement of feeding tubes. *Nutrition in Clinical Practice, 21*, 40–55.

Burns, S. M. (Ed.). (2014). *AACN essentials of critical care nursing.* McGraw Hill Education.

Cardinal Health. *Covidien: Kangaroo Nasogastric Feeding Tube.* (2018, December 29). http://mycardinalmsds. com/DFU/2011_11_15_8884710859_IFU.pdf

Hodin, R., & Bordeianou, L. (2020). *Inpatient placement and management of nasogastric and nasoenteric tubes in adults.* UpToDate Topic 15070 Version 18.0.

Numata, Y., Ishii, K., Seki, H., Yasui, N., Sakata, M., Shimada, A., & Matsumoto, H. (2018). Perforation of abdominal esophagus following nasogastric feeding tube intubation: A case report. *International Journal of Surgery Case Reports, 45*, 67–71. https://doi.org/10.1016/j.ijscr.2018.03.007

Powers, J., Luebbehusen, M., Aguirre, L., Cluff, J., David, M. A., Holly, V., Linford, L., Park, N., & Brunelle, R. (2018). Improved safety and efficacy of small-bore feeding tube confirmation using an electromagnetic placement device. *Nutrition Clinical Practice, 33*(2), 268–273. https://doi.org/10.1002/ncp.10062

Administering Local Anesthetics

Brooke Carpenter

INDICATIONS FOR THE PROCEDURE

Local anesthetics are used to block nerve transmission at the site of administration and thereby temporarily inhibit sensation to the area. There are a variety of techniques for administration, including topical anesthesia, peripheral nerve blocks, infiltrative (subcutaneous/submucosal), neuraxial (spinal/epidural), and IV regional anesthesia. This book focuses on administration of subcutaneous local anesthesia. A common technique is direct infiltration of the targeted site.

Indications for subcutaneous infiltration of local anesthetics are:

1. Open wound/laceration repair or abscess drainage
2. Vascular access procedures (IV placement, central lines, suturing)
3. Lumbar punctures

CONTRAINDICATIONS FOR THE PROCEDURE

Relative Contraindications

1. History of prior contact dermatitis or delayed localized swelling with a local anesthetic. It is important to note that most allergic reactions related to local anesthetics are likely secondary to the preservatives (methylparaben) or antioxidants (only used in anesthetics that contain epinephrine; Becker & Reed). Additionally, most patients with a prior reaction will likely be tolerant to an anesthetic from an alternate classification. If the drug is known, it is reasonable to proceed with a local anesthetic of a different classification (amide versus ester), preservative free, and without epinephrine. However, allergen testing before the patient receives a local anesthetic is ideal.

2. The use of epinephrine additives in patients with cardiac disease remains controversial. The provider should exercise caution in patients with unstable angina, uncontrolled diabetes, uncontrolled hypertension, uncontrolled hyperthyroidism, refractory dysrhythmias, recent myocardial infarction, or coronary bypass surgery within 6 months.

Absolute Contraindications

1. History of a prior true allergic reaction to a local anesthetic (i.e., anaphylaxis, generalized urticaria, or other life-threatening reaction). The provider should not proceed with the use of any local anesthetic until a thorough evaluation has been done by an allergist. If the procedure is urgent or emergent, an alternative anesthetic modality should be utilized.
2. The use of epinephrine additive should be avoided for digital and penile blocks, skin flaps, or procedures of the ear or nasal tip. The provider should avoid epinephrine to these areas owing to the potent vasoconstrictor properties and risk of localized ischemia.

EQUIPMENT NEEDED

The provider should first choose the local anesthetic agent depending on the procedure location, duration, and patient history. Local anesthetics are classified as amides or esters (Table 17.1). The most commonly used anesthetics for subcutaneous infiltration are all amide agents—lidocaine, bupivacaine, mepivacaine, and procain. Esters are less common and generally used for a patient with a history of a prior allergic reaction to an amide agent.

Lidocaine is most versatile and commonly used. It is typically given as a 1% solution with or without epinephrine. Epinephrine as an additive produces local vasoconstriction, reduces bleeding during the procedure, decreases anesthetic systemic toxicity,

TABLE 17.1 Local Anesthetic Drug Classifications

Esters	Amides
Benzocaine (Americaine, Lanacane)	Articaine (Septocaine, Zorcaine)
Chloroprocaine (Nesacaine)	Bupivacaine (Marcaine)
Cocaine	Levobupivacaine
Procaine (Novocaine)	Dibucaine (Nupercainal)
Proparacaine	Etidocaine (Duranest)
Tetracaine	Lidocaine (Xylocaine)
	Mepivacaine (Carbocaine)
	Prilocaine (Citanest)
	Ropivacaine (Naropin)

Data from Hsu, D. (2020). Subcutaneous infiltration of local anesthetics. In J. F. Wiley (Ed.), *UpToDate*. Retrieved March 28, 2021, from https://www.uptodate.com/contents/subcutaneous-infiltration-of-localanesthetics?search=infiltrative%20local%20anestheia&source=search_result&selectedTitle=5~150&usage_type=default&display_rank=5#H2694370

and prolongs numbing effects by 3 hours. Alternatively, bupivacaine has an intermediate onset with a longer duration of action and is useful for prolonged procedures where epinephrine is contraindicated. Equipment needed includes:

1. Chlorhexidine or povidone–iodine topical antiseptic
2. Sterile gloves
3. Sterile gauze
4. 25-gauge, 27-gauge, or 30-gauge 1.5-inch-long needle
5. Syringe (1, 3, 5, or 10 mL)
6. Local anesthetic agent

STEPS FOR THE PROCEDURE

1. Discuss the procedure (direct infiltration of local anesthetic) with the patient and/ or caregiver, including complications. Review patient allergies. Obtain consent as necessary.
2. Choose anesthetic agent according to technique, location, and clinical situation.
3. Assess area distal to wound/laceration/injection site to confirm there is no vascular compromise.
4. Clean site with chlorhexidine or povidone–iodine and allow to dry.
5. Put on sterile gloves.
6. *For intact skin:* rapidly insert needle at a 45° angle with the bevel up, directly into the subcutaneous layer (Figure 17.1). While withdrawing the needle, steadily inject small amounts of anesthetic. Aspiration prior to injecting can be considered but is not mandatory, unless injecting in a highly vascularized area. *For open wounds:* administer a few drops of anesthetic into the wound bed prior to inserting the needle into the subcutaneous layer, and then proceed with administration as described.
7. After a few minutes, test the site for adequate anesthesia by stimulating area with a sharp object.

COMPLICATIONS OF THE PROCEDURE

1. **Central nervous system or cardiovascular toxicity:** Symptoms can include metallic taste, tingling lips, dizziness, altered mental status, bradycardia, heart block, dysrhythmia, or cardiac arrest.
   Treatment:
   • Stop injection; while stabilizing the patient, prepare lipid emulsion bolus, manage airway, proceed with advanced cardiac life support (ACLS) if necessary; administer benzodiazepines for seizure activity.
   • Amiodarone is the first-line antiarrhythmic; avoid vasopressin, beta blockers, or calcium channel blockers. Administer epinephrine at less than 1 µg/kg.
2. **Vasovagal syncope:** Likely a response to the actual injection. If this occurs, the provider should place the patient in Trendelenburg position, assess vital signs, administer oxygen via nasal cannula, and stimulate reflexes using cold compresses.

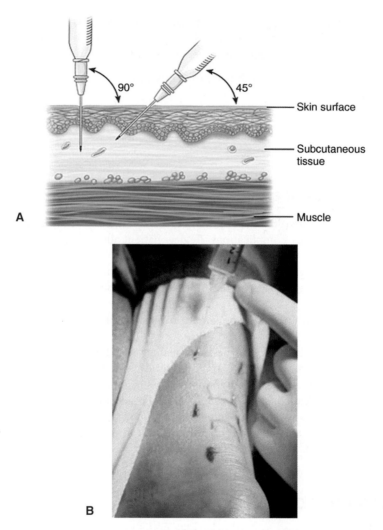

FIGURE 17.1. (A) Subcutaneous injection deposits medication in subcutaneous tissue at a 45° or 90° angle. (B) Local anesthetic used for the procedure. (A) Reprinted with permission from Craven, R. F., Hirnle, C. J., & Henshaw, C. M. (2016). *Fundamentals of nursing* (8th ed.). Wolters Kluwer. (B) Reprinted with permission from Easley, M. E., & Wiesel, S. W. (2010). *Operative techniques in foot and ankle surgery*. Wolters Kluwer.

3. **Allergic reaction:**
   - *Contact dermatitis and/or inflammation:* blistering and localized eczematous rash can occur up to 72 hours after administration. Follow treatment as indicated for contact dermatitis.
   - *Urticaria and anaphylaxis:* provider should proceed with emergent treatment of anaphylaxis and monitor for any signs of airway compromise (wheezing, oral swelling, stridor) or hypotension.

POSTPROCEDURE CARE

There is minimal postprocedure care following subcutaneous infiltration of local anesthesia. The key assessment factor is adequate pain control, which should be evaluated before, during, and after the procedure. Monitoring for the above complications is imperative, along with educating the patient on contacting their healthcare provider if they experience any delayed allergic reactions at the injection site (i.e., contact dermatitis).

BIBLIOGRAPHY

Achar, S., & Kundu, S. (2002). Principles of office anesthesia: part I. infiltrative anesthesia. *American Family Physician, 66*(1), 91–93. https://www.aafp.org/journals/afp.html

Becker, D. E., & Reed, K. L. (2012). Local anesthetics: Review of pharmacological considerations. *Anesthesia Progress, 59*(2), 90–102. https://doi.org/10.2344/0003-3006-59.2.90

Hsu, D. (2020). Subcutaneous infiltration of local anesthetics. In J. F. Wiley (ed.), *UpToDate*. Retrieved March 28, 2021, from https://www.uptodate.com/contents/subcutaneous-infiltration-of-localanesthetics?search=infiltrative%20local%20anestheia&source=search_result&selectedTitle=5~150&usage_type=default&display_rank=5#H2694370

Latham, J., & Martin, S. (2014). Infiltrative anesthesia in office practice. *American Family Physician, 89*(12), 956–962.

Roberts, J. R., & Hedges, J. R. (2010). *Clinical procedures in emergency medicine*. Saunders/Elsevier.

CHAPTER

18 Wound Closure—Sutures

Diana Filipek-Oberg

INDICATIONS FOR THE PROCEDURE

Suturing is warranted in the medical field when there is a need to bring tissue together, most likely related to wounds or surgical sites. A needle that is attached to a specific suture is used through various techniques to close the wound or surgical site. It is important to note that there are different options for the sutures with regard to both the technique of closing the wound as well as the specific suture material and size to choose (Figure 18.1). Prior to closing the wound, it is important to make sure you have cleansed the area and washed the wound out appropriately.

Indications for the procedure are:

1. Types of open wounds requiring closure include, but are not limited to, stab wounds, lacerations, most penetrating traumas
2. Offer support to strengthen wounds until the healing process increases their tensile strength
3. Decrease the risk of bleeding and infection within wounds
4. Approximating skin edges for both functional result as well as cosmetic result

It is important to note that if the wound appears to be complex or a facial wound, you can consider a consultation placed to plastic surgery for wound examination and closure. Complex wounds include wounds with multiple layers, not symmetrical, or complex locations (near eyes, eyebrow, hand/fingers, etc.).

CONTRAINDICATIONS FOR THE PROCEDURE

Relative Contraindications

1. **Facial wounds and complex wounds:** Consider a consultation to plastic surgery for repair.
2. **Tendon, nerve, joint, or other anatomic structure damage:** This wound should be explored prior to closure.
3. **Contaminated wounds:** Do not close a wound that appears dirty or to have a foreign body within it. You need to obtain imaging to confirm that there is a foreign body, then clean/debride the wound appropriately. If there is a foreign body, discuss the approach with your medical–surgical team.
4. **Overall factors:** Time from injury, tissue damage, contamination, and potential for foreign material prior to suture wound closure. Discuss any concerns or thoughts with the medical team to plan appropriate wound management.

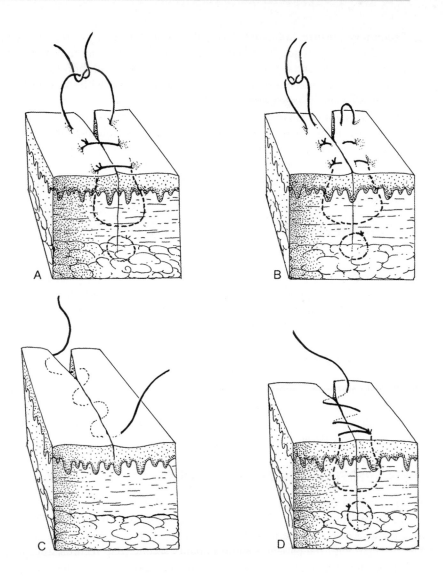

FIGURE 18.1. Techniques of skin closure: (A) Simple interrupted sutures. (B) Vertical mattress sutures. (C) Running intracuticular (subcuticular) sutures. (D) Continuous simple sutures. Reprinted with permission from Lawrence, P. F. (2007). *Essentials of surgical specialties* (3rd ed.). Lippincott Williams & Wilkins.

Absolute Contraindications

1. **Time outside the "golden period":** Chances of developing a wound infection increase with each hour that passes from the time of initial injury.
   a. **Time frame:** Generally speaking, 6 to 8 hours from the time of injury is a safe interval to repair the uncomplicated laceration by primary closure/intention.

b. **Secondary closure indicated:** Skin ulcerations, abscess cavities, punctures, partial thickness tissue losses, and small, noninfectious animal bites can be left to heal by secondary closure. For wound care, you will thoroughly cleanse, irrigate, and debride, but sutures are not required. Cover with sterile nonadherent dressing and change every 24 to 48 hours.

c. **Delayed primary closure:** Bite wounds and lacerations that go beyond the golden period of repair should be cleansed, irrigated, and debrided, then covered with a dry sterile dressing. Oral antibiotics should be provided over a course of 3 to 5 days, upon which the patient returns for a wound check. If the wound appears to be "fresh," closure with sutures or another adhesive can be considered.

EQUIPMENT NEEDED

1. Appropriate suture material: This depends on the location and size of the wound. Absorbable sutures lose tensile strength within 60 days of being placed, often used under casts, facial sutures, and oral mucosa. Most commonly used are Vicryl, Dexon, and PDS (polydioxanone). Nonabsorbable suture options are silk, nylon, polypropylene, and polybutester. Silk is frequently used to secure central lines, chest tubes, and other lines/medical equipment.
2. Sterile/nonsterile gloves
3. Needle
4. Needle holder/driver
5. Gauze
6. Normal saline or water for wound cleansing. Of note, hydrogen peroxide has been found to do more damage than positive outcomes.

STEPS TO PERFORMING THE PROCEDURE

1. Perform standard steps (see Preface).
2. Select the appropriate type of suture and size (as above) for the wound. Prepare the area for where you will perform the procedure and obtain all equipment needed. Discuss plan with the patient. Obtain patient's recent Tdap records, and order to be administered if necessary. Make sure to wear gloves and protective eyewear. Remove any jewelry or clothing/material if needed. Consider clipping hair that may get in the way of wound closure, but do not clip eyebrows, because they grow back occasionally.
3. Assess the wound. Obtain measurements to document. Examine whether wound is dirty or includes any foreign bodies. If so, obtain appropriate imaging to assess for foreign bodies, usually x-rays.
4. Administer appropriate pain medications for patient. Lidocaine may be given through an injection around the wound area. Do not use lidocaine with epinephrine at areas with terminal blood flow, such as fingers, ears, nose, or toes. Oral or intravenous pain medication can also be used.

5. Cleanse the wound. Use sterile water or saline to thoroughly cleanse the wound of dirt and debris. Wound irrigation can be completed with normal saline through a syringe, with catheter application, to provide a steady stream to the wound area to wash out debris and other contaminants (Figure 18.2).
6. Using appropriate suture type and size for the wound, begin to suture. There are multiple techniques for sutures to close wounds (Figure 18.3).
   a. **Simple interrupted suture:** This is the standard technique for closure of most uncomplicated wounds (Figure 18.4). With the needle loaded to the driver, insert the needle perpendicular to the epidermis, about one-half the needle distance to the wound edge, therefore allowing the needle to exit the wound on the contralateral side at an equal distance from the wound's edge. Rotate the needle through the dermis using your wrist in a fluid motion. The needle tip should exit the skin on the opposite side of the wound. Needle body should be grasped with surgical forceps and pulled upward with the forceps as the body of the needle is released from the needle driver. The number of sutures required to close

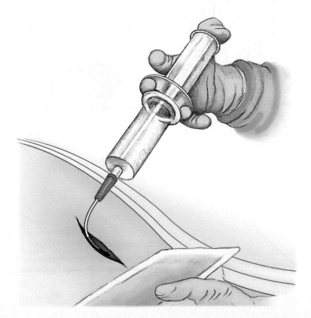

FIGURE 18.2. Irrigating a deep wound. When preparing to irrigate a wound, attach a 19-gauge needle or catheter to a 35-mL piston syringe. This setup delivers an irrigation pressure of 8 psi, which is effective in cleaning the wound and reducing the risk of trauma and wound infection. To prevent tissue damage or—in an abdominal wound—intestinal perforation, avoid forcing the needle or catheter into the wound. Irrigate the wound with gentle pressure until the solution returns clean. Position the emesis basin under the wound to collect remaining drainage. Reprinted with permission from *Lippincott's nursing advisor* (2014). Wolters Kluwer.

Over and over sutures
(interrupted and continuous)

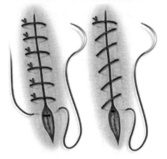

Subcuticular sutures
(interrupted and continuous)

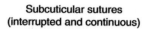
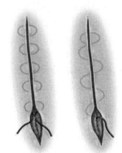

Horizontal mattress sutures
(interrupted and continuous)

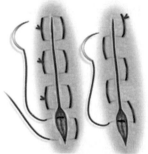

Vertical mattress sutures
(interrupted and continuous)

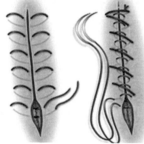

FIGURE 18.3. Suture closure techniques. Reprinted with permission from Chung, K. C., Disa, J. J., Gosain, A., Lee, G., Mehrara, B., Thorne, C. H., & van Aalst, J. (2019). *Operative techniques in plastic surgery*. Wolters Kluwer.

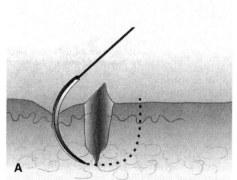
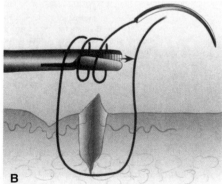

FIGURE 18.4. (A and B) A simple interrupted cuticular suture secured with an instrument tie. Reprinted with permission from Fleisher, G. R., Ludwig, S., & Baskin, M. N. (2004). *Atlas of pediatric emergency medicine*. Lippincott Williams & Wilkins.

a wound depends on the length, shape, and location of the wound/lacerations. Sutures should be placed just far enough from each other so that no gap appears within the wound edges. The fewest sutures should be used at all times. Suture material is then tied off, with care taken to minimize tension across the dermis and to avoid overly constricting the wound's edges.

b. **Running suture:** Used often for percutaneous closure of a longer wound, the same procedure is done as noted previously. However, instead of cutting the suture after the initial knot, the needle is used to make repeated bites at a 45° angle to the wound direction. This is continued until the final bite is taken at a 90° angle to the wound direction, and then it is knotted off (Figure 18.5).

7. Cover wound with appropriate dressing. Discuss plan for suture removal and post-suture care.

COMPLICATIONS OF THE PROCEDURE

1. **Infection:** Patient, nursing staff, and advanced practice providers should continuously monitor wounds that are both open and closed for any signs of infection. This includes redness in the area, swelling, pus-like drainage, fevers, malodorous drainage, and red streaks. If noticed, the patient will need oral antibiotics as discussed with the medical team. This is why the provider should apply an antibiotic ointment, such as topical bacitracin, and a nonadhesive dressing immediately after suture repair is complete.

2. **Delayed wound healing:** Monitor closely to see if the wound is healing appropriately, including looking for any outward signs of infection, well-approximated edges, full skin closure, and adherence. Sutures may need to be removed for appropriate wound exploration or different wound closure.

3. **Bleeding:** If bleeding occurs while suturing, apply direct pressure to the wound with 4 × 4 sponges. Continuous pressure must be maintained for a minimum of 10 minutes and, if possible, use an ace wrap to secure the sponges.

POSTPROCEDURE CARE

Once the wound is closed, it is important to make note of when the suturing is done so that appropriate removal can be scheduled or planned, whether inpatient, follow-up in clinic, or as an outpatient. Face sutures usually remain in for 4 to 5 days, scalp for 5 days, abdomen/trunk approximately 7 days, arm or leg approximately 7 to 10 days, and foot or hand approximately 7 to 10 days. While sutures are intact, monitor the wound daily for any signs or symptoms of infection such as redness, swelling, tenderness, pus-like drainage, or odor. Also, it is important to write a procedure note that states whether the wound was cleansed prior to closing, how many sutures were used, what size suture and material, as well as when they will be ready for removal.

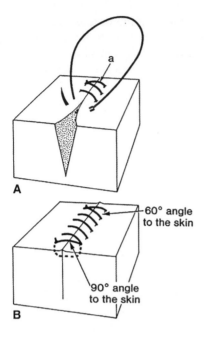

A

B

60° angle to the skin

90° angle to the skin

FIGURE 18.5. The continuous over-and-over suture. (A) Begin this continuous suture with a single suture that is tied to anchor the rest of the suture. Pass the needle perpendicular to the skin edge; the suture threads lie perpendicular to the wound margin to maximize the effect of the suture on extrinsic wound tension, as with the simple interrupted suture. (B) To finish and tie off this continuous suture, grab the loop formed at the free end after insertion of the needle through the skin at its midpoint with the needle holder, and pull on this loop. It will come together as if it were a single thread. Tie the needle end of the suture material and this "looped" free end as a simple interrupted suture would be tied. When one is proficient with this suture, eversion of the skin edges is quite adequate. Reprinted with permission from Simon, R. R., Ross, C. P., Bowman, S. H., & Wakim, P. E. (2012). *Cook county manual of emergency procedures.* Wolters Kluwer.

When sutures are ready for removal, first cleanse the area with an appropriate cleansing agent (Figure 18.6). Then remove, using tweezers to lift the suture and scissors to cut. Use the tweezers to gently pull the suture out of the wound area.

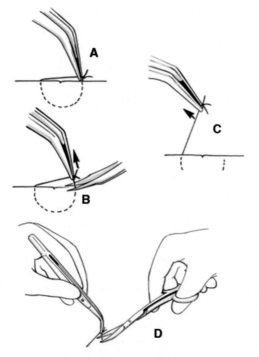

A

B

C

D

FIGURE 18.6. Suture removal. (A) Suture grasped by pliers near the entrance into tissue. (B) Suture pulled gently up while scissor is inserted close to the tissue. Suture is cut in the part previously buried in the tissue. (C) Suture is held up for vertical removal. (D) Suture is pulled gently to bring it out on the side opposite from where it was cut. The objective is to prevent the external part of the suture from passing through the tissue and introducing infectious material. Reprinted with permission from Wilkins, E. M. (2013). *Clinical practice of the dental hygienist* (11th ed.) Wolters Kluwer.

BIBLIOGRAPHY

Kantor, J. (Ed.). (2017). *Atlas of suturing techniques: Approaches to surgical wound, laceration, and cosmetic repair.* McGraw Hill.

Mackay-Wiggan, J. (2018). *Suturing techniques.* Medscape, Updated on July 10, 2018.

Trott, A. T. (2012). *Wounds and lacerations: Emergency care and closure.* Elsevier-Saunders.

UpToDate, Inc. (2020, June). *Closure of minor skin wounds with sutures.* Wolters Kluwer.

19 Wound Closure—Staples

Kristina Davis

INDICATIONS FOR THE PROCEDURE

A laceration often requires wound closure, which can be obtained by utilizing metal staples. Wound closure is performed to achieve hemostasis, minimize wound infection, preserve function, reduce pain, and improve cosmetic outcome. Staple closure is rapid, easily performed, does not require hair removal, and causes minimal tissue reaction. Staple placement is comparable with suture repair in regard to infection rates, cost, and tensile strength.

Location indications for the procedure are:

1. Scalp, arms, legs, or truck laceration
2. Shallow (through the dermis)
3. Noncosmetic areas
4. Linear laceration

CONTRAINDICATIONS FOR THE PROCEDURE

Relative Contraindications

1. Staples should not be used in hands or feet because of discomfort they may cause.
2. Any area that has cosmetic significance should not be closed with staples, owing to the inability to meticulously close a wound.

Absolute Contraindications

1. Staples should not be used in patients who may require magnetic resonance imaging (MRI) or computed tomography (CT) imaging acutely.
2. Acute allergy to metallic component of staple.

EQUIPMENT NEEDED

1. Stapler
2. Anesthetic
   a. Injectable—consider pain of an anesthetic injection versus the pain of staple placement. Discuss risks versus benefits with the patient.
      i. Lidocaine 1%, 2%, with/without epinephrine; bupivacaine 0.25%; diphenhydramine 1% for patients who are allergic to ester local anesthetic
      1. Small gauge needle 25 or 27
      2. Syringe

b. Topical
   i. Lidocaine/epinephrine/tetracaine
3. Forceps
4. Antibiotic ointment
5. Staple remover (in case a staple is misplaced)

STEPS TO PERFORMING THE PROCEDURE

1. Perform Standard Steps (see Preface for discussion of consent and patient identity).
2. Obtain a history
   a. Circumstance of injury
   b. Level of contaminating
   c. Past medical history that may influence healing
   d. Immunization status
3. Perform a wound assessment
   a. Anatomic location (Figure 19.1)
   b. Extent of injury (access closely for tendon and vascular injury)
   c. Exploration
   d. Consider imaging for foreign bodies or underlying fracture.
   e. Assess tetanus status
4. Perform wound cleaning
   a. The extent of wound cleansing is a clinical decision and should be based on the wound and level of contamination. High-pressure irrigation greater than 25 psi should be done only for highly contaminated wounds that need debridement.
   b. Irrigation with saline or a 1:10 diluted povidone/iodine solution with saline. May also wash wound under a running faucet with tap water.
5. Perform wound repair
   a. Align and evert wound edges (may be accomplished with an assistant), stapler centered while pressing gently against the skin, space staples evenly apart.
   b. The staple crossbar (cross member) should not be lying directly on the skin but rather a few millimeters above it.

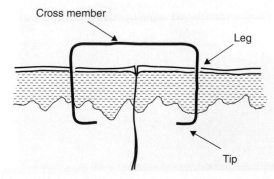

FIGURE 19.1. Cross section of a staple. Reprinted with permission from Mattu, A., Chanmugam, A. S., Swadron, S. P., Tibbles, Woolridge, D., & Marcucci, L. (2010). *Avoiding common errors in the emergency department.* Wolters Kluwer.

6. Considerations
    a. A deeper laceration may be closed with staples secondary to repair of the deep fascia and tension reductions with deep, absorbable sutures.
    b. Oral antibiotics should be considered for high-risk patients or contaminated wounds.

COMPLICATIONS OF THE PROCEDURE

1. **Infection:** Patient discharge instructions should include signs and symptoms of wound infection and strict return precautions.
2. **Poor cosmetic outcome:** Discuss with the patient and/or guardian the possibility of scarring.
3. **Retained foreign body:** For suspected foreign body (FB), imaging should be obtained prior to closure. There may be instances when an FB is left intentionally based on location, FB material, and risks versus benefits of removal. Include the patient and/or guardian in the decision-making process. If an FB is left intentionally, consider antibiotic prophylaxis and specialist follow-up.
4. **Tendon injury:** Inspect visually for tendon involvement. Assess musculoskeletal movement to include strength and range of motion (passive and active).
5. **Nerve injury:** Assess distal sensation including two-point discrimination.

POSTPROCEDURE CARE

Once staples are placed, a nonadherent dressing may be considered based on wound location. Antibiotic ointment may be applied with a warning to patients that bacitracin may cause dermatitis, and if this occurs patients should discontinue use. Patients need to follow up for staple removal in 7 to 10 days for scalp, 10 to 14 days for lower extremities, and 7 to 10 days for upper extremities. Removal must be done with a staple remover (Figure 19.2). Patients should be instructed to return for symptoms of infection.

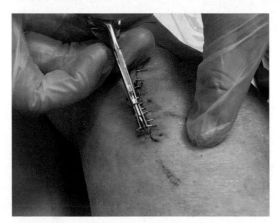

FIGURE 19.2. Staple removal. Note the staple remover's tip around the staple as pressure is applied to the handle to remove the staple. Reprinted with permission from Egol. K. (2017). *The orthopaedic manual: From the office to the OR.* Wolters Kluwer.

BIBLIOGRAPHY

Lammers, R., & Aldy, K. (2019). Methods of wound closure. In J. Roberts, C. Custalow, & T. W. Thomsen (Eds.), *Roberts and Hedges' clinical procedures in emergency medicine and acute care*. Elsevier. (7th ed., pp. 655–707).

Mankowitz, S. (2017). Laceration management. *Journal of Emergency Medicine, 53*(3), 369–382.

Miller, J., & Moake, M. (2018). Procedure. In *Harriet Lane handbook* (pp. 30–72).

Quinn, R., Wedmore, I., Johnson, E., Islas, A., Anglim, A., Zafren, K., Bitter, C., & Mazzorana, V. (2014). Wilderness medical society practice guidelines for basic wound management in the austere environment: 2014 Update. *Wilderness & Environmental Medicine, 25*, S118–S133. https://www.wemjournal.org/article/S1080-6032(14)00278-6/pdf

Shah, K., & Mason, C. (2015). *Essential emergency procedures* (2nd ed.). Wolters Kluwer Health.

Singer, A., Hollander, J., & Quinn, J. (1997). Evaluation and management of traumatic lacerations. *New England Journal of Medicine, 337*(16), 1142.

Wilson, J., & Diaz, C. (2017). Do not miss a foreign body in a wound. In A. Mattu, A. Chanmugam, S. Swadron, C. Tibbles, D. Woolridge, & L. Marcucci (Eds.), *Avoiding common errors in the emergency department*. Philidelphia, PA.

Incision and Drainage

Wesley Davis

INDICATIONS FOR THE PROCEDURE

An incision and drainage (I&D) is the gold standard for treatment of soft tissue abscesses, including pilonidal and Bartholin abscesses. Abscesses are a type of skin and soft tissue infection that results from microbial invasion of the skin and the subcutaneous tissues. The diagnosis of a superficial abscess is based on physical examination findings. Superficial abscesses that are amenable to I&D outside of the surgical suite present as fluctuant and tender masses in the dermal and subdermal tissues. Abscesses are usually erythematous, hot to the touch, swollen, and painful (Figure 20.1). Special consideration should be given to detect foreign bodies if the abscess involves trauma, drug use, or abscess recurrence.

CONTRAINDICATIONS FOR THE PROCEDURE

Relative Contraindications

1. Complex abscesses, abscesses with deep foreign bodies, and perirectal abscesses may require drainage under general anesthesia in the operating room for debridement.

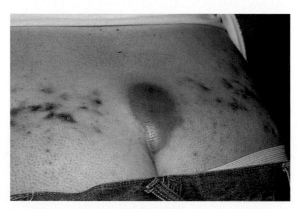

FIGURE 20.1. Abscess. This walled-off lesion began as folliculitis, which later became a furuncle and then an abscess. Reprinted with permission from Goodheart, H. P. (2003). *Goodheart's photoguide of common skin disorders* (2nd ed.). Lippincott Williams & Wilkins.

Perirectal abscesses can have complex involvement of the tissues surrounding the rectum that may not be apparent on physical examination.

2. Consider specialty consultation for abscesses located on cosmetically challenging areas, such as the face, breasts, and hands.

Absolute Contraindications

1. Abscesses of the nasolabial folds and areas of the face that drain into the cavernous sinus should be managed by an otorhinolaryngologist or other specialist trained to manage complex infectious conditions of the face.
2. Periurethral abscesses should be managed by a urologist.

EQUIPMENT NEEDED

1. Universal precaution materials (gloves, protective eyewear)
2. Scalpel with a no. 11 blade
3. Hemostat
4. Forceps
5. Irrigation syringe
6. Normal saline solution for irrigation
7. Gauze packing material, iodoform or plain ribbon gauze
8. Local anesthetic such as lidocaine with epinephrine or bupivacaine
9. Culture swab

STEPS TO PERFORMING THE PROCEDURE

1. Wear protective eyewear and gloves.
2. Prepare the skin surface with either betadine or chlorhexidine solution.
3. Administer the local anesthetic to the region using a 27-guage needle. Using a field block technique (Figure 20.2), the anesthetic should be injected into the skin overlying the abscess where the incision will be made. Do not inject the anesthetic

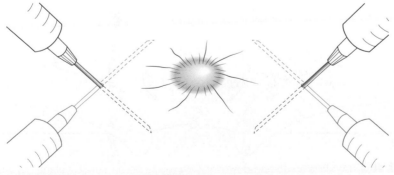

FIGURE 20.2. Administer a field block with local anesthetic. Reprinted with permission from Zuber, T. J., & Mayeaux, Jr., E. J. (2004). *Atlas of primary care procedures.* Lippincott Williams & Wilkins.

into the abscess cavity because this will increase pain and will not anesthetize the wound. In certain instances, and depending on the location of the abscess, a nerve block may be used for regional anesthesia.

4. Use the scalpel to make a linear incision over the total length of the abscess (Figure 20.3). Care should be taken to make the incision along natural skin lines to minimize scar formation.

5. If a culture is necessary, it should be obtained immediately after the incision is made (Figure 20.4).

6. Probe the depth of the abscess with a hemostat, breaking open any loculations.

7. Irrigate the abscess cavity with normal saline solution. Although irrigation has not been proven to improve treatment success of abscesses, some providers advocate the use of irrigation to remove any residual debris.

8. Gently pack the abscess cavity with gauze packing material (Figure 20.5), leaving approximately 2 cm extruding and taped to the skin. Packing is typically indicated for abscesses measuring greater than 5 cm in diameter or abscesses in immuno-compromised or diabetic patients. Overpacking may impede proper healing.

9. Cover the area with an absorbent gauze dressing.

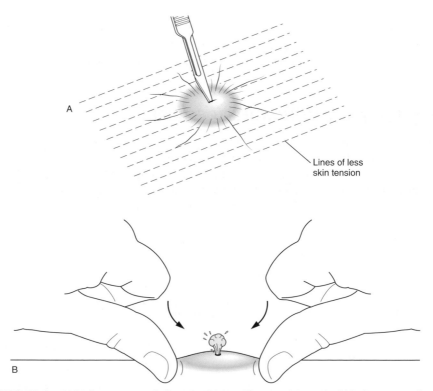

A

Lines of less skin tension

B

FIGURE 20.3. (A) Make an up-and-down incision with a no. 11 surgical blade. (B) Apply pressure around the abscess to expel the pus from the wound. Reprinted with permission from Zuber, T. J., & Mayeaux, Jr., E. J. (2004). *Atlas of primary care procedures.* Lippincott Williams & Wilkins.

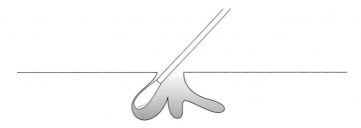

FIGURE 20.4. Insert a probe through the opening, and draw it back and forth to break adhesions and dislodge necrotic tissue. Reprinted with permission from Zuber, T. J., & Mayeaux, Jr., E. J. (2004). *Atlas of primary care procedures.* Lippincott Williams & Wilkins.

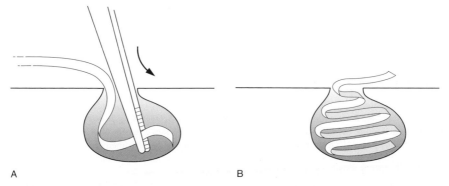

A   B

FIGURE 20.5. If the cavity is large enough, pack it with plain or iodoform gauze to promote drainage and prevent premature closure. Reprinted with permission from Zuber, T. J., & Mayeaux, Jr., E. J. (2004). *Atlas of primary care procedures.* Lippincott Williams & Wilkins.

COMPLICATIONS OF THE PROCEDURE

1. **Inadequate anesthesia:** Abscesses are acidic and can cause local anesthetics to lose effectiveness. Avoid injecting the anesthetic into the abscess cavity.
2. **Abscess recurrence:** One of the most common causes of abscess recurrence is inadequate drainage resulting from an incision that is too small.
3. **Bleeding and damage to nerves or blood vessels:** Be aware of underlying vascular structures and nerves. Consult a specialty service such as general surgery when necessary.
4. **Fistula formation**: Any abscess that forms a fistula after I&D should be referred to general surgery for possible repair.
5. **Scarring:** Before the procedure, inform the patient that scarring is possible, and obtain informed consent. The incision should be made in the precise location of the lesion.

POSTPROCEDURE CARE

For uncomplicated subcutaneous abscesses, including those caused by methicillin-resistant *Staphylococcus aureus*, I&D is considered curative. Antibiotics are only beneficial for patients with an abscess surrounded by cellulitis, an abscess associated with signs of systemic infection such as fever, a single abscess greater than 2 cm, or multiple abscesses. Additionally, antibiotics should be prescribed for patients with certain comorbidities, including diabetes, an immunosuppressed state, valvular heart disease, or the presence of an indwelling medical device. Empiric intravenous antibiotic therapy should be considered for patients with perioral or perirectal abscesses, abscesses with a potential connection to a pressure ulcer, and abscesses with prominent skin necrosis.

Most cutaneous abscesses that are treated with I&D require a follow-up visit within 2 to 3 days. Immunocompromised patients, such as diabetics, may warrant closer monitoring. If a packing was placed in the abscess, it should be removed within 2 to 3 days. With successful I&D, the patient will report a decrease in pain and minimal drainage from the incision. Incisions for abscess drainage usually heal within 1 to 2 weeks. If the abscess has continued drainage, repacking at 2- or 3-day intervals may be needed. If the patient has continued pain, an undrained cavity or loculation should be considered.

BIBLIOGRAPHY

Ambrose, G., & Berlin, D. (2019). Incision and drainage. In J. R. Roberts, C. B. Custalow, & T. W. Thomsen (Eds.), *Roberts and Hedges' clinical procedures in emergency medicine and acute care* (7th ed.). Elsevier.

Chinnock, B., & Hendey, G. W. (2016). Irrigation of cutaneous abscesses does not improve treatment success. *Annals of Emergency Medicine, 67(3)*, 379–383. https://doi.org/10.1016/j.annemergmed.2015.08.007

Coffman, D. (2016). *Incision and drainage of an abscess.* https://www-clinicalkey-com.libproxy.usouthal.edu/#!/content/medical_procedure/19-s2.0-mp_FM-006

Marco, C. A. (2018). Dermatologic presentations. In R. M. Walls, R. S. Hockberger, & M. Gausche-Hill (Eds.), *Rosen's emergency medicine: Concepts and clinical practice* (9th ed.). Elsevier.

Rajendran, P. M., Young, D., Maurer, T., Chambers, H., Perdreau-Remington, F., Ro, P., & Harris, H. (2007). Randomized, double-blind, placebo-controlled trial of cephalexin for treatment of uncomplicated skin abscesses in a population at risk for community-acquired methicillin-resistant *Staphylococcus aureus* infection. *Antimicrobial Agents and Chemotherapy, 51(11)*, 4044–4048. https://doi.org/10.1128/AAC.00377-07

Ramakrishnan, K., Salinas, R. C., & Agudelo Higuita, N. I. (2015). Skin and soft tissue infections. *American Family Physician, 92(6)*, 474–483. https://www.aafp.org/afp/2015/0915/p474.html

Spelman, D., & Baddour, L. M. (2018). *Cellulitis and skin abscess in adults: Treatment.* https://www.uptodate.com/contents/cellulitis-and-skin-abscess-in-adults-treatment?topicRef=6336&source=see_link

Stevens, D. L., Bisno, A. L., Chambers, H. F., Dellinger, E. P., Goldstein, E. J., Gorbach, S. L., & Wade, J. C. (2014). Practice guidelines for the diagnosis and management of skin and soft tissue infections: 2014 update by the infectious diseases society of America. *Clinical Infectious Disease, 59(2)*, 147. https://doi.org/10.1093/cid/ciu296

Usatine, R. P. (2019). Abscess. In R. P. Usatine, M. A. Smith, E. J. Mayeaux, & H. S. Chumley (Eds.), *The color atlas and synopsis of family medicine* (3rd ed.). McGraw-Hill.

Usatine, R. P., Stulberg, D., Pfenninger, J., & Small, R. (2012). *Dermatologic and cosmetic procedures in office practice.* Elsevier/Saunders.

Wimberly, H. (2019). *Incision and drainage of abscesses.* 5 Minute Consult. https://5minuteconsult.com/collectioncontent/30-156244/procedures/incision-and-drainage-of-abscesses

Paronychia

Allison Rusgo
Patrick C. Auth

INDICATIONS FOR THE PROCEDURE

An acute paronychia is one of the most common hand infections. It is defined as a localized and superficial infection of the lateral aspect of the nail fold, also known as the perionychium. Typically, there is a traumatic disruption in the natural seal between the nail fold and the nail plate; this compromises the tissue and allows for bacteria to colonize the space. The infection usually spreads around the nail plate, but it can also effect the eponychium or cuticle (Figure 21.1).

With respect to etiology, paronychial infections occur because of minor trauma such as nail-biting, manicures, application of artificial nails, or embedded lateral nails ("hangnails"). These infections are also common in children who suck their fingers. The bacterial culprits in paronychial infections can be aerobic or anaerobic, with the most common affecting organisms noted as *Staphylococcus* aureus, streptococcal species, and *Pseudomonas aeruginosa*.

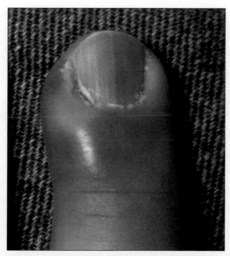

FIGURE 21.1. Example of paronychia. Reprinted with permission from Sherman, S. C., Ross, C., Nordquist, E., Wang, E., & Cico, S. (2015). *Atlas of clinical emergency medicine*. Wolters Kluwer Health.

Indications for the procedure are:

1. Similar to the treatment of other types of fluctuant abscesses, the indication for this procedure is the drainage of the affected area, which releases the infectious material and promotes healing.

   - Patient presentation with tenderness, erythema, edema, warmth, fluctuance, and possible purulent drainage around the affected eponychial tissue.
   - To treat the majority of acute paronychial infections, local anesthesia is not required. This is particularly true when the affected area has turned yellow or white, indicating that the nerves have died secondary to the infection.

Techniques

There are two common techniques that can be used: the elevation method or the simple incision method:

- In the elevation procedure, the provider will utilize an instrument such as a blunt probe or an elevator to separate the perionychium and eponychium and express the purulent material for drainage.
- In the simple incision method one can utilize the bevel of an 18-gauge needle. The needle is placed horizontally on the nail surface and inserted at the point of maximal fluctuance to release the infectious material.
- For more extensive infections that do not directly involve the nail fold, one should anesthetize the affected digit and utilize a #11 blade scalpel to incise over the area of maximal fluctuance. This will promote drainage of the infection (Figures 21.2 and 21.3).

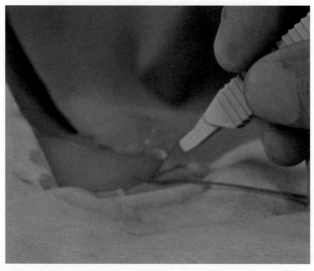

FIGURE 21.2. A #11 blade scalpel. Reprinted with permission from Herzog, E. (2017). *Herzog's CCU book.* Wolters Kluwer Health.

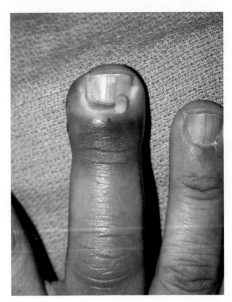

FIGURE 21.3. Acute paronychia and follow-up showing postincision drainage at the affected area. Reprinted with permission from Thorne, C. H., Gurtner, G. C., Chung, K., Gosain, A., Mehrara, B., Rubin, P., & Spear, S. L. (2014). *Grabb and Smith's plastic surgery* (7th ed.). Lippincott Williams & Wilkins.

- It should also be noted that if there is concern for a more proximal infection that extends into the finger, a portion of the lateral nail fold may need to be excised for complete healing.

CONTRAINDICATIONS FOR THE PROCEDURE

Relative Contraindications

1. **Acute paronychia without abscess**: For patients with a localized cellulitis of the affected area without fluctuance, surgical drainage is not recommended. For these patients, conservative management with warm water soaks several times a day, elevation, and oral antibiotic therapy should be employed. Patients should follow up with a healthcare provider to determine whether the infection has resolved or a collection of pus has formed, thus necessitating surgical drainage.

Absolute Contraindications

1. **Deep space infections**: If there is concern that the infection is fulminant and involves the deeper structures of the hand, simple incision and drainage should not be performed. The patient should be referred to a hand specialist for further treatment and management.

2. **Chronic paronychia infections**: Chronic paronychial infections differ from acute infections in that they last longer than 6 weeks and are caused by fungal infections. They do not present with fluctuance or respond to surgical drainage. Patients with chronic paronychial infections should be educated on the importance of avoiding contact irritants and keeping hands dry. These patients may also benefit from antifungal medications and referred to hand specialists for additional management.

EQUIPMENT NEEDED

1. Alcohol or povidone-iodine (Betadine) wipes
2. Three or four towels for drapes
3. 4 × 4-inch gauze pads
4. Sterile gloves
5. Normal saline solution
6. Blunt probe or elevator tool
7. 18-gauge needle (if utilizing 18-gauge needle technique)
8. #11 blade scalpel (if incision is required)
9. ¼-inch packing material
10. 19 to 22-gauge needle (for digital anesthesia)
11. 1% to 2% lidocaine without epinephrine (for digital anesthesia)
12. Bandage scissors
13. Dressing of choice to cover wound

STEPS TO PERFORMING THE PROCEDURE

Blunt-tool technique (Figure 21.4):
1. **Skin preparation**: Apply a single layer of povidone-iodine solution to the affected area and allow to air dry before performing the procedure.
2. **Sterile draping**: Place drapes around the affected area and don sterile gloves.
3. **Drainage**: Utilize a blunt metal probe or elevator tool to separate the eponychial fold from the nail. This should be performed at the area between the perionychium and the eponychium and extend to the proximal aspect of the nail to allow for drainage of the infection.
4. **Irrigation**: Affected area should be sufficiently irrigated with normal saline solution and dried.
5. **Packing:** A small amount of ¼-inch packing material can be inserted under the nail fold to promote further drainage if necessary (not required in all instances, can be helpful to ensure complete drainage of purulent material).
6. **Dressing**: Dressing of choice can be lightly applied to wound.
   Alternative method utilizing the simple incision technique:
7. **Skin preparation**: Same as noted previously.
8. **Sterile draping**: Same as noted previously.

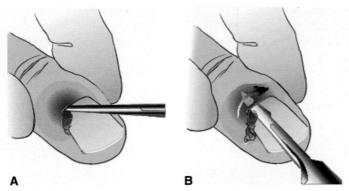

A   **B**

FIGURE 21.4. Drainage of the paronychia by the elevation method using a blunt probe to separate the perionychium and eponychium and express the purulent material. Reprinted with permission from Henretig, F. M. (1997). Incision and drainage of a paronychia. In F. M. Henretig, & C. King (eds.), *Textbook of pediatric emergency procedures*. Lippincott Williams & Wilkins.

9. **Drainage:** Place the bevel-end of an 18-gauge needle horizontally on the surface of the nail and insert it at the junction between the lateral nail fold and the nail plate; this should occur at the point of maximal fluctuance, lifting the skin around the nail fold and opening the infectious cavity for drainage.
10. **Drainage:** If necessary, one can gently expand the size of the cavity created by the 18-gauge needle for increased drainage.
11. **Drainage**: Light pressure can be applied to the external skin around the affected area to release any remaining infectious material.
12. **Irrigation**: Affected area should be sufficiently irrigated with normal saline solution and dried.
13. **Packing**: A small amount of ¼-inch packing material can be inserted into the newly created cavity to promote further drainage (not required in all instances, can be helpful to ensure complete drainage of purulent material).
14. **Dressing**: Dressing of choice can be lightly applied to wound.

Additional Considerations for Complex Infections

If a paronychial infection extends proximally into the finger, portions of the lateral aspect of the nail plate may need to be removed (Figure 21.5). This should be completed after anesthesia of the affected digit via a digital block, and packing should be used at the end of the procedure to allow for maximal drainage of the purulent material.

Alternatively, a small incision can be made with a #11 scalpel into the lateral aspect of the affected finger over the point of maximal fluctuance to express the pus. This should also be completed once the digit has been properly numbed.

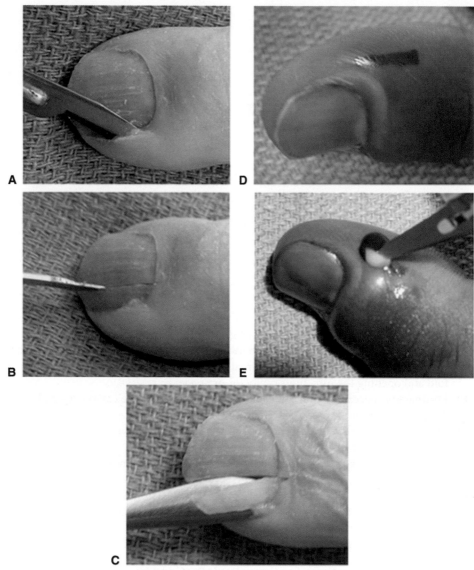

FIGURE 21.5. (A) Incision to drain the paronychia; (B, C) Incision and removal of a portion of the nail plate; (D, E) Alternative incision to drain the paronychia. Reprinted with permission from Wiesel, S. (2015). *Operative techniques in orthopaedic surgery*, four volume set (2nd ed.). Wolters Kluwer Health.

COMPLICATIONS OF THE PROCEDURE

1. **Excess bleeding**: If an incision is made during the procedure and excess bleeding is encountered, direct pressure should be applied to the wound until bleeding has ceased.
2. **Insufficient drainage**: If the procedure was performed without significant expression of pus, the affected area should be cleaned sufficiently and packed with ¼-inch gauze to promote further drainage of infectious material.

3. **Deep space infection**: If during the procedure, it is determined that the infection has spread to deeper structures of the upper extremity, provider should complete the localized procedure and refer patient to hand specialist for further surgical management.

POSTPROCEDURE CARE

Following the successful drainage of an acute paronychia, there is rarely a need for admission unless there are extenuating circumstances. Some indications for hospitalization are a deep space infection, severe surrounding cellulitis, or a patient who is significantly immunocompromised with systemic symptoms secondary to the infection.

For patients who are discharged with a simple paronychia, oral antibiotic therapy is not required; however, there are instances where a 7-day course of antibiotics can be used. Providers should consider the use of oral antistaphylococcal agents (i.e., cephalexin 500 mg three times/day for 7 days) in patients who are immunocompromised or diagnosed with vascular insufficiency or in cases where there is mild/moderate cellulitis surrounding the affected site. It should also be noted that in instances where a paronychial infection is secondary to nail-biting or finger-sucking, antibiotics such as clindamycin or amoxicillin-clavulanic acid should be used to cover for flora originating from the oral cavity.

Following the procedure, all patients should be instructed to elevate the area, immobilize/protect the wound, and perform warm soaks three to four times per day for several days. This process will promote cleanliness and healing and will allow the cavity to remain open for additional drainage. Providers should also ensure that patients understand the importance of seeking immediate medical attention if new or worsening symptoms of infection develop. Patients should return for a follow-up appointment within two days of the initial procedure to assess healing and remove the packing.

Patient education is also an important component of this diagnosis, especially to prevent reoccurrences. Providers should help patients understand the importance of keeping fingernails clean, moisturizing fingers to prevent cracking/breaks in the skin, avoiding nail-biting and finger-sucking, trimming hangnails with a clean nail-trimmer, wearing gloves when exposed to contact irritants, and thoroughly drying hands after excessive exposure to moisture.

BIBLIOGRAPHY

Auth, P. C., & Bottomley, G. S. (2007). Incision and drainage of an abscess. In R. W. Dehn & D. P. Asprey (Eds.), *Essential clinical procedures* (2nd ed., pp. 369–379). Saunders Elsevier.

Billingsley, E. M., & Vidimos, A. T. (2017, September 11). *Paronychia* (W. D. James, Ed.). Retrieved from Medscape website https://emedicine.medscape.com/article/1106062-overview

Germann, C. A. (2016). Nontraumatic disorders of the hand. In J. T. Tintinalli, J. Stapczynski, O. Ma, D. M. Yealy, G. D. Meckler, & D. M. Cline (Eds.), *Tintinalli's emergency medicine: A comprehensive study guide* (8th ed.). McGraw-Hill.

Lifchez, S. D., & Kelamis, J. A. (2015). Surgery of the hand and wrist. In F. C. Brunicardi, D. K. Andersen, T. R. Billiar, D. L. Dunn, J. G. Hunter, J. B. Matthews, & R. E. Pollack (Eds.), *Schwartz's principles of surgery* (10th ed.). McGraw-Hill.

Rockwell, P. G. (2001). Acute and chronic paronychia. *American Family Physician, 63*(6), 1113–1117.

Usatine, R. P. (2013). Paronychia. In R. P. Usatine, M. A. Smith, H. S. Chumley, & E. J. Mayeaux, Jr. (Eds.), *The color atlas of family medicine* (2nd ed.). McGraw-Hill.

CHAPTER 22   Nail Hematoma Release

Megan E. Schneider

INDICATIONS FOR THE PROCEDURE

1. The purpose of nail hematoma release is to decrease the pain and pressure on the nail bed from a subungual hematoma (Figure 22.1).
2. A subungual hematoma is the collection of blood beneath the nail plate from a direct injury to the nail bed (Figure 22.2). Crush injuries are the most common cause.
3. The procedure of creating a small hole in the nail plate to release the trapped blood is known as trephination. Trephination of the nail drains the hematoma and, therefore, reduces the pressure and the pain of the nail bed. If the pressure is not relieved, the nail plate may avulse from the nail bed, causing delayed regrowth and a poor cosmetic outcome. Trephination is often the definitive management for a subungual hematoma.

CONTRAINDICATIONS FOR THE PROCEDURE

Relative Contraindications

1. Trephination is more effective for acute (<48 hours) subungual hematoma. After that, the hematoma may coagulate and be less amenable to drainage.

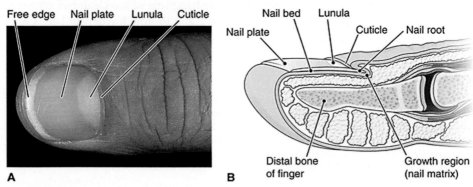

FIGURE 22.1. Anatomy of the distal finger. (A) Photograph of a nail, superior view. (B) Midsagittal section of a fingertip. Reprinted with permission from Cohen, B. J., & Hull, K. L. (2016). *Memmler's structure and function of the human body* (11th ed.); A, from Bickley, L. S. (2003). *Bates' guide to physical examination and history taking* (8th ed.). Lippincott Williams & Wilkins.

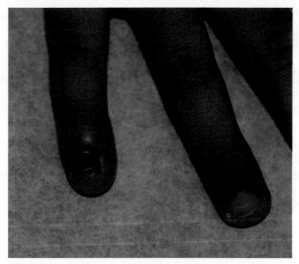

FIGURE 22.2. Typical appearance of a large subungual hematoma. From Chung, E. K., Atkinson-McAvey, L. R., Boom, J. A., & Matz, P. S. (2010). *Visual diagnosis and treatment in pediatrics* (2nd ed.). Originally, courtesy of Julie A. Boom, MD. Wolters Kluwer Health.

2. Subungual hematomas that involve more than 50% of the nail may indicate a possible laceration of the nail bed. Some clinicians recommend removal of the nail plate to search for and repair potential nail bed lacerations. However, complete removal adds to the risk of a poor cosmetic outcome. If the nail plate is intact (not fractured) and well adherent at all nail borders, large hematomas may be released through trephination with good patient outcomes.
3. Patients with subungual hematomas typically require an x-ray to rule out an underlying fracture. A fracture of the distal phalanx may inadvertently be converted to an open fracture through the trephination process. In the presence of a minimally displaced fracture, such as a tuft fracture, subungual hematomas should still be treated with decompression of the collected blood. However, clinicians should consider the principles of management for open fractures, which may include antibiotic therapy.
4. Nontraumatic subungual hematomas, which may be the result of subungual tumors, may not be relieved by trephination and require follow-up to evaluate the cause.
5. If the subungual hematoma is not painful or if blood is spontaneously draining, then trephination is unlikely to be of additional benefit.

Absolute Contraindications

There are no absolute contraindications.

EQUIPMENT NEEDED

1. Personal protective equipment such as a face mask with eye shield and gloves
2. Cleansing antiseptic solution such as betadine or chlorhexidine

3. Trephination device such as an electrocautery unit, an 18-gauge needle, or a Number 11 scalpel
4. Sterile gauze and bandaging material

STEPS TO PERFORMING THE PROCEDURE

1. Obtain informed consent from the patient or appropriate surrogate decision maker.
2. Perform hand hygiene.
3. Patient should be in the sitting or supine position. Apply the personal protective equipment.
4. Cleanse the patient's nail with the antiseptic solution. Note that alcohol is flammable and should be washed off with sterile water or allowed to dry completely before performing electrocautery, if using alcohol as an antiseptic.
5. Bore a hole through the center of the hematoma *avoiding the lunula and its associated nail matrix. Avoid contact with the nail bed.*
   a. Electrocautery devices are the preferred tools for this procedure, because they are sterile, minimize patient discomfort, and effectively drain the hematoma. Providers should familiarize themselves with their electrocautery device by reading the manufacturer's instructions. Heat the tip until it is red hot, hold the unit at 90° to the nail, and then apply it to the center of the hematoma with gentle pressure to the nail plate. Repeat as needed at the same location until completely through the nail plate. The hole should be large enough (3–4 mm) for continued drainage. When performed correctly, the heat dissipates when the device reaches the hematoma, preventing injury to the nail bed and pain for the patient.
   b. A sterile 18-gauge needle or a #11 scalpel are alternative trephination devices. These are used without additional heat and are the preferred methods for patients with artificial nails because acrylic nails are considered flammable. The needle or the scalpel is held at 90° to the nail and rotated between the thumb and the index finger in a drill-like fashion. A 3- to 4-mm hole is preferred to provide adequate drainage. This method requires the use of more pressure to get through the nail plate, which will increase the pain of the procedure to the patient. Providers utilizing this method should consider performing a digital block for pain control. There is also an increased risk of injuring the nail bed with the needle or scalpel.
6. Once through the nail, the hematoma often drains spontaneously. Gentle pressure may be applied to completely release the entire collection of blood.
7. After the hematoma is released, the patient's pain should improve significantly. Consider additional injuries if the patient's pain does not improve.
8. Cleanse the nail and apply a sterile bandage. A nonadherent dressing is useful, as blood may continue to ooze from the drainage site for 1 to 2 days (Figure 22.3).

COMPLICATIONS OF THE PROCEDURE

1. Permanent nail loss or deformity is the most likely complication from the treatment of a subungual hematoma, especially if there is an underlying nail bed injury. There is also risk of an iatrogenic injury to the nail bed if the procedure is not performed

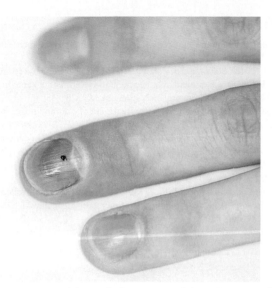

FIGURE 22.3. Appearance of the nail after successful trephination of the sub-ungual hematoma. Reprinted with permission from Fleisher, G. R., Ludwig, S., & Baskin, M. N. (2004). *Atlas of pediatric emergency medicine*. Lippincott Williams & Wilkins.

correctly. However, the patient may lose the nail if the hematoma is not drained. Therefore, this risk should be explained to the patient, while noting that treatment with trephination is preferred.

2. Infection is a rare complication. Use of sterile technique and applying a postprocedure bandage can minimize the risk further. Routine use of prophylactic antibiotics is not recommended. Antibiotics, such as cephalexin, may be used if the patient has a concomitant distal phalanx fracture and there is concern that it is an open fracture or was converted into an open fracture during the hematoma release.

3. Heat-induced coagulation may result in incomplete evacuation of the hematoma. If this occurs, a second drainage site may be attempted.

POSTPROCEDURE CARE

The patient should be instructed to keep the affected finger clean and dry. A bandage should be reapplied daily until the drainage site closes. The patient should notify the provider of increased pain, warmth, erythema, swelling, purulent discharge, or fever because these may indicate an infection. The patient should also seek care if the hematoma reaccumulates, because this may be a sign of a more extensive nail bed injury.

Patients with a tuft fracture or minimally displaced fracture of the distal phalanx must be placed in an extension splint for 3 to 4 weeks. They should also be referred to a hand specialist for follow-up.

Finally, patients should also be advised that the nail will likely fall off but that regrowth can be expected to occur in 8 to 12 weeks.

BIBLIOGRAPHY

Brown, D. (2007). Draining subungual hematomas. In R. W. Dehn & D. P. Asprey (Eds.), *Essential clinical procedures* (2nd ed., pp. 417–423). Elsevier.

Fastle, R., & Bothner, J. (2018). *Subungual hematoma*. UpToDate Topic 6335 Version 13.0.

Kearney, A., & Canty, L. (2016). Assessment, management and treatment of acute fingertip injuries. *Emergency Nurse, 24*(3), 29–34. https://doi.org/10.7748/en.24.3.29.s28

Oetgen, M. E., & Dodds, S. D. (2008). Non-operative treatment of common finger injuries. *Current Review of Musculoskeletal Medicine, 1*, 97–102. https://doi.org/10.1007/s12178-007-9014-z

Patel, L. (2014). Management of simple nail bed lacerations and subungual hematomas in the emergency department. *Pediatric Emergency Care, 30*(10), 742–748. https://doi.org/10.1097/PEC.0000000000000241

Pingel, C., & McDowell, C. (2018). *Subungual hematoma drainage*. In *StatPearls*. https://www.ncbi.nlm.nih.gov/books/NBK482508/

Salter, S. A., Ciocon, D. H., Gowrishankar, T. R., & Kimball, A. B. (2006). Controlled nail trephination for subungual hematoma. *The American Journal of Emergency Medicine, 24*, 875–877. https://doi.org/10.1016/j.ajem.2006.03.029

Neurological and Musculoskeletal Procedures

CHAPTER

23

Lumbar Puncture

Damon Toczylowski

INDICATIONS FOR THE PROCEDURE

Lumbar puncture (LP) is performed to obtain a sample of cerebral spinal fluid (CSF) from the subarachnoid space in the lumbar cistern (located near the end of the spinal cord and dura mater of the coccygeal ligament). Anatomically, the spinal cord ends near the L1/L2 interspace in adults and L2/L3 in infants, making the interspace at L4/L5 the safest for LP. An imaginary line, called the supracristal plane or Tuffier line (found while laying a patient lateral/decubitus and visualizing a line from the iliac crests), will help identify the safest area for LP. If a patient is rich with adipose or muscle tissue, bedside ultrasound (US) may be indicated to help identify L4/L5. As the needle enters the L4/L5 space, several layers of skin, tissue, fat, and dura will be traversed while attempting to reach the subarachnoid space or lumbar cistern. Although an invasive procedure done in an area that can have catastrophic outcomes, LP, if done correctly and safely, can give rich clinical information.

Indications for the procedure are:

1. Diagnostically, an LP can help identify subarachnoid hemorrhage (SAH), central nervous system (CNS) infection, CNS autoimmune processes, or malignancies. If considering LP for diagnostic evaluation, it should be done early if warranted to help establish objective data.
2. Therapeutically, an LP can help treat hydrocephalus, cerebrospinal fistulas, and pseudomotor cerebri; deliver contrast or medications to the subarachnoid space; measure CSF pressures; and evaluate the subarachnoid space for placement of a lumbar subarachnoid drain.

CONTRAINDICATIONS FOR THE PROCEDURE

Relative Contraindications

1. Evaluation of papilledema on physical examination in a setting of altered mental status with suspected increased intracranial pressure (herniation) or SAH, infection near puncture site, coagulation disorders (where the international normalized ratio (INR) <1.4 or platelet count [PLT] $<100,000/mm^3$ and not corrected

with fresh frozen plasma [FFP]/platelets), recent surgical instrumentation, spinal tumors, or if myelography or pneumoencephalography is planned.

2. It is important to remember that LP done with coagulopathy can cause an epidural hematoma compressing the caudae equina.

3. If there is suspicion of SAH with altered mental status, focal neurologic deficits, or papilledema, a computed tomography (CT) head should be obtained prior to LP to reduce the risk of herniation/complications).

Absolute Contraindications

There are no absolute contraindications.

EQUIPMENT NEEDED

1. Sterile disposable LP kit or minor procedure tray with 21 gauge (adults) or 22 gauge (children)
2. Spinal needle
3. Sterile gloves and other protective personal equipment (PPE)
4. Specimen labels or laboratory forms
5. Glucometer/phlebotomy supplies for testing of serum or whole blood glucose.
6. Two over-bed tables (one sterile and one to position the patient)
7. Rolled towel or small pillow
8. A longer spinal needle may be required for persons with increased adipose or muscle tissue.

STEPS TO PERFORMING THE PROCEDURE

1. Prior to the procedure, obtain consent, perform an assessment looking for subjective/objective indicators that may indicate a possible complication (nuchal rigidity, photophobia, +Brudzinski/Kernig signs, fever, headache).
2. Assess for allergies to the anesthetics, analgesia, or possible medications to be used.
3. Ensure the patient is correct per institutional standards (time out).
4. In obtaining consent for the procedure, ensure that positioning, purpose, and complications of the procedure are discussed.
5. Obtain vital signs, look for nuchal rigidity, photophobia, Brudzinski and Kernig signs, fever, headache, nystagmus.
6. Position the patient in the lateral decubitus position with the knees pulled up toward the stomach and the head flexed to the chest. If a patient cannot lie flat, have them lean over a bedside table while sitting up. Proper positioning widens the intervertebral spaces between the spinous process, allowing for better access into the spinal cistern (Figure 23.1).
7. Palpate the supracristal plane and determine the location of the L4 to L5 interspace (in most adults, the spinal cord ends at L1, making the L4–L5 interspace the safest for access) (Figure 23.2).

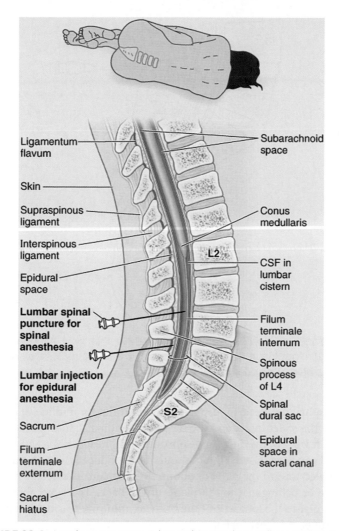

Ligamentum flavum

Skin

Supraspinous ligament

Interspinous ligament

Epidural space

Lumbar spinal puncture for spinal anesthesia

Lumbar injection for epidural anesthesia

Sacrum

Filum terminale externum

Sacral hiatus

Subarachnoid space

Conus medullaris

L2

CSF in lumbar cistern

Filum terminale internum

Spinous process of L4

Spinal dural sac

S2

Epidural space in sacral canal

FIGURE 23.1. Lumbar puncture. A long, thin sterile needle is inserted between lower lumbar vertebrae in the region of the cauda equina of the spinal cord. Reprinted with permission from McConnell, T. H. (2014). *Nature of disease* (2nd ed.). Wolters Kluwer.

8. Once a favorable site has been identified, clean the site with betadine or chlorhexidine, then don your sterile gloves and drape.
9. With a 25-gauge needle, make a small wheal with 1% lidocaine, then deeper with a 22-gauge needle.
10. When the patient is properly anesthetized, examine the 20- or 22-gauge needle for defects prior to insertion.

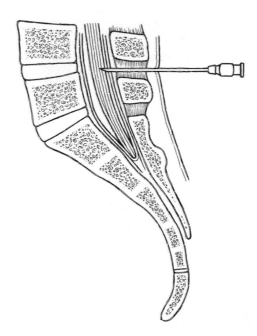

FIGURE 23.2. Spinal needle positioning in the spinal canal. Reprinted with permission from Agur, Anne, M. R., & Dalley, A. F. (2014). *Moore's essential clinical anatomy* (5th ed.). Wolters Kluwer.

11. Hold the spinal needle at 15° cephalad and introduce it midline to the plane of the back with the stylet intact and the bevel perpendicular to the axis of the body to minimize tearing of the dura (and subsequent LP headaches).

12. The spinal needle with stylet intact should be introduced through the skin in a tract that is angled toward the navel or about 15° cephalad. The needle must be entered at midline or orthogonal to the plane of the back. The bevel should initially be perpendicular to the long axis of the body to minimize tearing of the dura and the subsequent post-LP headache.

13. The needle will pass through several layers before reaching the subarachnoid space, where a "pop" will be felt. Once the pop is felt, remove the stylet to evaluate for the presence of CSF. If no fluid appears, rotate the needle slightly; if no fluid appears and you are certain that you are in the subarachnoid space, you can try to instill 1 mL of air, which may dislodge tissue from your needle.

14. ***Never*** instill normal saline or distilled water. If you hit bone while inserting, you may be at an incorrect angle or you entered off midline.

15. After several attempts at L4 to L5, it is appropriate to use Tuffier line (L3–L4); however, going any higher would risk puncturing the spinal cord.

16. Should the spinal needle be inserted to the hub without CSF, the needle was not long enough and needs to be replaced (seen in obese/muscular patients). Fluoroscopic or US utilization may be required if the patient is obese or muscular. US

guidance improves the rate of success and decreases complications; also, the angle of entrance can be improved. Additionally, consider using an atraumatic spinal needle, which will likely reduce the risk of spinal headaches or other complications.

17. Once CSF is successfully obtained, attach a manometer and stopcock to measure the pressure. Normal opening pressure is 7 to 18 cm H_2O. Increased pressure may be caused by congestive heart failure (CHF), ascites, SAH, infection, a space occupying lesion, or a tense patient. Decreased pressure may be caused by a CSF leak, needle position, or obstructed flow. If the opening pressure is greater than 50 cm H_2O, obtain only as much fluid as necessary for specimens.

18. Be sure to collect 0.5 to 2 mL fluid in the four vials provided in the LP kit. Send the vials for labs as follows:
    - 1-Culture (bacteriology)
    - 2-Glucose and protein
    - 3-Complete blood count w/differential
    - 4-Venereal Disease Research Laboratory (VDRL) test (neurosyphilis)
    - Counter immuno-electrophoresis
    - bacterial antigens

19. See Table 23.1 for reference ranges for fluid analysis. If CSF appears bloody and then clears, the tap is traumatic where the needle punctured a vein during puncture. Yellow CSF or xanthochromia is indicative of old blood (>12–24 hours) in the subarachnoid space or elevated protein levels.

TABLE 23.1 CSF Reference Values

Condition	CSF Color	CSF Opening Pressure CM H_2O	CSF Protein (mg/mL)	CSF Glucose (mg/mL)	CSF Cell Count
Adult normal	Clear	7–18	12–45	45–80	0–5 Lymph
Newborn	Clear	7–18	20–120	2/3 Serum	40–60 Lymph
Infection					
Viral	Clear/opal	Normal/⇑	Normal/⇑	Normal	10–500 PMN
Bacterial	Opal/yellow may clot	⇑⇑⇑	50–100k	⇓ <20k	25–100k PMN
Granuloma-tous	Clear/opal	⇑-Often	⇑ <500k	⇓ <20–40	10–500 Lymph
Neurologic					
Guillain-Barré	Clear/cloudy	Normal	⇑⇑⇑	Normal	Normal/⇑ lymph
Multiple sclerosis	Clear	Normal	Normal/⇑	Normal	0–20 Lymph

(continued)

TABLE 23.1 CSF Reference Values (*continued*)

Condition	CSF Color	CSF Opening Pressure CM H$_2$O	CSF Protein (mg/mL)	CSF Glucose (mg/mL)	CSF Cell Count
Psuedomotor cerebri	Clear	⇑	Normal	Normal	Normal
Miscellaneous					
Neoplasm	Clear/xanth	⇑	Normal/⇑	Normal//⇓	Normal/⇑lymph
Traumatic tap	Bloody	Normal	Normal	⇑	RBC=peripheral fewer in tube 4 than tube 1
SAH	Bloody or xanth after 2–8 hours	⇑-Usually	⇑	Normal	WBC/RBC ratio same in tubes 1 and 4

Data from Gomella, L. G., & Haist, S. A. (2007). *Clinician's pocket reference* (11th ed., pp. 289-296.). McGraw Hill.

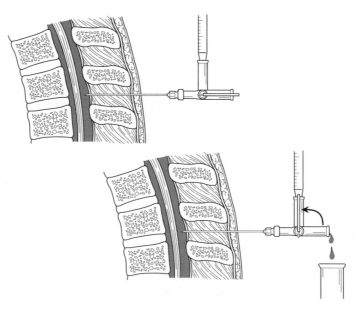

FIGURE 23.3. Spinal fluid drainage with stop cock. Reprinted with permission from Saint, S. (2004). *Saint-Frances guide to inpatient medicine* (2nd ed.). Wolters Kluwer.

20. After all vials are collected, remove the needle with stylet and dress the site.
21. Ensure the patient lies flat for 6 to 12 hours to reduce the possibility of spinal headache.

CSF tests to consider include:

- CBC w/differential
- CSF glucose + protein levels
- Gram stain and bacterial/fungal/mycobacterial cultures
- Cytology and wet mount inspection
- Spectrophotometer for xanthochromia
- Polymerase chain reaction (PCR) tests for herpes simplex virus (HSV), varicella zoster virus (VZV), BV, cytomegalovirus (CMV), enterovirus, tuberculosis, arboviruses, and toxoplasmosis
- Tests for syphilis (VDRL or fluorescent treponemal antibody absorption [FTA-ABS]), cysticercosis, histoplasmosis, coccidioidomycosis, and malaria

COMPLICATIONS OF THE PROCEDURE

During the procedure, patients may complain of paresthesia to one leg caused by impingement of the nerve root. If this occurs, the spinal needle should be retracted and repositioned toward the midline and reinserted.

POSTPROCEDURE CARE

Following the procedure, post-LP headaches may develop, so ensure that the patient lies flat for 6 to 12 hours. Treat with nonsteroidal anti-inflammatory drugs (NSAIDs) or acetaminophen by mouth, fluids, or caffeine. If the symptoms persist more than 5 days, a peripheral blood patch (peripheral blood injected into the dural space to seal the leak) may need to be instilled by an anesthesia team. Herniation syndromes (seen in coagulopathy/liver dysfunction) and trauma to the nerve root/paresthesia/paralysis (owing to anatomic variability or traumatic insertions) are typically not seen.

BIBLIOGRAPHY

Gomella, L. G., & Haist, S. A. (2007). *Clinician's pocket reference* (11th ed., pp. 289–296). McGraw Hill.

Kollef, M., & Isakow, W. (2012).) *The Washington manual of critical care* (2nd ed., pp. 600–604). Wolters Kluwer Health/Lippincott Williams & Wilkins.

Millington, S. J., Marcos, S. R., & Koeing, S. (2018). Better with ultrasound: Lumbar puncture. *Chest, 154*(5), 1223–1229. https://doi.org/10.1016/j.chest.2018.07.010

Nath, S., Koziarz, A., Badhiwala, J. H., Alhazzani, W., Jaeschke, R., Sharma, S., Banfield, L., Shoamanesh, A., Singh, S., Nassiri, F., Oczkowski, W., Belley-Côté, E., Truant, R., Reddy, K., Meade, M. O., Farrokhyar, F., Bala, M. M., Alshamsi, F., Krag, M., ... Almenawer, S. A. (2018). Atraumatic versus conventional lumbar puncture needles: A systemic review and meta-analysis. *The Lancet, 391*(10126), 1197–1204. https://doi.org/10.1016/S0140-6736(17)32451-0

Weigand, D. L. (2011). *AACN procedure manual for critical care* (6th ed., pp. 880–881). Elsevier-Sanders.

24 Compartment Pressure Monitoring

Kudret Usmani
Salina Wydo

Acute compartment syndrome is a rare but devastating condition that carries with it significant morbidity and mortality, especially in the context of delayed diagnosis. It is most commonly associated with fractures, especially fractures of the tibial shaft and distal radius (resulting in compartment syndrome of the distal leg and forearm, respectively). Cases have also been reported as having been caused by vascular injury, burns, emboli, iatrogenic injury, and soft tissue injury without fracture (e.g., crush injuries).

Compartment syndrome develops when the arteriovenous gradient (inflow) cannot meet the local metabolic demands of the tissue; an absolute difference between compartment pressures and the mean arterial pressure or diastolic BP dictates whether the intracompartmental pressure overwhelms local circulation. When the fascial compartment pressures exceed the body's ability to provide arterial inflow, there is irreversible local tissue ischemia and death. As the cells die, the result is the release of osmotically active substances (e.g., myoglobin), which causes edema of the local tissue. The ability of the tissue to expand as it swells is impaired by the relatively noncompliant native fascia. As a result, the pressure in the compartment increases, inflow to the tissue is further compromised, and the cycle of tissue destruction continues. Downstream, life-threatening effects of cell lysis include myoglobinuria, metabolic acidosis, renal insufficiency/failure, hyperkalemia, and other electrolyte disturbances that can result in cardiac dysrhythmias.

Irreversible damage occurs within 6 to 8 hours of elevated intracompartmental pressures. One study showed that irreversible ischemic tissue damage occurred when the difference between the compartment and mean arterial pressure was less than 30 mmHg and when the difference between the compartment and diastolic BP was less than 20 mmHg.

The timing of onset of compartment syndrome is variable, but it most commonly occurs in the first 24 hours after injury. Delayed onset compartment syndrome can be seen as late as 2 to 4 days after the initial insult. Good outcomes are dependent on early detection and treatment.

INDICATIONS FOR THE PROCEDURE

1. The diagnosis of compartment syndrome is based primarily on clinical examination. Providers should have a high index of suspicion based on history; initial evaluation includes performing serial physical examinations and following patient symptoms. In most patients, pain out of proportion to the injury is one of the *earliest* clinical signs of compartment syndrome. Pain with passive stretch is one of the

most sensitive physical examination signs for compartment syndrome. Other signs such as compartment tightness or compartment compressibility (to palpation) may be useful in serial examinations, but have historically shown poor reliability. Late signs, such as loss of palpable pulses, poikilothermia (coldness to touch), and paresis, may be seen only in truly advanced compartment syndrome and indicate that irreversible tissue damage and loss of function have occurred.

2. Ultimately, tracking serial laboratory values (i.e., creatine kinase, urine myoglobin) supports the diagnosis of compartment syndrome and should not be relied on to make the diagnosis. In clear cases, compartment pressure measurement may not be necessary. The use of compartment pressure measurements is particularly helpful in the obtunded patient or in any patient in whom a clinical examination cannot be obtained.

3. Another indication for compartment pressure measurement can be in the setting of polytrauma, when a patient has multiple distracting injuries and is unable to provide an accurate subjective pain assessment.

CONTRAINDICATIONS FOR THE PROCEDURE

Relative Contraindications

1. Broken or compromised skin (e.g., cellulitis, abscess, blisters) overlying site of optimal measurement
2. Coagulopathy

Absolute Contraindications

1. There are no absolute contraindications to measuring compartment pressures.
2. The risk–benefit ratio of measurement should be evaluated prior to measurement. If the clinical concern for compartment syndrome exists, but the practitioner is not comfortable with the attendant risks, surgical consultation should be obtained.

MEASUREMENT TECHNIQUES AND ANATOMY

There are various methods of measuring compartment pressures, the two most common being the slit catheter and side port needle techniques (Figure 24.1). There is no clinically significant difference between the use of the slit catheter and side port needle for reliable compartment measurements. The advantage of the slit catheter technique over simple manometry is that the former system is designed for continuous serial measurements. Historically, or in areas of low resource availability, an 18-guage needle connected to manometry (commonly, an arterial line setup) has been used to measure compartment pressures. Although this method will generate a numerical value, it has been shown to be consistently higher (by 18–19 mmHg) than either the side port needle or slit catheter technique and is no longer recommended for routine compartment pressure measurements. A review of compartmental anatomy is pertinent prior to performing the procedure, because it is important to be reliably able to measure the pressures in each compartment. Elevated pressures in any of the compartments should prompt urgent

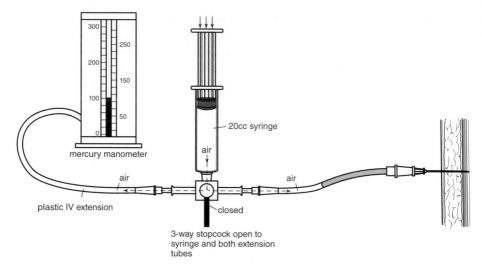

FIGURE 24.1. Principle of compartment pressure monitoring. To measure tissue pressures, the apparatus is assembled as shown to aspirate a column of sterile saline into the extension tubing. The tissue pressure is measured by determining the amount of pressure within this closed system that is required to overcome the pressure within the closed compartment. The column of saline transmits this pressure back to the transducer for display and interpretation. Reprinted with permission from Bucholz, R. W., & Heckman, J. D. (2001). *Rockwood & Green's fractures in adults* (5th ed.). Lippincott Williams & Wilkins.

surgical consultation. As lower extremity compartment syndrome is the most common location, our discussion will focus on the distal lower extremity.

There are four compartments to the distal lower extremity, each containing muscular and neurovascular structures, bounded by stiff, noncompliant fascia (Figure 24.2). Each compartment consists of structures that generally share a common function, as well as neural and blood supply. The anterior compartment contains structures generally responsible for dorsiflexion and eversion of the foot (tibialis anterior, deep peroneal nerve); it is the compartment most commonly affected by compartment syndrome. The lateral compartment contains the fibularis longus and brevis and is primarily responsible for eversion of the foot. The deep superficial and posterior compartments contain the soleus and gastrocnemius, which serve as the primary flexors of the foot and ankle.

Heckman et al. found differences in compartment pressures right at the fracture site versus 5 cm proximal and distal to the fracture site and recommended multiple measurements in multiple compartments to accurately track the development of compartment syndrome in the four leg compartments (further description of compartmental anatomy is beyond the scope of this manual). Laboratory tests include serial measurements of serum creatine phosphokinase and urine measurements of myoglobin in the form of positive urine benzidine test for occult blood without red blood cells, but these measurements are often used more to trend the success of a decompression rather than to actually characterize the severity of disease.

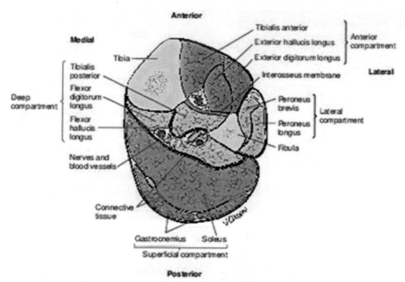

FIGURE 24.2. Cross-sectional anatomy of the distal lower extremity. These illustrations demonstrate how compartment syndrome of the lower extremity develops: cross-section of the lower leg with the compartments, nerves, and blood vessels; swelling of the muscles (in this case from bleeding) causing compression of the nerves and blood vessels. Reprinted with permission from Agur, Anne, M. R., & Dalley, A. F. (2016). *Grant's atlas of anatomy* (14th ed.). Wolters Kluwer.

EQUIPMENT NEEDED

1. Commercial system such as the C2Dx STIC™ (Figure 24.3, previously Stryker Pressure Monitor™), containing:
   - Prefilled syringe of sterile normal saline
   - 18-gauge stainless-steel needle with 1.5 mm side port, 2.5″ long
   - Tapered chamber stem/diaphragm chamber
   - Handheld calibrated tested digital manometer
   - Topical antiseptic (e.g., isopropyl alcohol or chlorhexidine) to clean anticipated site of measurement

STEPS TO PERFORMING THE PROCEDURE

Per the manufacturer's instructions, or generally (Figure 24.4):
1. Power-on the device and place the needle firmly onto the tapered chamber stem/diaphragm.
2. Remove cap on prefilled syringe and connect syringe to chamber stem; take care to preserve sterility of needle and syringe contents.

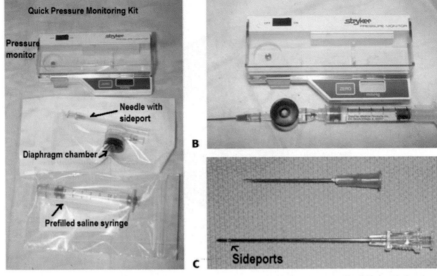

FIGURE 24.3. Stryker intracompartmental pressure monitor. Reprinted with permission from Wiesel, S. (2015). *Operative techniques in orthopaedic surgery, four volume set* (2nd ed.). Wolters Kluwer Health.

3. Open the cover of the monitor; place needle/diaphragm/syringe into place, black side down.
4. Turn on the monitor; prime the system by purging air from needle/syringe and zeroing the device.
5. Determine the location and the angle of insertion for the needle.
6. Introduce the needle directly into the muscular compartment at a right angle to the skin.
7. Inject saline (<3cc) into the muscular compartment; hold the device still.
8. Check display for pressure reading.

COMPLICATIONS OF THE PROCEDURE

1. Local discomfort
2. Infection, including cellulitis and/or abscess (minimized with appropriate sterile technique)
3. Bleeding or hematoma formation
4. Possible damage to underlying blood vessels or nerves

POSTPROCEDURE CARE

Local wound care to puncture sites (i.e., keep clean and dry). If pressures are consistent with compartment syndrome or clinical concern persists, urgent surgical consultation is required. If pressures are not consistent with compartment syndrome but clinical concern persists, continue clinical examinations and consider surgical consultation.

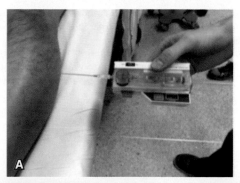

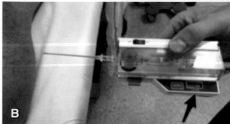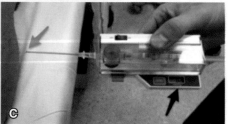

FIGURE 24.4. Use of assembled side-port needle device (A, B, C). Note that the device is held still and needle inserted at 90° angle to the skin. Reprinted with permission from Ahmad, C. S., & Romeo, A. A. (2018). *Baseball sports medicine.* Lippincott Williams & Wilkins.

BIBLIOGRAPHY

Agur, M. R. A., & Lee, M. J. (1999). *Grant's atlas of anatomy* (10th ed.). Lippincott Williams & Wilkins.

Ahmad, C. S., & Romeo, A. A. (2019). *Baseball sports medicine.* Lippincott Williams & Wilkins.

Boody, A. R., & Wongworawat, M. D. (2005). Accuracy in the measurement of compartment pressures: A comparison of three commonly used devices. *Journal of Bone and Joint Surgery, 87*(11), 2415–2422. https://doi.org/10.2106/JBJS.D.02826

Bucholz, R. W., & Heckman, J. D. (2001). *Rockwood & Green's fractures in adults* (5th ed.). Lippincott Williams & Wilkins.

Garner, M. R., Taylor, S. A., Gausden, E., & Lyden, J. P. (2014). Compartment syndrome: Diagnosis, management, and unique concerns in the twenty-first century. *HSS Journal, 10*(2), 143–152. https://doi.org/10.1007/s11420-014-9386-8

Hammerberg, E. M., Whitesides, T. E., & Seiler, J. G. (2012). The reliability of measurement of tissue pressure in compartment syndrome. *Journal of Orthopaedic Trauma, 26*(9), e166. https://doi.org/10.1097/BOT.0b013e31822908cf

Heckman, M. M., Whitesides, T. E. Jr, Grewe, S. R., Judd, R. L., Miller, M., & Lawrence, J. H. 3rd. (1993). Histologic determination of the ischemic threshold of muscle in the canine compartment syndrome model. *Journal of Orthopaedic Trauma, 7*(3), 199–210. https://doi.org/10.1097/00005131-199306000-00001

McQueen, M. M., Duckworth, A. D., Aitken, S. A., & Court-Brown, C. M. (2013). The estimated sensitivity and specificity of compartment pressure monitoring for acute compartment syndrome. *Journal of Bone and Joint Surgery, 95*(8), 673–677. https://doi.org/10.2106/JBJS.K.01731

Moed, B. R., & Thorderson, P. K. (1993). Measurement of intracompartmental pressure: A comparison of the slit catheter, side-ported needle, and simple needle. *Journal of Bone and Joint Surgery, 75*(2), 231–235.

Olson, S. A., & Glasgow, R. R. (2005). Acute compartment syndrome in lower extremity musculoskeletal trauma. *Journal of the American Academy of Orthopaedic Surgeons, 13*(7), 436–444. https://doi .org/10.5435/00124635-200511000-00003

Premkumar, K. (2003). *Massage connection* (2nd ed.), Lippincott Williams & Wilkins

Wiesel, S. W. (2015). *Operative techniques in orthopaedic surgery (four volume set)* (2nd ed.). Lippincott Williams & Wilkins.

Arthrocentesis

Kristopher Jackson

INDICATIONS FOR THE PROCEDURE

The practice of therapeutically draining excess joint fluid is as old as Western medicine itself. In fact, medical texts authored more than 400 years ago describe the symptomatic relief experienced by patients with painful, swollen joints who underwent therapeutic drainage of their excess joint fluid. Today, the indication for arthrocentesis is not dissimilar to the procedural indication centuries ago: to offer patients relief from painful, swollen joints. However, the clinical benefits of this procedure extend beyond merely providing pain relief.

A painful, swollen joint can be attributed to many physiologic processes. Laboratory analysis of a patient's synovial fluid can help providers determine the etiology of a patient's joint effusion and ensure prompt treatment when clinically indicated. Laboratory testing of synovial fluid can assist providers in discerning between an acute infectious process (e.g., a septic joint), crystalline arthropathies (e.g., gout, pseudogout), osteoarthritis, inflammatory conditions (e.g., rheumatoid arthritis, systemic lupus erythematosus), hemarthrosis (e.g., coagulopathy, trauma), and some neoplastic conditions.

Indications for the procedure are as follows:

1. Determine the etiology of pain or swelling in a single joint (e.g., monoarthritis)
2. Evaluate for suspected infection (e.g., septic joint)
3. Administer intra-articular medications
4. Provide symptomatic relief of recurrent, large joint effusions of a known etiology

CONTRAINDICATIONS FOR THE PROCEDURE

Relative Contraindications

1. **Cellulitis and impaired skin integrity:** Providers should not perform arthrocentesis if the procedure requires introducing a needle into the joint space through potentially infected soft tissue, because this would contaminate the otherwise sterile joint space. However, if the patient's physical examination findings are suggestive of septic arthritis, a potentially life-threatening condition, synovial fluid collection is critical to patient management and should therefore be performed. Extra care should be taken to avoid performing the arthrocentesis in areas of skin affected

by ulcerated or inflamed skin owing to psoriasis or eczema. These areas are felt to represent sites of increased bacterial colonization that may, in turn, increase the patient's risk of infection following arthrocentesis.

2. **Coagulopathy:** Providers should carefully consider the risks and benefits of arthrocentesis among patients with inherited or acquired bleeding disorders. Performing arthrocentesis in patients with coagulopathy does carry a risk of causing iatrogenic hemarthrosis. Although there are data to suggest that the risk of hemarthrosis is low, even among therapeutically anticoagulated patients (see, e.g., Thumboo & O'Duffy), providers should carefully weigh the risks of arthrocentesis in this patient population against the value of the clinical information they stand to gain by performing it. According to Zayat et al., the risk of iatrogenic hemarthrosis in patients with coagulopathy undergoing arthrocentesis can be further mitigated by avoiding deeper joints (e.g., those with less palpable landmarks) and the use of large-bore needles. Reversal agents or blood products to correct a patient's coagulopathy should also be considered based on the individual patient, medical history, and the reason for the underlying coagulopathy.

3. **Prosthetic joint:** If the patient has undergone prior joint replacement surgery, providers should consult an orthopedic surgeon prior to performing arthrocentesis. If there is concern for infection in a prosthetic joint, an orthopedic surgeon may: (a) recommend observation or conservative management, (b) wish to perform the procedure themselves because scar tissue and abnormal anatomy may make the procedure more technically complex, and/or (c) perform an operative incision and débridement procedure in lieu of arthrocentesis.

Absolute Contraindications

Although there are no absolute contraindications to performing an arthrocentesis, providers should consider carefully each of the relative contraindications listed previously. Providers should also consider their skill set and familiarity with the procedure before attempting deeper anatomic sites that may be more technically challenging.

EQUIPMENT NEEDED

Before performing an arthrocentesis procedure, the provider should gather the supplies necessary for the joint on which the procedure will be performed.

1. Chlorhexidine or povidone–iodine solution
2. Sterile gloves
3. Fenestrated drape
4. Skin marking pen
5. Syringes
   a. For smaller joints (e.g., wrist, foot), obtain two 2 to 5 mL syringes.
   b. For larger joints with large effusions (e.g., knee), obtain one 10 cc syringe for the administration of local anesthesia as well as one 60 cc syringe for fluid aspiration (or multiple smaller syringes if a 60 cc syringe is not available).

   c. If planning to administer a corticosteroid following joint fluid aspiration, obtain an additional syringe in which to draw up additional anesthetic and corticosteroid.
6. 25g or 27g needle for administering local anesthesia
7. 18 to 25g needle for aspiration
   a. Note: Needle selection warrants careful consideration of the size and depth of the joint undergoing aspiration. In the following step-by-step instructions, a 1.5 inch, 18 to 21g needle is used for arthrocentesis in the knee based on recommendations by Stephens et al. A 0.5 to 1.5 inch, 23 to 25g needle is used for the wrist. These are suggestions, but suitable adjustments should be made based on patient's size and clinical presentation.
8. Untreated specimen tubes or sterile screw cap containers
9. Lidocaine (1% or 2%) or bupivacaine (0.25% or 0.5%).
   a. Note: Lidocaine is shorter acting and has a more rapid onset of action, whereas bupivacaine has a slower onset but may provide longer anesthetic effects in the postprocedure period.
10. If available, ethyl chloride spray or prilocaine/lidocaine topical cream can provide additional analgesia in patients who are particularly squeamish or needle averse.
11. If clinically warranted, obtain a corticosteroid for injection into the joint space such as methylprednisolone or triamcinolone acetonide.
   a. Note: The dose of methylprednisolone or triamcinolone to be administered tends to correspond with the size of the joint. As described by Stephens et al., the dose of methylprednisolone or triamcinolone acetonide for intra-articular administration to the shoulder, wrist, and ankle joints is typically in the 20 to 40 mg range. The dose of intra-articular methylprednisolone or triamcinolone delivered to the knee is generally greater, 20 to 80 mg.

STEPS TO PERFORMING THE PROCEDURE

1. Obtain informed consent.
2. If available and/or clinically indicated, apply topical anesthetic ointment (e.g., prilocaine/lidocaine topical cream).
3. Position the patient.
   a. *Knee*: Position the leg with the knee fully extended or slightly flexed. If necessary, support the knee with a towel roll.
   b. *Wrist*: Position the patient with the palm facing upward. If necessary, support the wrist with a towel roll.
4. Palpate the joint for anatomic landmarks (Figure 25.1A-C).
   a. *Knee*: Palpate the medial and lateral borders of the patella. If desired, mark the possible points of entry, most commonly the suprapatellar approach (1 cm lateral and 1 cm superior to the patella) or the midpoint approach (1 cm medial or lateral to the patella) (Figure 25.2A-C).
   b. *Wrist*: Palpate the radiocarpal joint line. If desired, mark the planned point of entry just distal to Lister tubercle and on the ulnar aspect of the extensor pollicis longus tendon.

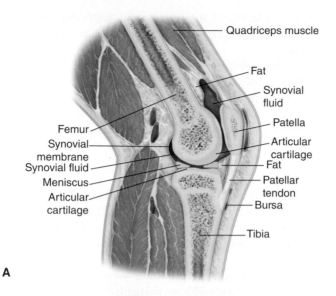

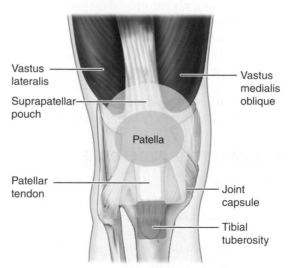

FIGURE 25.1. Structure of the knee. (A) Anatomy of the knee; (B) Anterior view of knee and surrounding structures; (C) Bony anatomy of the knee. (A) Reprinted with permission from Freer, J. M. (2016). *The Washington Manual of Bedside Procedures*. Wolters Kluwer. Modified with permission from Creason, C. (2010). *Stedman's Medical Terminology*. Wolters Kluwer; (B) Reprinted with permission from Freer, J. M. (2016). *The Washington Manual of Bedside Procedures*. Wolters Kluwer. Modified with permission from Anderson, M. K. (2012). *Foundations of Athletic Training* (5th ed.). Wolters Kluwer;

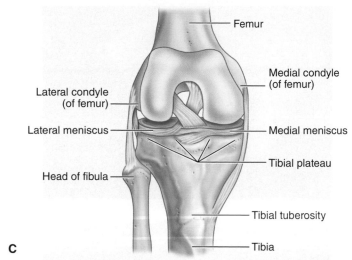

Femur

Medial condyle
(of femur)

Lateral condyle
(of femur)

Lateral meniscus

Medial meniscus

Tibial plateau

Head of fibula

Tibial tuberosity

Tibia

C

FIGURE 25.1. (*continued*) (C) Reprinted with permission from Freer, J. M. (2016). *The Washington Manual of Bedside Procedures.* Wolters Kluwer. Modified with permission from Anderson, M. K. (2012). *Foundations of Athletic Training* (5th ed.). Wolters Kluwer.

5. Prepare the skin using chlorhexidine or povidone–iodine solution.
6. Apply sterile fenestrated drape.
7. Draw up 5 to 10 cc of local anesthetic and, if planning to administer a corticosteroid injection following aspiration of synovial fluid, draw up 3 to 5 mL of local anesthetic and the appropriate dose of corticosteroid for the anatomic location.
8. If available or desired, administer ethyl chloride spray.
9. Using a 25 to 27g needle, create a subcutaneous wheal at the planned point of entry. If there is a lot of redundant tissue, you may wish to anesthetize deeper layers of tissue for patient comfort.
   Knee:
10. Remove the 25 to 27g needle, and apply the larger needle selected for joint aspiration to the syringe of remaining anesthetic.
11. Place the nondominant hand on the knee joint and displace the patella.
12. With the patella gently displaced, use the dominant hand to introduce the needle one cm lateral or medial (depending on the approach) to the patella and direct the needle behind the patella toward the intercondylar notch of the femur.
13. Once in the joint space, fluid should flow freely into the syringe. With the nondominant hand, the practitioner may wish to apply gentle pressure to both sides of the joint to assist with fluid evacuation.
14. Note the appearance of the fluid. If it appears purulent or unusually turbid and a corticosteroid injection was planned, consider forgoing corticosteroid administration. This may be a sign of infection.

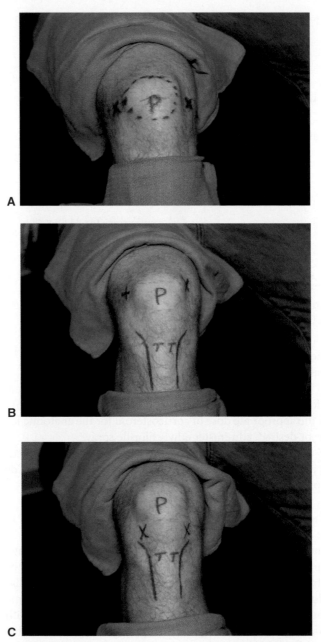

FIGURE 25.2. Patellar approaches for arthrocentesis. (A) Lateral or medial midpatellar insertion approach. Points of insertion are marked with an X. (B) Superolateral or superomedial (i.e., suprapatellar) insertion approach. Points of insertion are marked with an "X." (C) Inferolateral or inferomedial (i.e., infrapatellar) approach. Points of insertion are marked with an "X." Reprinted with permission from Freer, J. M. (2016). *The Washington Manual of Bedside Procedures*. Wolters Kluwer.

15. If fluid appears as expected and a corticosteroid infection was planned following synovial fluid evacuation, remove the syringe used for drainage while stabilizing the needle introduced into the joint space. With the needle stabilized, attach the syringe containing the remaining anesthetic and corticosteroid mixture and administer accordingly.
16. Withdraw the needle and apply an adhesive bandage.
17. Transfer synovial fluid to sterile specimen cup for fluid analysis, as indicated.
    Wrist:
18. Through the subcutaneous wheal, introduce the 25g needle attached to a syringe perpendicular to the skin (Figure 25.3). Continue to aspirate back on the syringe as the needle is advanced into the joint space. A popping sensation is common when the needle enters the joint space. Should the needle strike bone, retract the needle and adjust the angle of approach.
19. Continue to aspirate fluid until drainage ceases.

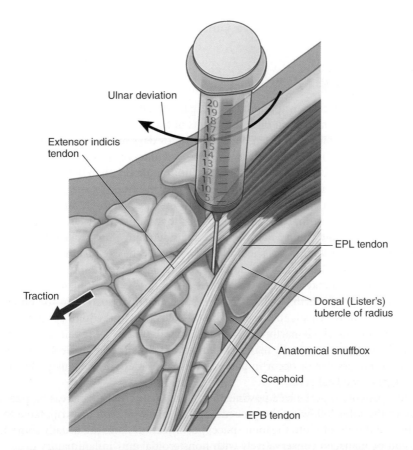

FIGURE 25.3. Through the subcutaneous wheal, introduce the 25g needle attached to a syringe perpendicular to the skin.

20. If fluid appears as expected and a corticosteroid injection was planned following synovial fluid evacuation, remove the syringe used for drainage while very carefully stabilizing the needle introduced into the joint space.
21. Carefully attach the syringe containing the remaining anesthetic and corticosteroid mixture and administer accordingly. If the needle remains in the joint space, there should be no resistance when the solution is administered.
22. Withdraw the needle and apply an adhesive bandage.
23. Transfer synovial fluid to sterile specimen cup for fluid analysis, as indicated.

COMPLICATIONS OF THE PROCEDURE

Complications from arthrocentesis are relatively uncommon but can be from the procedure itself as well as the intra-articular medications administered during the procedure.
  a. Local trauma, tendon injury, or hemarthrosis
  b. Postprocedural pain or a "postinjection flare"
  c. A "dry tap" or failure to aspirate joint fluid
  d. Infection

POSTPROCEDURE CARE

If a corticosteroid injection was administered, patients should be advised that (1) their pain and discomfort may return once the effects of the local anesthetic subside, (2) the peak effect of the steroid administered may not be for days following administration of the medication, and (3) while the effects of intra-articular corticosteroid injections may be short-lived, weight-bearing joints should not undergo more than three corticosteroid injections per year. If the patient is under the care of an orthopedic surgeon or is undergoing evaluation for an arthroplasty procedure in the affected joint, the patient should be advised that some orthopedic surgeons prefer that patients not have corticosteroid injections for some time, often 3 months, prior to undergoing joint replacement surgery. Patients with large joint effusions should be advised that these effusions are oftentimes prone to recurrence. These patients should be counseled that a compression sleeve or compression stocking may help slow the rate at which fluid reaccumulates.

Hemarthrosis after arthrocentesis is rare but is usually apparent in the hours following the procedure. This is the result of blood collecting in the joint space following injury to a blood vessel. Hemarthrosis is usually manifested by joint pain, swelling, and stiffness. Hemarthrosis is usually managed conservatively, although patients with symptoms that do not resolve or occur in patients with an underlying coagulopathy should seek emergency medical care.

A few patients experience a postinjection flare manifested by increasing pain and stiffness in the joint following the procedure. This phenomenon is attributable to the instillation of the steroid into the joint space; postinjection flares are usually short-lived and should be managed conservatively with nonsteroidal anti-inflammatory drugs. Patients should be advised that if these symptoms do not subside in several days, this could indicate that the joint space has become infected. However, infection as a complication of arthrocentesis is very rare, assuming that the practitioner who performs the procedure prepares the site properly and maintains the appropriate aseptic technique during the procedure. Should the synovial fluid collected during the procedure appear infected, the patient should be hospitalized and started on empiric antimicrobials while awaiting synovial fluid culture data. A septic joint is a potentially life-threatening condition.

BIBLIOGRAPHY

Aceves-Avila, F. J. (2003). The first descriptions of therapeutic arthrocentesis: A historical note. *Rheumatology, 42*(1), 180–183. https://doi.org/10.1093/rheumatology/keg001.

Akbarnia, H., Saber, A. Y., & Zahn, E. (2020). *Knee arthrocentesis. StatPearls*. Retrieved from https://www.ncbi.nlm.nih.gov/books/NBK470229/.

Bettencourt, R., & Linder, M. (2010). Arthrocentesis and therapeutic joint injection: An overview for the primary care physician. *Primary Care: Clinics in Office Practice, 37*(4), 691–702. https://doi.org/10.1016/j.pop.2010.07.002.

Claiborne, J. R., Branch, L. G., Reynolds, M., & Defranzo, A. J. (2017). An algorithmic approach to the suspected septic wrist. *Annals of Plastic Surgery, 78*(6), 659–662. https://doi.org/10.1097/sap.0000000000000974.

Ferrand, J., El Samad, Y., Brunschweiler, B., Grados, F., Dehamchia-Rehailia, N., Séjourne, A., Schmit, J.-L., Gabrion, A., Fardellone, P., & Paccou, J. (2016). Morbimortality in adult patients with septic arthritis: A three-year hospital-based study. *BMC Infectious Diseases, 16*(1). https://doi.org/10.1186/s12879-016-1540-0.

Patel, A., & Punnapuzha, S. (2020). *Wrist arthrocentesis. StatPearls*. Retrieved from https://www.ncbi.nlm.nih.gov/books/NBK559228/.

Purcell, D., Terry, B. A., & Sharp, B. R. (2019). *Joint arthrocentesis. In Emergency orthopedics handbook* (pp. 87–104). Springer International Publishing. https://doi.org/10.1007/978-3-030-00707-2_4.

Stephens, M. B., Beutler, A. I., & O'Connor, F. G. (2008). Musculoskeletal injections: A review of the evidence. *American Family Physician, 78*(8), 971–976.

Thomsen, T. W., Shen, S., Shaffer, R. W., & Setnik, G. S. (2006). Arthrocentesis of the knee. *New England Journal of Medicine, 354*(19), e19. https://doi.org/10.1056/nejmvcm051914.

Thumboo, J., & O'Duffy, J. D. (1998). A prospective study of the safety of joint and soft tissue aspirations and injections in patients taking warfarin sodium. *Arthritis & Rheumatism, 41*(4), 736–739. https://doi.org/10.1002/1529-0131(199804)41:4<736::aid-art23>3.0.co;2-p

Villa-Forte, A. (2020). *How to do wrist arthrocentesis*. Merck Manuals Professional Version. Retrieved February 27, 2020 from https://www.merckmanuals.com/professional/musculoskeletal-and-connective-tissue-disorders/how-to-do-arthrocentesis/how-to-do-wrist-arthrocentesis.

Zayat, A. S., Buch, M., & Wakefield, R. J. (2017). *Arthrocentesis and injection of joints and soft tissue*. In Firestein, G. S., Budd, R., Gabriel, S. E., McInnes, I. B., & O'Dell, J. R (Eds.), *Kelley and Firestein's textbook of Rheumatology* (pp. 802–816). Elsevier.

Zuber, T. J. (2002). Knee joint aspiration and injection. *American Family Physician, 66*(8), 1497–1500.

26 Negative Pressure Wound Therapy Application

Diana Filipek-Oberg

INDICATIONS FOR THE PROCEDURE

Wound vacuum-assisted closure (3M™ V.A.C.® Therapy), or negative pressure wound therapy (NPWT), is done to promote healing of complex acute or chronic wounds by preparing the wound bed for closure through granulation tissue formation (Figure 26.1). NPWT will apply controlled negative pressure directly to the wound bed, which allows

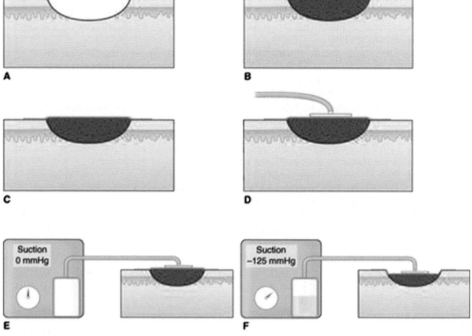

FIGURE 26.1. Principles of negative pressure wound therapy. The wound (A) and a foam, cut to fit the wound geometry, which is placed inside the wound (B). The wound is sealed airtight with a thin, adhesive drape (C) with the attached "suction pad" (connecting pad), including the drainage tube (D). The wound is hermetically sealed with a thin, adhesive drape and connected to the vacuum source by means of the attached "suction pad" (suction strength 0 mmHg) (E). At suction strength—125 mmHg—the foam has collapsed, and the exudate collection reservoir is already partly filled (F). Reprinted with permission from Lynn, P. (2018). *Taylor's clinical nursing skills* (5th ed.). Wolters Kluwer.

for a reduction of edema, thereby improving nutrient and oxygen delivery as well as granulation tissue stimulation. This will, in turn, promote wound healing. Other goals of NPWT include increased perfusion to marginally viable flaps, skin graft preparation of wound bed, decrease in wound size as well as full wound closure of both simple and complex wounds.

Indications for NPWT, both chronic (C) (30 days or more) and acute (A), are:

1. Diabetic foot ulcers (C) (Figure 26.2)
2. Stage III and IV pressure ulcers (C)
3. Venous and arterial insufficiency ulcers (C)
4. Partial thickness burns (A)

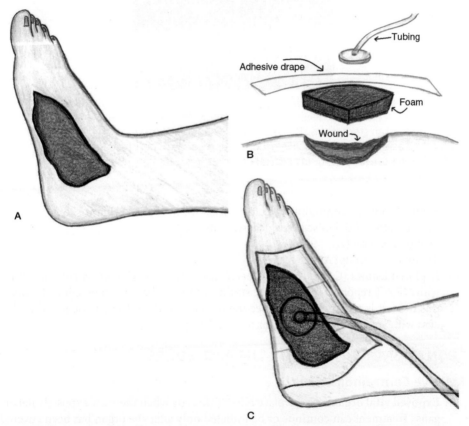

FIGURE 26.2. Schematic illustration of a medial foot ulceration with granulation tissue (A) being covered by a negative pressure wound therapy (NPWT) device (B, C). The adhesive dressing material is placed over the selected foam and overlapping the skin at the periphery of the wound to provide an airtight seal. In some cases, adhesive products such as Mastisol or tincture of benzoin can be used around the wound to further secure the dressing material. The tube is then connected to a collection canister in the NPWT device and set in the desired pressure (mmHg). Reprinted with permission from Zgonis, T. (2017). *Surgical reconstruction of the diabetic foot and ankle* (2nd ed.). Wolters Kluwer Health.

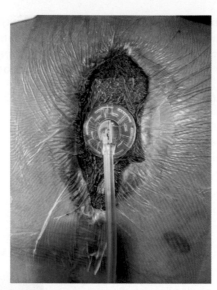

FIGURE 26.3. An example of negative-pressure wound therapy after sternal dehiscence and development of osteomyelitis following cardiac surgery via median sternotomy. This modality is commonly used in the modern management of chest wall infections. Reprinted with permission from LoCicero, J. (2018). *Shields' general thoracic surgery* (8th ed.). Wolters Kluwer.

5. Surgical wounds, commonly infected sternal wounds (C/A) (Figure 26.3)
6. Postoperative and dehisced surgical wounds (C/A)
7. Skin grafts, flaps (A)
8. Traumatic wounds (A)
9. Explored fistulas (C/A). There has been successful management of enteric fistulae with NPWT reported through case studies, but there have been no clinical trials at this time. It is recommended to see the manual for the NPWT system and to discuss with your medical team prior to initializing therapy.

CONTRAINDICATIONS FOR THE PROCEDURE

Relative Contraindications

1. **Exposed vital organs:** *Never* place NPWT directly when there are exposed vital organs. Treatment can continue or be initiated only after the organ has been covered by protective mesh and you have discussed this with the medical/surgical team.
2. **Active bleeding and difficult wound hemostasis:** Stop NPWT immediately if active bleeding is noticed.
3. **Patients undergoing anticoagulation therapy:** It is important to closely monitor patients who are on anticoagulation therapy, antiplatelet therapy, and who have bleeding disorders. Follow their complete blood count and coagulation studies as well as have nursing monitor the system output and record closely.

4. **Special considerations**: As a provider, there are a few things one must consider and discuss with the medical/surgical team prior to starting NPWT:
   a. Sharp edges within the wound, i.e., bone fragments
   b. Spinal cord injury
   c. Enteric fistulas: Confirm that they are explored with the medical team.
   d. Patients who will likely require magnetic resonance imaging (MRI), defibrillation, and hyperbaric oxygen chamber. Consider how they will transport and go through the scanners, as well as whether the electrical components can travel within the hyperbaric chamber.

Absolute Contraindications

1. **Allergy to required components:** Confirm with patient any allergies prior to beginning NPWT.
2. **Malignancy:** NPWT can lead to cellular proliferation. Consider hematology/oncology consult if NPWT is clinically indicated.
3. **Necrotic tissue with eschar present**: If present, it will not form granulation tissue, and therapy will therefore not be able to perform to its goal. After debridement of necrotic tissue and complete removal of eschar, NPWT may be used.
4. **Untreated osteomyelitis or sepsis within the wound area:** Wounds with infection should have been treated with systemic antibiotics prior to initialization of NPWT. If one notices continued deterioration of the wound and/or infection continuation, then one must consider a surgical consult for debridement/wound evaluation.
5. **Nonenteric and unexplored fistulas**

EQUIPMENT NEEDED

Remember to follow your healthcare system's policies for NPWT. The following is a list of generic equipment for the majority of NPWT:

1. Gloves, gown: remember to follow institution's policy, as it may call for sterile approach
2. Normal saline for wound cleansing, gauze to dry skin
3. Protective barrier wipe to protect skin around the wound
4. Device specific: NPWT dressing, tubing, transparent draping kit
   a. 3M™ V.A.C.® Therapy Dressings
      i. Black polyurethane foam (3M™ V.A.C.® Granufoam™ Dressing) is most frequently used. This has larger pores and is therefore effective with stimulation of granulation tissue.
      ii. White polyvinyl chloride (3M™ Whitefoam™ Dressing) is dense, premoistened foam. It has a higher density and therefore requires a higher pressure to obtain the same granulation rate as V.A.C.® Granufoam™ Dressing. Can be used with tunneling and shallow undermining owing to the higher tensile strength.
      iii. 3M™ V.A.C.® Granufoam Silver™: same as black polyurethane foam but reduces infection in wounds caused by the antimicrobial silver it contains. This requires additional precautions to be taken. Be sure to follow the specific product instructions.

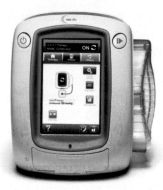 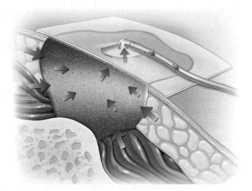

FIGURE 26.4. A vacuum-assisted wound closure device (3M™ V.A.C.® Ulta Therapy System) assists wound closure by providing localized negative pressure to the wound bed and wound margins. Courtesy of 3M. © 2021, 3M. All rights reserved. 3M and the other marks shown are marks and/or registered marks. Unauthorized use prohibited.

5. Scissors, sterile cotton swabs for wound measurements, exploration of tunneling, and to provide support with foam dressing
6. 3M™ V.A.C.® Ulta Therapy Unit or other NPWT vacuum unit (Figure 26.4)
7. Wound measuring ruler
8. Towel or absorbent pad to go under the wound area to prevent soiled linens

STEPS TO PERFORMING THE PROCEDURE

1. Order the appropriate equipment. Remember either to base on prior NPWT dressing change or to assess wound beforehand to confirm that you have ordered the appropriate equipment.
2. Prepare the equipment and patient. Confirm with the patient understanding of the procedure. Make sure to assess the patient and provide appropriate pain management for the patient in preparation for the procedure. Remember to have completed a thorough physical examination and focused examination on the specific wound. Make sure you have assistance if required.
3. Prepare the clean field needed to complete the dressing change. Position the patient for wound cleansing and dressing application. Try to find the best position for both patient comfort as well as best visualization of the wound.
4. Remove prior dressing and assess the wound. Always count the total number of pieces of foam removed from the wound and ensure the same number of foam pieces was removed as placed. Measure length, width, and depth to record (Figures 26.5 and 26.6). Obtain a picture to use for documentation of progression if warranted. Remember to follow institution's policies and practice Health Insurance Portability and Accountability Act (HIPAA) guidelines here.
5. Cleanse wound using institution's policy/protocol. This cleansing and irrigation will allow for the wound to be prepared for application of the dressing. Prepare the periwound area and clip hair if necessary. Dry skin using gauze and use barrier preparation to the skin around the wound.

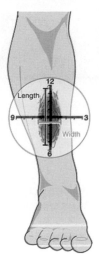

FIGURE 26.5. Wound measurement (length × width). Reprinted with permission from Doughty, D. B., & McNichol, L. L. (2015). *Wound, Ostomy and Continence Nurses Society® core curriculum: Wound management.* Wolters Kluwer Health.

6. Open an intact NPWT dressing package. Cut the foam to fit the wound as per your measurements and assessment. Remember to include tunneling and undermining in your foam dressing—if undressed, tunneling can result in an abscess or cyst when pressure closes off the wound entrance owing to granulation. The 3M™ V.A.C. Whitefoam™ Dressing is recommended for use in tunnels. Do not place foam into blind or unexplored tunnels. Cover any exposed sutures, ligaments, nerves with nonadherent dressing.

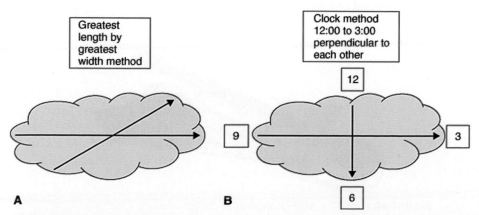

FIGURE 26.6. Two wound measurement methods. (A) Greatest length by greatest width method; (B) clock method 12:00 to 3:00, perpendicular to each other. Reprinted with permission from Sussman, C., & Bates-Jensen, B. (2011). *Wound care* (4th ed.). Wolters Kluwer Health.

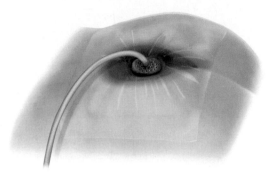

FIGURE 26.7. 3M™ V.A.C.® Dressing placement. An appropriately sized 3M™ V.A.C.® Granufoam™ Dressing black foam is placed into the wound cavity, covered to ensure proper seal, and connected to 125 mmHg pressure. Reprinted with permission from Wexner, S. D., & Fleshman, J. W. (2018). *Colon and rectal surgery: Anorectal operations* (2nd ed.). Wolters Kluwer Health.

7. Foam should be placed into the wound without force (Figure 26.7). Confirm that the foam is covering all of the wound areas and does not overlap onto intact skin. Foam that is directly placed onto intact skin can cause skin breakdown. Remember to count how many pieces of foam you use and place into the wound. Document this to confirm how many pieces are removed at the next wound NPWT dressing change.

8. Place the transparent drape over the foam in the wound to cover the foam as well as an additional 3 to 5 cm of intact skin. To bridge wounds, see specific manufacturer instructions (Figure 26.8).

9. Cut a hole approximately the size of quarter or 2.5 cm into the drape. Then apply the 3M™ SensaT.R.A.C.™ Pad with the tubing connected over the hole. Connect the SensaT.R.A.C.™ Pad tubing to the canister tubing. Ensure that the canister is attached to the 3M™ V.A.C.® Therapy Unit or other NPWT unit as well as all the tubing connected and that clamps are undone.

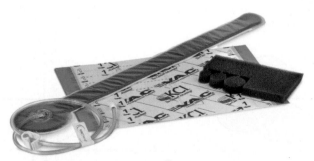

FIGURE 26.8. 3M™ V.A.C.® Granufoam™ Bridge Dressing. Courtesy of 3M. © 2021, 3M. All rights reserved. 3M and the other marks shown are marks and/or registered marks. Unauthorized use prohibited.

10. Turn the power on to the NPWT unit and enter the appropriate NPWT settings. If applicable, use the 3M™ Seal Check™ Feature to confirm that you have an appropriate seal. Assess the dressing integrity and seal integrity because the dressing and foam will collapse and appear wrinkly when done correctly. If there appears to be a leak, check the tubing and dressing/drape for leaks. Use an additional drape for sealing leaks as needed.
    a. Pressure settings: The 3M™ V.A.C.® Therapy default setting is continuous suction at-125 mmHg but these settings may be individualized and adjusted to the patient's needs. The 3M™ V.A.C.® Therapy Clinical Guidelines recommend to consider titrating up by 25 mmHg for wounds that have excessive drainage, large wound volume, when using 3M™ V.A.C. Whitefoam™ Dressings in wound/tunneling, and a tenuous seal. Consider titrating down by 25 mmHg for extremes of age, risk of excessive bleeding, pain/discomfort not relieved by appropriate analgesia, wound bed/periwound ecchymosis, and circulatory compromise.
11 Discard used supplies and clean up the area and patient.
12. Remember to record the wound size, characteristics, imaging, as well as supplies used and procedure in the patient chart.

COMPLICATIONS OF THE PROCEDURE

1. **Infection:** If present, increase the frequency of NPWT wound dressing changes to 12 to 24 hours. Obtain a wound culture in order for appropriate antibiotics to be initiated. Consider infectious disease consult if warranted. Trend complete blood count (CBC) to monitor white blood cells (WBC).
2. **Bleeding:** If active bleeding suddenly occurs, or large amounts of frank red blood are noted in the tubing or within the canister, immediately stop negative pressure wound therapy. Leave dressing intact and take measures to stop bleeding.
3. **Fistula formation:** Wounds with enteric fistulas require special precautions to optimize negative pressure wound therapy. If enteric fistula effluent management or containment is the sole goal of therapy, negative pressure wound therapy is not recommended. Consider discussing with medical/surgical team to see plan of action.
4. **Pain:** Monitor pain before, during, and after NPWT dressing changes. If patient complains of pain during the therapy, consider switching to the 3M™ V.A.C. Whitefoam™ Dressing. Confirm patient receives adequate analgesia for dressing change procedures. If there is a sudden increase or change in pain, one must look for the cause.
5. **Tissue loss and disruption of underlying tissues/structures:** Assess for osteomyelitis, check for small leaks and cover, change dressing often, clean wound more thoroughly, evaluate for signs and symptoms of infection, examine the wound and debride as necessary.
6. **Ischemia, necrosis—stop negative pressure wound therapy:** Assess patient and wound with the medical/surgical team. May warrant surgery for wound exploration and debridement.
7. **Lack of improvement within 1 to 2 weeks:** If there is no improvement during the therapy, consider the following actions: (1) confirm that the patient is receiving adequate pressure relief; (2) changing the therapy settings from continuous to

intermittent or vice versa; (3) providing a therapeutic pause by interrupting negative pressure wound therapy for 1 to 2 days and then resuming; (4) evaluate nutritional status and consult nutrition; (5) assess wound for infection; and (6) check therapy history log to ensure that the actual number of therapy hours a day matches the recommendation of 22 hours a day. Also consider cutting the foam slightly smaller than the wound edges to promote inward epithelial migration.

POSTPROCEDURE CARE

Once the procedure is completed, turn on the 3M™ V.A.C.® Therapy Unit and enter the appropriate settings of negative pressure as well as continuous versus intermittent therapy. Confirm that there are no leaks and that the foam dressing is obtaining appropriate suction (see earlier in procedure). Remember to document a procedure note including wound measurements, a picture of the wound, supplies used, and whether and how the patient tolerated the procedure. Document if any preprocedure pain medication was warranted. NPWT dressings should be changed 48 hours after the initiation of NPWT and then two to three times a week, as indicated by the wound's response to the NPWT. Make sure you place NPWT orders for nursing to monitor and record output, as well as what settings to maintain the on the V.A.C.® Therapy Unit. If nursing is to change the dressings, place appropriate orders indicating timing, supplies, and preprocedure pain medication. If the patient is to leave the hospital with a V.A.C.® Therapy Unit, remember to coordinate with home care so the patient can be set up with home nursing and appropriate supplies. Home care services will likely need a script for the appropriate supplies as well as NPWT settings. Remember to include pressure setting and intermittent or continuous setting.

BIBLIOGRAPHY

Baranoski, S., & Ayello, E. A. (2011). *Wound care essentials.* http://ebookcentral.proquest.com
Hess, C. T. (2012). *Clinical guide to skin & wound care.* http://ebookcentral.proquest.com
Woods, L. (2017). Negative-pressure wound therapy. In D. L. Wiegand (Ed.), *AACN procedure manual for high acuity, progressive and critical care (1200–1209).* Elsevier.
3M™ V.A.C.® Therapy Clinical Guidelines: A Reference Source for Clinicians (2021). Retrieved from https://hcbgregulatory.3m.com

CHAPTER 27

Cast Application

Angela Grochowski
Angela McGill

INDICATIONS FOR THE PROCEDURE

A cast is an immobilizing device that can be used on extremities. It is circumferential and prevents motion so as to allow an injured area to heal. This is in contrast to a splint, which is not circumferential and is hard on only one side. A splint is used when significant swelling is expected, as in acute injuries. It is usually a bridge to a cast, although sometimes it is used as definitive treatment.

Although individual indications for a cast are beyond the scope of this book, the following are some broad general indications.

1. Closed fractures that have been successfully reduced or fractures that are in acceptable alignment of the hand, wrist, forearm, elbow, knee, leg, ankle, and foot.
2. Unstable dislocations of the ankle, wrist, or elbow can be immobilized in a cast after reduction.
3. Severe sprains of ankles and wrists sometimes feel better, and heal more quickly, with short periods of immobilization in a cast.
4. Surgeons sometimes choose to immobilize a joint after surgeries to protect repairs. For example, a cast is sometimes applied following a patellar tendon repair or after a thumb carpometacarpal joint arthroplasty.

CONTRAINDICATIONS TO THE PROCEDURE

Relative Contraindications

Swelling, poor tissue, diabetes, and neuropathy are relative contraindications. If the area to be casted is very swollen, applying a cast could cause compartment syndrome. In addition, the cast will likely become loose in a few days as the swelling improves. If there is significant swelling, casting should be delayed. Older adult patients often have poor skin quality that tears and breaks down easily. They are at an increased risk for complications from a cast. Diabetics with neuropathy or patients with neuropathy for other reasons are also at increased risk for complications. They may not be able to feel whether there is a pressure point in the cast causing skin issues.

Absolute Contraindications

Open fractures and an active infection in area to be casted are absolute contraindications. If there is a wound from an open fracture, this area needs to be monitored for signs of infection. Also, there is typically more significant soft tissue injury in open fractures, which results in more severe swelling. If there is an active infection in the extremity to be casted, you would not want to place a cast, as you would then be unable to monitor the infection.

EQUIPMENT NEEDED

1. Gloves
2. Scissors
3. Basin with water (temperature will affect working time, lukewarm is best, cold if more working time is needed)
4. Tube dressing/stockinet
5. Cast padding
6. Rigid synthetic splinting material (fiberglass cast tape/orthoglass, or plaster)
7. Optional useful equipment: finger traps, foot casting stand
8. An extra set of hands. Although these casts can be applied by one solo practitioner, it is much easier to have an assistant to help position the patient and hold him or her in the proper position.
9. Cast saw (you need to be able to remove the cast, if necessary, after application). This can also sometimes be necessary to modify the cast after you have applied it (i.e., cutting back an edge that is impeding motion of fingers or toes)

STEPS TO PERFORMING THE PROCEDURE

Short arm cast:

1. Gather necessary materials: gloves, scissors, stockinette, webril, casting material, foot holder, and water source. Apply gloves.
2. Position patient for procedure. Patient can be lying in a bed with elbow flexed to 90° or sitting in a chair with the arm on a table (Figure 27.1).

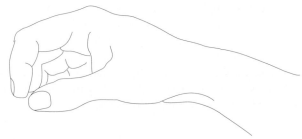

FIGURE 27.1. Arm positioning for casting. Reprinted with permission from Zuber, T. J., & Mayeaux, E. J. (2004). *Atlas of primary care procedures* (2nd ed.). Figure 66.3, Patricia Gast, Medical Illustrator. Lippincott Williams & Wilkins.

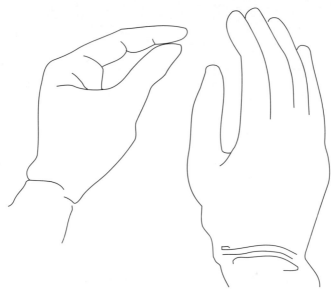

FIGURE 27.2. Forearm stockinette prior to casting material application. Reprinted with permission from Zuber, T. J., & Mayeaux, E. J. (2004). A*tlas of primary care procedures* (2nd ed.). Figure 67.4, Patricia Gast, Medical Illustrator. Lippincott Williams & Wilkins.

   a. If the patient is unable to maintain the proper position for casting, finger traps can he used to suspend the arm from an intravenous (IV) pole. If using this method, be sure to do step 3 (applying stockinette) prior to applying finger traps and hanging arm.

3. Measure stockinet to the appropriate size (Figure 27.2). Cut a hole for the thumb and place stockinet over the arm. Care should be taken to avoid any wrinkles as these can cause pressure ulcers on the skin. Stockinet should extend past the area your cast will be beginning and ending so you have room to fold it over and create a clean edge.

4. Wrap the area to be casted with webril cast padding. Be cautious not to pull this too tight because it can be constricting. Start distal and work proximal. Cover 50% of the previously covered area as you wrap. Make sure the webril layer is at least two to three layers thick. Apply extra padding at areas of bony prominence (radial styloid, metacarpal heads), as well as at edges of cast (Figure 27.3).

5. Moisten the casting material, using cold water to give yourself the longest working time.

6. Apply fiberglass roll, starting at the wrist to have an anchor point and then working up to hand and back proximal. Care should be taken around the thumb to make sure the thumb can move freely without rubbing in the cast. This can be achieved by cutting the extra cast material, creating arches around the thumb, by bending the fiberglass in half through the web space or by twisting the casting material. Apply the fiberglass tape in the same way that you did the webril, covering 50% of the material with your new layer as you come down the forearm. Two rolls of fiberglass tape are adequate to provide stabilization.

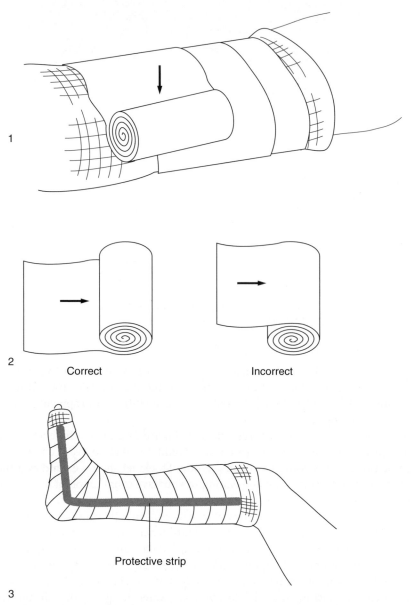

1

2   Correct   Incorrect

3

Protective strip

FIGURE 27.3. Steps to padding application prior to casting. Reprinted with permission from Zuber, T. J., & Mayeaux, E. J. (2004). *Atlas of primary care procedures* (2nd ed.). Figure 68.3a-c, Patricia Gast, Medical Illustrator. Lippincott Williams & Wilkins.

7. Once fiberglass is applied, mold the cast to fit and to stabilize the fracture. You want to give the cast an interosseous mold (essentially a slightly triangular shape) on the forearm. Unless instructed otherwise by the orthopedist, the wrist should be neutral, in approximately 20° of extension (Figure 27.4).
8. Wet your gloves with water and smooth all the layers over the cast.

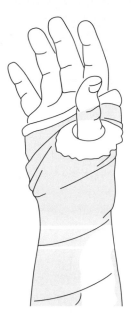

FIGURE 27.4. Wrist in neutral position. Reprinted with permission from Zuber, T. J., & Mayeaux, E. J. (2004). *Atlas of primary care procedures* (2nd ed.). Figure 67.8, Patricia Gast, Medical Illustrator. Lippincott Williams & Wilkins.

Short leg cast:

1. Gather necessary materials: gloves, scissors, stockinet, webril, casting material, foot holder, and water source.
    a. Select a tube dressing size that is appropriate for the patient's leg size; generally, a 3 to 4 inch works for an adult leg. Always err on the side of it being larger, because using a tube dressing that is too small can cause compression.
2. Position patient for casting (Figure 27.5).
    a. If able, the patient should sit at side of bed with knees bent to 90°.
    b. If casting stand available, have the patient place the ball of the foot on edge of stand, and position stand so that the ankle is in a neutral position (90° angle).
3. Place the tube dressing over the foot. The tube dressing should extend out further than the cast padding will go so that you have material left to fold over and created a padded edge (Figure 27.6). (For a short leg cast, the tube dressing should extend out past toes and up to the knee.)
4. Apply cast padding, starting distally at toes, and work your way proximal. Apply the padding using a technique in which you cover half of the previous laid padding with the next pass. Use a figure 8 technique around the ankle.
    a. Use extra care around bony prominences. Be sure to apply extra padding over the metatarsal heads, malleoli, and proximally.
    b. In general, if appropriate for the injury, end the cast 2 cm proximal to the fibular head to prevent compression of the peroneal nerve.

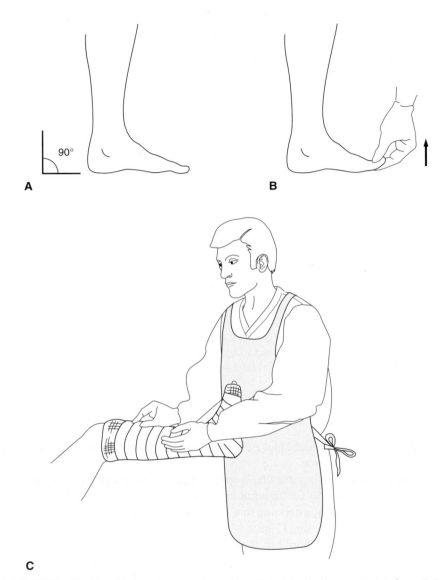

90°

A

B

C

FIGURE 27.5. Position for lower extremity casting. Reprinted with permission from Zuber, T. J., & Mayeaux, E. J. (2004). *Atlas of primary care procedures* (2nd ed.). Figure 67.8, Patricia Gast, Medical Illustrator. Lippincott Williams & Wilkins.

5. Wet your rigid splinting material and apply in the same manner as cast padding, starting distally and working proximally.
   a. 90° and neutral. Be sure not to pronate or supinate the foot.
6. After two layers of rigid material are applied, fold over the ends of your tube dressing and apply a final layer (Figure 27.7).
   a. If patient will be permitted weight bearing in the cast, be sure to add at least one additional layer to give the cast more strength.

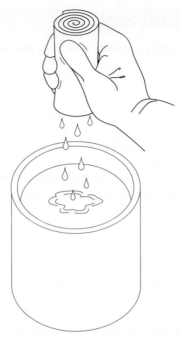

FIGURE 27.6. Place the plaster or fiberglass roll in lukewarm water and allow it to sit for a few seconds until the bubbling ceases. Reprinted with permission from Zuber, T. J., & Mayeaux, E. J. (2004). *Atlas of primary care procedures* (2nd ed.). Figure 68.4, Patricia Gast, Medical Illustrator. Lippincott Williams & Wilkins.

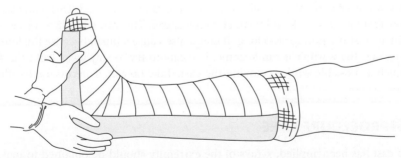

FIGURE 27.7. Full-leg cast. Reprinted with permission from Zuber, T. J., & Mayeaux, E. J. (2004). *Atlas of primary care procedures* (2nd ed.). Figure 68.6, Patricia Gast, Medical Illustrator. Lippincott Williams & Wilkins.

7. Wet your gloves and then smooth over the layers of rigid casting material. Gently mold the cast to the shape of the leg.
8. Allow cast to dry completely.
   a. Be sure to warn the patient that the cast material will slip on floors. If allowing weight bearing, give them a cast shoe if available.

COMPLICATIONS OF THE PROCEDURE

Complications can occur during application of cast, during cast wear, or during cast removal.

During Application

1. Casting materials harden by an exothermic reaction. Plaster creates more heat than fiberglass. If water was already warm, and now you have the additional heat as the material hardens, the patient could get burned. Water should be tepid, or even cold if a long working time is desired.
2. If you select the wrong size tube dressing, or pull the padding or cast material too tight, this could also result in a cast that is too tight, compressing the injured extremity. Any concern about tightness of the cast should be addressed immediately, because these problems can lead to compartment syndrome in the patient.

During Cast Wear

1. A cast that is too tight, because of either application error or the injury swelling can cause compartment syndrome. As stated previously, any complaints after applications, whether it be on the first day or weeks later, need to be addressed.
2. If water gets down into the cast, the cast padding holds this moisture against the skin. This can cause skin breakdown and/or infection. Patient's placing things inside the cast (i.e., a pencil to try to scratch an itch) can also cause lacerations that lead to infections.

During Cast Removal

1. A saw is used to break through a cast so that it can be removed. This is an oscillating saw that vibrates back and forth at a high speed. This can still cause a laceration if left against the skin for too long. It could also cause a burn, because the longer the cast saw, the warmer it can become. Use care to try to stay away from the skin as much as possible while removing the cast. Take breaks, if necessary, to allow the saw to cool.

POSTPROCEDURE CARE

After a cast has been applied, x-rays of the extremity should be obtained to make sure there is still satisfactory alignment and no loss of reduction of the fracture. In addition, the patient needs to be educated on how to care for the cast. The cast must remain dry and should be covered for showers/bathing. Nothing should be placed inside the cast. Patients also need to be made aware of concerning signs/symptoms of any potential complications. For example, they need to be made aware that they should seek emergent treatment should they have significant pain that is unrelieved by position change or medication. Color change in their toes/fingers is also something they should seek expert advice for immediately. Should water accidentally get inside the cast, or if the patient places something in it, a provider needs to be seen to have the cast changed.

BIBLIOGRAPHY

Dresing, K., Trafton, P., & Engelen, J. (2021). *Casting of lower limb for pediatric fracture*. Surgeryreference .aofoudnation.org. Retrieved April 1, 2021, from https://surgeryreference.aofoundation.org/further-reading/casting-of-lower-limb-for-pediatric-fractures?searchurl=%2fSearchResults#videos-from-casts-splints-and-support-bandages-nonoperative-treatment-and-perioperative-protection-

Monsell, F., & Sepulveda, D. (2016). *Short arm cast*. Surgeryreference.aofoundation.org. Retrieved April 1, 2021, from https://surgeryreference.aofoundation.org/orthopedic-trauma/pediatric-trauma/distal-forearm/basic-technique/short-arm-cast

Tank, J. (2014, March). *Closed reduction, traction, and casting techniques*. Ota.org. Retrieved April 1, 2021, from https://ota.org/sites/files/2018-06/G09-Closed%20Reduction%2C%20Traction%20and%20Casting%20Techniques.pdf

Casting Techniques (2019, March 19). *Casting techniques*. Retrieved from https://musculoskeletalkey.com/casting-techniques/

Dawn M. Specht

INDICATIONS FOR THE PROCEDURE

1. Allowing access to the venous system while avoiding access to the arterial system
2. Obtaining blood specimens
3. Gaining access for IV administration of medications and fluid

CONTRAINDICATIONS FOR THE PROCEDURE

Relative Contraindications

1. Accessing the venous system on the side of a mastectomy may result in lymphedema.
2. Accessing the venous system in the arm with a hemodialysis fistula or graft may damage the hemodialysis access device.
3. Accessing the vessels of the lower extremities may increase the risk of deep vein thrombosis. This is supported by expert opinion only.
4. Placing peripheral catheters in limbs with decreased sensation may increase risk because impaired sensation requires more frequent observation to protect the patient from unnoticed infiltration or extravasation.

Absolute Contraindications

1. Accessing a gangrene, burned or infected limb
2. Unnecessary request for IV catheter when therapy may be administered orally
3. Competent patient refuses procedure
4. Changing a catheter because it is "routine" or due despite its being functional without signs of complications. Cochrane systematic review by Webster et al. found no support for routine changing of peripheral IV catheters as a method to prevent phlebitis, infiltration, or infection.

EQUIPMENT NEEDED

For laboratory samples:

1. Handwashing supplies
2. Gloves

3. Skin disinfectant, common choices include alcohol, betadine, and chlorhexidine. Chlorhexadine preparation in alcohol is preferred because of 30-second dry time and no skin staining: 2% chlorhexidine in 70% alcohol. The Infusion Therapy Standards recommend use of a skin aseptic with a greater than 50% chlorhexidine solution. Note whether skin visibly soiled will also need soap and water.
4. Tourniquet (disposable, nonlatex)
5. Vacutainer
6. Vacutainer straight needle or attaching butterfly needle. Note well: Needle should be self-retracting or designed for use with a needless system.
7. Laboratory tubes, tube stopper colors vary based on diagnostic ordered.
8. Labels with two unique patient identifiers
9. Band-Aid or gauze for post access site care
10. Needle disposable box

For peripheral IV catheter placement:

1. Handwashing supplies
2. Gloves
3. Skin disinfectant (see above)
4. Tourniquet (disposable, nonlatex)
5. Two IV catheters, smallest gauge appropriate for therapy. For instance, a 20-gauge IV catheter will suffice for both blood and IV fluid administration.
6. Extension tubing
7. Saline flush
8. Clear adhesive dressing and catheter securing device
9. Needle (sharps) disposal box

For IV catheter placement and laboratory samples:

1. Handwashing supplies
2. Gloves
3. Skin disinfectant (see preceding discussion)
4. Tourniquet (disposable, nonlatex)
5. IV catheter smallest gauge appropriate for therapy. For instance, a 20 gauge IV catheter will suffice for both blood and IV fluid administration.
6. Vacutainer
7. Vacutainer needleless connector, also known as leur lock connector
8. Laboratory tubes, tube stopper colors vary based on diagnostic ordered.
9. Labels with two unique patient identifiers
10. Extension tubing
11. Saline flush
12. Clear adhesive dressing and catheter securing device
13. Needle (sharps) disposal box

Note: Some institutions have composed prepackaged kits that include gloves, skin antiseptic, tourniquets, tape, clear dressings. This IV start kit may vary at each institution (Figure 28.1).

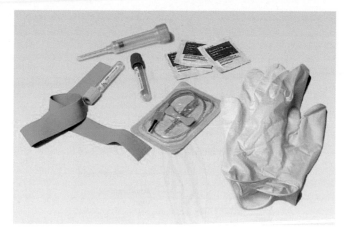

FIGURE 28.1. Some of the items needed to obtain a blood specimen are shown here (clockwise, from bottom left): tourniquet, Vacutainer (vacuum) blood tubes, safety syringe with needle, alcohol sponges, and gloves. Also shown is a butterfly needle pack with a needleless Vacutainer adaptor, used to puncture a Vacutainer blood tube. Also needed are 2 × 2 gauze squares and tape or a Band-Aid, identification stickers, and a red biohazard bag. A Vacutainer sleeve and/or needle system may also be used. (If the butterfly needle is used, the syringe and needle are not required.) Additional items are needed to initiate an IV infusion. Reprinted with permission from Rosdahl, C. B., & Kowalski, M. T. (2012) *Textbook of basic nursing* (10th ed.). Wolters-Kluwer. Photo © Keith Bunker Rosdahl.

STEPS TO PERFORMING THE PROCEDURE

1. Explain the purpose of the procedure to the patient as well as risks/benefits and obtain verbal consent to proceed.
2. Wash your hands with soap and water.
3. Dry hands and put on gloves.
4. Palpate veins. Note that when deciding on the venipuncture site the purpose of access will influence the site selection (Figure 28.2). Venipuncture for lab samples commonly occurs in the antecubital fossa at the median cubital vein. IV catheter placement avoids areas of flexion and typically should occur in the forearm at the median, basilica, or cephalic vein (Figure 28.3). These venous sites are most likely to last the full duration of the infusion therapy.
5. Apply tourniquet above area identified for puncture, usually halfway between the shoulder and elbow. Tourniquet time should be limited to less than 1 minute. If more time is required, release and reapply. Tighten to allow veins to fill but verify radial pulse remains.
6. Palpate through the skin for a spongy vessel that is without pulsation.
7. Disinfect selected site with antiseptic, allow to dry. Do not palpate after antiseptic application because this increases the risk of contamination, false blood culture results, and prolonged hospitalization.

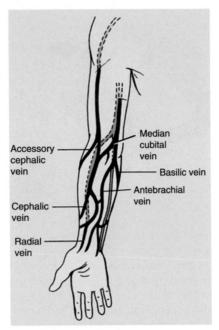

FIGURE 28.2. Common venipuncture sites. Reprinted with permission from Lippincott. (2018). *Lippincott's nursing procedures* (8th ed.). Wolters Kluwer.

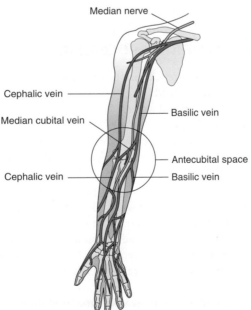

FIGURE 28.3. The antecubital space is the most common site for performing venipuncture because it contains several large veins that are easy to find in most people. The median cubital, cephalic, and basilic veins are all good veins to use for venipuncture. From Carter, P. (2019). *Lippincott acute care skills for advanced nursing assistant*. Wolters Kluwer.

8. Insert the device (needle or catheter) with the bevel side up at a 15° angle to the skin until a flash of blood is viewed. A flash will be visible in butterfly needle or IV catheters only. The Vacutainer straight needle will be inserted until a tug is followed by a decrease in resistance, then a tube is inserted in the Vacutainer body, and the vacuum in the tube will pull blood into the tube (Figures 28.4 and 28.5).

9. A. *Inserting IV and drawing blood*:

   Once the IV catheter has a flash, advance the plastic catheter, remove the tourniquet, retract the needle while occluding the insertion site, apply the extension tubing, and stabilize with clear dressing and tape. Hadaway notes the need to secure and dress and then draw samples. Apply leur adapter and Vacutainer to extension tubing with tourniquet reapplied to the arm. Insert lab tubes. The first tube is usually a blood culture; if not required, then a blue tube for the coagulation studies is first. It will self-fill to the appropriate level. When it stops filling, remove, rotate tube to mix additives in the tube, and place the next tube in the Vacutainer hub. Repeat until all tubes are filled.

   B. *Drawing blood via a butterfly needle*:

   Once the blood is visualized in the tubing, connect the leur adapter Vacutainer system to the end. The first tube is usually a blood culture; if not required, then a blue tube for the coagulation studies is first. It will self-fill to the appropriate level. When it stops filling remove, rotate tube to mix additives in the tube, and place the next tube in the Vacutainer hub until all tubes are filled.

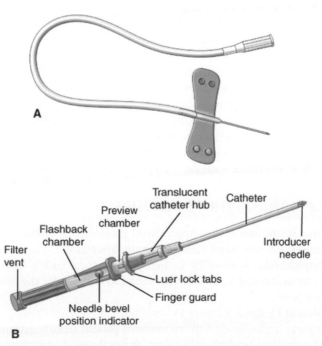

FIGURE 28.4. Examples of venipuncture devices. (A) Butterfly needle. (B) Over-the-needle catheter. Reprinted with permission from Timby, B. K., & Smith, M. E. (2017). *Introductory medical-surgical nursing* (12th ed.). Wolters Kluwer.

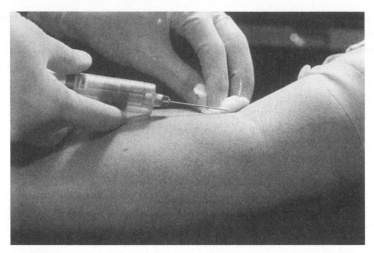

FIGURE 28.5. Venipuncture with a vacutainer straight needle. Reprinted with permission from Procop, G. W., & Koneman, E. W. (2016). *Koneman's color atlas and textbook of diagnostic microbiology* (7th ed.). Wolters-Kluwer.

    C. *Drawing blood via a straight needle:*
       The first tube is usually blue for the coagulation studies. It will self-fill to the appropriate level. When it stops filling, remove and rotate tube to mix additive, and place the next tube in the Vacutainer hub until all tubes are filled.
10. A. *After drawing blood with a straight needle or butterfly*:
       After the last tube has filled, remove the tourniquet, remove the needle, and apply direct pressure with gauze until bleeding has ceased. Apply Band-Aid or clean gauze with tape. Place needles in the needle disposal box. Label tubes at the bedside.
    B. *After drawing blood from IV catheter*:
       Remove the tourniquet, scrub the extension set hub with alcohol, and flush system with 0.9% normal saline until no blood is visible in the line. Make sure no fluid leaks from the catheter system or collects under the skin surrounding the insertion site. Date, time, and initial V site dressing and document in the medical record.

COMPLICATIONS OF THE PROCEDURE

1. **Hematoma formation at site:** Apply direct pressure to the site.
2. **Failed access:** Remove needle and reattempt procedure.
3. **Thrombophlebitis:** Remove IV catheter. Apply local care if circumferential extremity edema is noted. Consider ultrasound to evaluate for the presence of a deep vein thrombosis.
4. **Infiltration of IV fluid:** Remove IV catheter.
5. **Nerve injury:** Immediately remove needle if patient reports extreme pain, electrical shock sensation, tingling or burning, or numbness during the needle insertion. Hadaway identifies high-risk nerve injury sites as the dorsal hand, radial wrist, and volar wrist areas.

6. **Extravasation:** If a vesicant has infused, consider administration of an appropriate agent, e.g., dopamine extravasation may require regitidine administration prior to catheter removal.
7. **Bloodstream infection:** Remove device, culture blood, and administer appropriate antibiosis.
8. **Arterial access:** Remove catheter, then hold direct pressure for 10 minutes until bleeding has stopped, and apply a pressure dressing. Monitor frequently.

POSTPROCEDURE CARE

Postprocedure site assessment after blood draw will allow for the assessment of the puncture site. Document any noted hematoma and ensure the size is not expanding. IV catheters should be secured and have routine flushing with 0.9% normal saline solution to prevent occlusion. This requires an order in the electronic health record.

Note: The use of local anesthetics such as 1% lidocaine, EMLA cream, and LMX should be considered when difficult access is expected; however, the use is not routine and typically increases the procedure time by about 30 minutes.

BIBLIOGRAPHY

Aziz, A.-M. (2009). Improving peripheral IV cannula care: Implementing high-impact interventions. *British Journal of Nursing, 18*(20), 1242–1246. https://doi.org/10.12968/bjon.2009.18.20.45116

Centers for Disease Control (CDC). (2011). *Guidelines for the prevention of intravascular catheter-related infections.* https://www.cdc.gov/hai/pdfs/bsi-guidelines-2011.pdf

Frank, R. (2019). *Peripheral venous access in adults.* Retrieved from UptoDate.

Gorski, L. A. (2017). The 2016 infusion therapy standards of practice. *Home Healthcare Now, 35*(1), 10–18. https://doi.org/10.1097/nhh.0000000000000481.

Hadaway, L. (2019). *Infusion Therapy Standards 2016: Focusing on vascular access devices.* https://cdn.ymaws.com/www.avainfo.org/resource/resmgr/files/networks/avacny/Infusion_Therapy_Standards_2.pdf

Webster, J., Osborne, S., Rickard, C. M., & Marsh, N. (2019). Clinically-indicated replacement versus routine replacement of peripheral venous catheters. *Cochrane Database of Systematic Reviews, 1*(1), CD007798. https://doi.org/10.1002/14651858.CD007798.pub5

World Health Organization (WHO). (2010). *WHO guidelines on drawing blood: Best practices in phlebotomy.* https://www.ncbi.nlm.nih.gov/books/NBK138665/

Dawn M. Specht

INDICATIONS FOR THE PROCEDURE

A femoral venipuncture is an uncommon procedure, as the addition of ultrasound technology and line placement may precede the need for specimens. However, in life-threatening situations, where time is of the essence and laboratory specimens are of utmost importance to the differential diagnoses, the procedure will occur. The femoral venipuncture is performed to obtain specimens for laboratory analysis that cannot be obtained via peripheral venipuncture.

The femoral area is easily accessed during cardiopulmonary resuscitation. The femoral triangle refers to an area in the groin that is produced by the inguinal ligament superiorly and bordered on either side by the sartorius and adductor longus muscles (Figure 29.1). The components from the outer to the inner aspect are the femoral nerve, femoral artery, femoral vein, and lymphatics. Using the pneumonic NAVY will assist in locating the vein. Palpation of the femoral artery pulsation indicates that the outer side toward the femur contains the nerve and the inner side toward the perineum contains the vein (Figure 29.2). The anatomic location of the venipuncture, below the waist, may increase the risk of infection, so care must be taken to provide as clean an area as possible.

Indications for the procedure are:

1. Obtain venous specimens during an emergency situation when no other avenue for collection is available.
2. Obtain a venous specimen when all other avenues have failed.

CONTRAINDICATIONS FOR THE PROCEDURE

Relative Contraindications

1. Coagulopathy may increase the risk of bleeding after venipuncture; however, this may be followed by direct pressure at the site for 5 to 10 minutes to prevent active bleeding.
2. Absence of femoral artery pulsation may make it difficult to locate the femoral vein, which lies medial to the femoral artery; however, utilizing the midinguinal point halfway between the anterior superior iliac spine and the pubic tubercle provides a reference point for locating the vein.

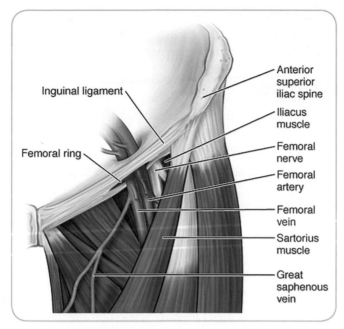

FIGURE 29.1. Femoral triangle. The triangle is bounded by the inguinal ligament superiorly, the adductor longus medially, and the sartorius laterally. The femoral artery, vein, and nerve pass through this area to enter the thigh. Reprinted with permission from Anderson, M. K. (2016). *Foundations of athletic training* (6th ed.). Wolters-Kluwer.

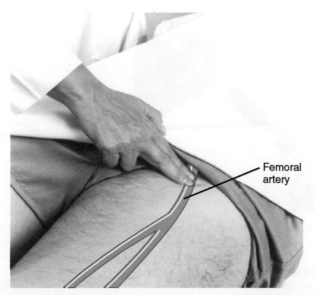

FIGURE 29.2. Palpation of the femoral artery. Reprinted with permission from Jones, R. M., & Rospond, R. M. (2009). *Patient assessment in pharmacy practice* (2nd ed.). Wolters-Kluwer.

Absolute Contraindications

1. Femoral vein thrombosis on side of access
2. Alternate peripheral site is available for specimen

EQUIPMENT NEEDED

The advanced practice provider should gather equipment prior to the procedure. Some clinical sites may have kits available, whereas others will require the manual gathering of equipment. The following equipment is needed:

1. Chlorhexidine prep stick or betadine and gauze (chlorhexidine preferred)
2. Drape
3. Vacutainer with 19-gauge needle or a large syringe (30cc) with an 18-gauge needle and a vacutainer transfer device for syringe attachment after needle removal (Figure 29.3)
4. Laboratory tubes (Figure 29.4)
5. Labels for tubes
6. Laboratory tube bag
7. Personal protective equipment: gown, gloves, and eye shield
8. Gauzes: 2 × 2 or 4 × 4, for direct pressure application after blood draw
9. Band Aid or dressing for puncture site

STEPS TO PERFORMING THE PROCEDURE

1. Check laboratory studies for coagulopathy if available.
2. Obtain verbal consent in nonemergency situations.

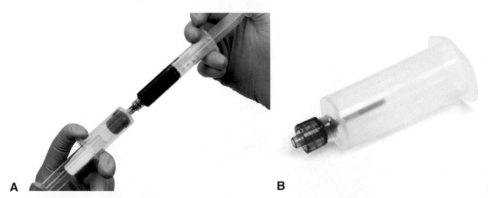

A   **B**

FIGURE 29.3. (A) Vacutainer with 19-gauge needle or a large syringe (30cc) with an 18-gauge needle and a vacutainer transfer device for syringe attachment after needle removal. From Becton, Dickinson and Company, 2021. (B) BD Vacutainer® Luer-Lok™ access device provides the security of a threading locking luer connection, replacing the need for a luer slip device. It can be used for accessing blood or urine directly from catheters or Foley ports. Courtesy and © Becton, Dickinson and Company.

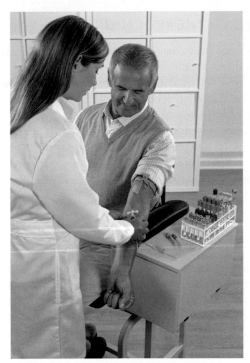

FIGURE 29.4. BD Vacutainer® blood collection tubes. Courtesy and © Becton, Dickinson and Company.

3. Gather supplies, consider having extra needles and laboratory tubes.
4. Explain procedure to the patient.
5. Position the patient supine with the inguinal area exposed. The target side may require abducting and rotating the leg 15° to open the femoral triangle.
6. Palpate the area to identify femoral arterial pulsation; remember to puncture medially from the pulsation. Pal states femoral venous access site is located 1 cm below the inguinal ligament and 0.5 to 1 cm medial to the femoral arterial pulsation.
7. Don personal protective equipment (sterility is preferred).
8. Drape the inguinal area.
9. Cleanse the insertion site with a chlorhexidine preparation stick for at least 30 seconds. If betadine is utilized, paint the area and allow to dry before proceeding.
10. Puncture the femoral vein with a syringe and needle or a vacutainer system with needle, needle bevel up on a 20 to 30° angle aimed toward the head of the patient. If a syringe is utilized, maintain a small amount of negative suction by elevating the plunger of the syringe. As the vein is punctured, a flash of dark venous blood will return. If a vacutainer is utilized, a laboratory tube will need to be inserted after vessel puncture to create suction and will fill with dark venous blood. Stabilize the vacutainer system as tubes are changed until all necessary tubes are obtained.
11. Remove the needle and hold direct pressure for at least 3 minutes.

COMPLICATIONS OF THE PROCEDURE

1. **Failed venous access:** Reevaluate need and retry if benefit outweighs risk.
2. **Bleeding:** Apply direct pressure.
3. **Infection:** Best prevented by sterile procedure, but culture, then treat for organism
4. **Arterial puncture:** If arterial blood is sampled, hold pressure for 5 to 10 minutes at the site (samples can still be sent to the laboratory).
5. **Femoral hematoma, potential arteriovenous fistula formation:** These are most common with femoral line placement but can occur in low groin punctures. Ultrasound the groin to determine fistula or pseudoaneurysm presence; consult surgery.
6. **Deep vein thrombosis:** Doppler ultrasound if newly developed edema on the side of the puncture

POSTPROCEDURE CARE

The advanced practice provider must document the procedure in the electronic health record. Document the patient's response to the procedure as well as the puncture site and distal circulation assessment postprocedure. The results of the laboratory studies should be given to the provider. Place follow-up assessment orders of the extremity that includes circulation and motor assessment in addition to groin checks for the general nursing care.

BIBLIOGRAPHY

Androes, M., & Heffner, A. (2018). *Placement of femoral venous catheters: General preparation.* https://www.uptodate.com/contents/placement-of-femoral-venous-catheters?search=femoral%20venipuncture&source=search_result&selectedTitle=1~150&usage_type=default&display_rank=1

Pal, N. (2018). *Femoral central venous access technique.* https://emedicine.medscape.com/article/80279-technique

30 Arterial Blood Gas

Janice K. Delgiorno

INDICATIONS FOR THE PROCEDURE

An arterial blood gas (ABG) is one of the most common tests ordered/performed in the critical care setting. An ABG measures gases in the arteries, specifically oxygen and carbon dioxide. An ABG requires blood to be drawn from an artery (usually the radial, but sometimes the femoral or brachial). The blood can also be drawn from an arterial catheter, frequently placed in critical care for close hemodynamic supervision and frequent sampling. An ABG will measure the pH of the blood, the bicarbonate level, and the partial pressure of oxygen and carbon dioxide. Some blood gas analyzers can also measure carboxyhemoglobin, methemoglobin, and hemoglobin.

Indications for the procedure are:

1. Acute or chronic respiratory failure
2. Patients on mechanical ventilation to assess effectiveness of ventilator settings
3. To assess carboxyhemoglobin toxicity
4. Patients with a serious illness that can affect acid/base status such as trauma, burns, sepsis, renal failure, diabetic ketoacidosis, and multisystem organ failure
5. To assess the need for oxygen in patients with chronic obstructive pulmonary disease

CONTRAINDICATIONS FOR THE PROCEDURE

Relative Contraindications

The need for the arterial puncture should be assessed for the patient with increased risk of bleeding. If arterial puncture is needed, pressure will need to be held on the puncture site after the puncture is completed. Relative contraindications are:

1. Severe coagulopathy
2. Use of thrombolytics
3. Local infection at the intended puncture site: an alternative puncture site should be selected.

Absolute Contraindications

No absolute contraindications exist; however, a sampling site may be deemed inappropriate owing to lack of collateral flow, peripheral vascular disease, or Raynaud syndrome. In cases of contraindication of the radial site, consider brachial or femoral sites with the use of ultrasound.

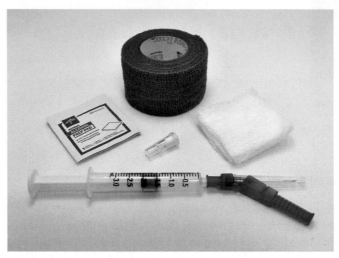

FIGURE 30.1. Sample arterial blood gas kit. Reprinted with permission from Carter, P. (2020). *Lippincott essentials for nursing assistants* (5th ed.). Wolters Kluwer.

EQUIPMENT NEEDED

1. 22-gauge needle with cap
2. 2 to 3 mL heparinized syringe
3. Specimen bag (with ice depending on institutional protocol)
4. Patient label for the specimen
5. Chlorhexidine or alcohol wipe
6. Personal protective equipment (gloves, mask/face shield if indicated)
7. 2 × 2 gauze for holding pressure post procedure
8. Sharps container

Note: many institutions have ABG kits that contain the needle and syringe (Figure 30.1).

STEPS TO PERFORMING THE PROCEDURE

1. Perform the Standard Steps in the Preface.
2. Explain the procedure to the patient.
3. Gather the equipment.
4. Determine the intended puncture site and position the patient appropriately. If you are performing a radial artery puncture, hyperextend the wrist approximately 30° to 40°. You can place a small roll (washcloth, gauze, etc.) under the wrist to assist with positioning (Figure 30.2).
5. If you are performing a radial artery puncture, perform a modified Allen test to assess for collateral circulation. This ensures that there will still be blood supply to the hand should the ABG cause a blockage in the radial artery (Figure 30.3).

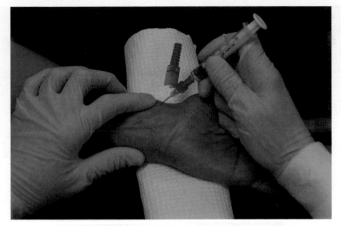

FIGURE 30.2. Arterial puncture technique. Note that the wrist is supported on a small roll. Reprinted with permission from Lippincott. (2018). *Lippincott's nursing procedures* (8th ed.). Wolters Kluwer.

In the conscious, cooperative patient:
- Compress both ulnar and radial arteries at the wrist to obliterate pulses.
- Have patient clench and release a fist until blanching of the hand occurs.
- With radial artery still compressed, release pressure on ulnar artery.

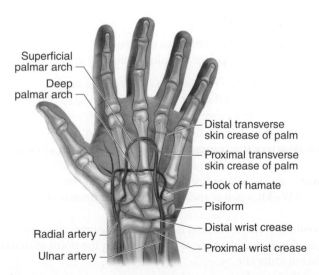

FIGURE 30.3. Arterial flow, underlying bony structures, and anatomic structures of the hand. Left hand supinated position. Blood supply to the hand provided by radial and ulnar artery. Reprinted with permission from Freer, J. (2016). *Washington manual of bedside procedures*. Wolters Kluwer Health and Pharma.

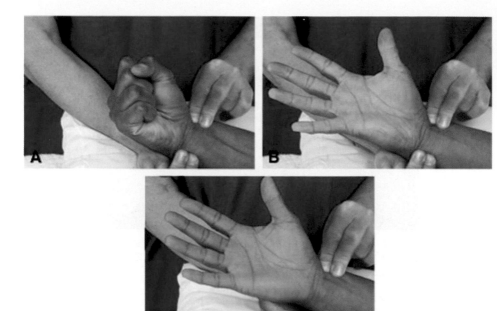

FIGURE 30.4. Performing Allen test. (A) Compressing the arteries with the patient's fist closed. (B) Maintaining compression as patient unclenches fist. (C) Compressing only the radial artery. Collateral flow is indicated by normal flow returning to the hand. Reprinted with permission from Lynn, P. (2014). *Taylor's handbook of clinical nursing skills* (2nd ed). Lippincott Williams & Wilkins.

- Watch for normal color to return to the hand.
- Always document the presence of ulnar collateral flow (Figure 30.4).

In the unconscious patient or patient unable to cooperate:
- Compress both ulnar and radial arteries at the wrist to obliterate pulses.
- Elevate patient's hand above level of their heart.
- Lower patient's hand below the level of their heart.
- With radial artery still compressed, release pressure on ulnar artery.
- Note: If normal color fails to appear, collateral circulation may be assumed to be inadequate, and an alternative puncture site should be chosen.

6. If using an ABG kit, open it and remove preheparinized syringe, needles, and syringe cap.
7. Attach needle to syringe, keeping needle in sterile protective cap.
8. Palpate the chosen radial artery as before, noting the point of maximal pulse. This will be the puncture site.
9. Clean the puncture site.
10. Remove the needle cap, and, at a 35° to 40° angle with bevel in upward position, pierce the skin at the puncture site and slowly advance the needle. Once the artery is punctured, blood will enter the syringe. If the needle goes through the artery, slowly withdraw the needle until blood again appears in the syringe (Figure 30.5).

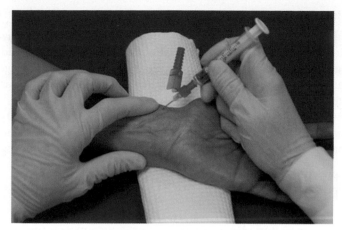

FIGURE 30.5. Blood for arterial blood gas analysis is usually drawn from the radial artery in the wrist. Reprinted with permission from Lippincott. (2018). *Lippincott's nursing procedures* (8th ed.). Wolters Kluwer.

11. After enough blood has been obtained for testing, withdraw the needle and immediately apply pressure directly on the puncture site with sterile gauze.
12. Do not recap the needle. Place the needle in the rubber square or close shield before needle removal.
13. Remove air from the syringe and cap with the black cap.
14. Label the syringe and place in a bag of ice.
15. Make sure the order contains the patient's temperature and any current oxygen settings.
16. Dispose of waste and sharps into appropriate receptacles.

COMPLICATIONS OF THE PROCEDURE

- Local hematoma
- Arterial vasospasm
- Arterial occlusion
- Air or thrombus embolism
- Local anesthetic anaphylactic reaction
- Infection at the puncture site
- Needle stick injury to healthcare personnel
- Vessel laceration
- Vasovagal response
- Hemorrhage
- Local pain

POSTPROCEDURE CARE

After the procedure, continue to monitor the site for bleeding and/or hematoma formation. If needed, apply additional pressure to the puncture site.

Test Results

Results are usually available within 5 to 15 minutes. Aberrant results may result from contamination with room air, resulting in abnormally low carbon dioxide and near-normal oxygen levels. Delays in analysis of the blood tube allow for ongoing cellular respiration and may lead to errors with inaccurately low oxygen and high carbon dioxide levels reported in the results.

The ABG sample may be used to determine more than pH, PCO_2, PO_2, and HCO_3, depending on the analyzer and testing ordered; e.g., electrolytes, lactate, and carboxyhemoglobin may be analyzed. Normal values at sea level include the following:

- Partial pressure of oxygen (PaO_2)—75 to 100 mmHg
- Partial pressure of carbon dioxide ($PaCO_2$)—35 to 45 mmHg

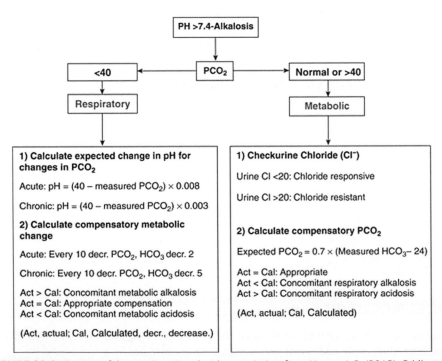

FIGURE 30.6. Review of the pH. Reprinted with permission from Yunen, J. R. (2012). *5-Minute ICU consult*. Wolters Kluwer.

- Arterial blood pH—7.35 to 7.45
- Oxygen saturation (SaO_2)—94% to 100%
- Bicarbonate (HCO_3^-)—22 to 26 mEq/L

A quick interpretation of the ABG begins with a review of the pH (Figure 30.6). If it is less than 7.35, acidosis is indicated. Acidosis may be caused by too much carbon dioxide (CO_2) or too little buffer bicarbonate (HCO_3). If the pH is greater than 7.45, alkalosis is indicated. Alkalosis may be caused by too little CO_2 or too much HCO_3.

BIBLIOGRAPHY

Kaufman, D. (2021). *Interpretation of arterial blood gases (ABG's)*. https://www.thoracic.org/professionals/clinical-resources/critical-care/clinical-education/abgs.php

Medistudent. (2018). *OSCE skills: Arterial blood gas.* Retrieved November 2, 2020, from https://www.medistudents.com/en/learning/osce-skills/cardiovascular/arterial-blood-gases/

Theodore, A. (2020). *Arterial blood gas.* https://www.uptodate.com/contents/arterial-blood-gases

CHAPTER

31 12-Lead Electrocardiogram Interpretation

Joshua Thornsberry

INDICATIONS FOR THE PROCEDURE

The 12-lead electrocardiogram (ECG) is the most commonly performed cardiovascular diagnostic procedure in clinical practice. It remains an essential tool for expeditious recognition of acute coronary syndromes, malignant dysrhythmias, and conduction system disorders. Accurate interpretation can provide diagnostic information for structural, functional, and electrical cardiac abnormalities, cardiotoxicities, and electrolyte imbalances. Findings from a 12-lead ECG may also support the diagnosis of acute pericarditis, pericardial effusion, acute pulmonary embolism, and other systemic pathologies. Interval analysis of a 12-lead ECG is imperative for monitoring specific pharmacotherapies as well as assessment of implanted cardiac device function.

Indications for the procedure are:

1. new or worsening chest discomfort (i.e., pain, pressure, or tightness)
2. epigastric discomfort
3. heartburn dyspnea
4. palpitations
5. syncope
6. stroke
7. cardiac arrest
8. A patient's clinical condition may change rapidly and a repeat 12-lead ECG may be indicated to rule out life-threatening etiology.
9. A patient's clinical condition may also improve, and obtaining a repeat 12-lead ECG to document resolution of previously seen abnormalities is essential for future 12-lead ECG comparisons.
10. Ultimately, a 12-lead ECG should be obtained anytime there is clinical uncertainty.

CONTRAINDICATIONS FOR THE PROCEDURE

Relative Contraindications

1. During advanced cardiovascular life support (ACLS), 12-lead ECG analysis should be deferred until return of spontaneous circulation (ROSC) to minimize interruption in high-quality cardiopulmonary resuscitation (CPR).

213

2. Sensitivity and irritation secondary to hair removal and abrasive skin preparation, for optimal electrode-to-skin contact, are self-limiting and not considered contraindications for performing a 12-lead ECG. The adhesive backing of some electrodes may also cause skin irritation; however, many manufacturers offer hypoallergenic alternatives.

Absolute Contraindications

There are no absolute contraindications to performing a resting 12-lead ECG if the patient is agreeable.

EQUIPMENT NEEDED

1. 12-lead ECG machine with acquisition module (i.e., lead wires)
2. 12-lead ECG paper
3. Disposable skin electrodes
4. Hair removal tools and skin preparation agents

INITIAL REVIEW OF THE 12-LEAD ELECTROCARDIOGRAM

The following information is presented for the Advanced Practice Nurse to guide interpretation procedures. The 12-lead may be obtained by assistive personnel; however, the clinician will perform the interpretation. After obtaining a 12-lead ECG, manual interpretation is preferred, because limitations to computer-generated analysis exist. To ensure thorough and accurate interpretation, a systematic analysis is recommended and should include a comprehensive review of rate, rhythm, axis, waves, intervals, and segments. Analysis should also include comparison with a prior (baseline) 12-lead ECG, if available, to determine the acuity of findings. It should be noted that a normal 12-lead ECG does not exclude the possibility of underlying heart disease or clinical pathology.

STEPWISE APPROACH TO 12-LEAD ELECTROCARDIOGRAM INTERPRETATION

1. Identify the baseline rhythm.
2. Evaluate the p-wave.
   a. Present or absent
   b. Upright, flattened, or inverted
   c. Monophasic or biphasic
3. Evaluate the t-waves.
   a. Upright or inverted
   b. Peaked
4. Evaluate the axis (Lead AVF and Lead I).
   a. Both upright = good axis
   b. Both inverted = severe right axis deviation
   c. Lead I upright and Lead AVF inverted = left axis deviation
   d. Lead I inverted and Lead AVF upright = right axis deviation

5. Evaluate R-wave progression.
   a. Constant progression should be seen from V1 to V4.
6. Evaluate for the presence or absence of Q-waves.

COMMON 12-LEAD ELECTROCARDIOGRAM FINDINGS AND THEIR CLINICAL SIGNIFICANCE

Axis Deviation

Axis refers to the overall direction of electricity through the heart and is a representation of the average of all ventricular depolarization (from the atrioventricular node through the left and right ventricles). In general, axis, in the frontal plane, is determined from the dominant deflection of the QRS complexes in leads I and aVF (Table 31.1). Normal axis is measured between −30° and 90° and represents a downward and leftward movement of depolarization. Axis measured beyond −30° and 90° is considered deviated and is termed left axis deviation (LAD), right axis deviation (RAD), or extreme axis deviation (Figure 31.1). Determining axis remains an important part of overall 12-lead ECG interpretation, as a shift from normal axis may represent new or worsening pathology (Table 31.2).

Atrial Enlargement

Left atrial enlargement (LAE), right atrial enlargement (RAE), and interatrial block occur primarily from atrial dilatation, hypertrophy, scar, or conduction delay and may cause abnormalities in P-wave morphology, duration, or amplitude. Although a 12-lead ECG may suggest atrial abnormality, findings are best correlated with echocardiography. The P-waves in leads II and V1 are used primarily for assessing the possibility of atrial abnormality (Figure 31.2).

Ventricular Hypertrophy

Left ventricular hypertrophy (LVH) is an increase in left ventricular muscle mass and occurs primarily from long-standing uncontrolled hypertension or high-grade aortic valve stenosis; however, LVH may also occur secondary to sustained mitral or aortic regurgitation as well as dilated and hypertrophic cardiomyopathies. As conduction occurs through the thickened left ventricle, the QRS complex amplitude is increased (Figure 31.3). A similar 12-lead ECG pattern may exist in young patients with thin chests with no LVH and is considered nonpathological. Other 12-lead ECG findings may also accompany

TABLE 31.1 Degrees of Axis

Axis	Lead I	Lead aVF
Normal axis (between −30° and 90°)	+	+
Left axis deviation (between −30° and −90°)	+	-
Right axis deviation (between 90° and 180°)	−	+
Extreme axis deviation (between 180° and −90°)	−	−

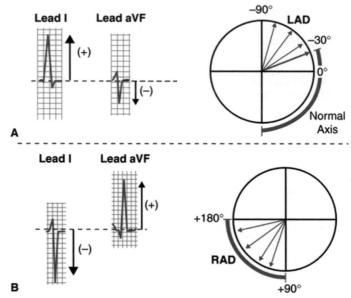

FIGURE 31.1. Axis deviations. Panel A includes QRS complexes from lead I (positive) and lead aVF (negative). The overlapping quadrant, therefore, is between 0° and −90°. The range of normal mean electrical axis extends from +90° to −30° (shown in panel A). If the vector lies between −30° and −90°, however, it represents a left-axis deviation (LAD). Panel B includes QRS complexes from lead I (negative) and lead aVF (positive). The overlapping quadrant, therefore, is between 90° and 180°, and represents a right-axis deviation (RAD). Reprinted with permission from Courneya, C., Parker, M. J., & Schwartzstein, R. M. (2010). *Cardiovascular physiology*. Wolters Kluwer.

TABLE 31.2 Common Causes of Left, Right, and Extreme Axis Deviation

Left Axis Deviation (Between −30° and −90°)	Right Axis Deviation (Between 90° and 180°)	Extreme Axis Deviation (Between 180° and −90°)
• Normal variant • Horizontal heart • Left anterior fascicular block • Left bundle branch block • Left ventricular hypertrophy • Mechanical shifts in the thorax • Inferior wall infarction • Chronic lung disease • Hyperkalemia • Wolff–Parkinson–White syndrome with right-sided accessory pathway • Congenital heart defects	• Normal variant • Vertical heart • Right posterior fascicular block • Right bundle branch block • Right ventricular hypertrophy • Mechanical shifts in the thorax • Dextrocardia • Lateral wall infarction • Chronic lung disease • Pulmonary embolism • Wolff–Parkinson–White syndrome with left-sided accessory pathway • Congenital heart defects	• Improper lead placement • Hyperkalemia • Paced rhythms • Ventricular dysrhythmias

	Lead II	Lead V$_1$
Normal	RA - - -⌒- - - - LA - - -⌒- - - - Combined ⌒	- - -⌒- - - - - - -⌣- - - - ⌒⌣
RA enlargement (P height > 2.5 mm in lead II)	RA ⌒ LA	RA ⌒⌣ LA
LA enlargement (Negative P in V$_1$ >1 mm wide and >1 mm deep)	RA ⌒ LA	RA ⌣ LA

FIGURE 31.2. The P wave represents superimposition of right atrial (RA) and left atrial (LA) depolarization. RA depolarization occurs slightly earlier than LA depolarization, because of the proximity of the RA to the sinoatrial node. In RA enlargement, the initial component of the P wave is prominent (>2.5 mm tall) in lead II. In LA enlargement, there is a large terminal downward deflection in lead V1 (>1 mm wide and >1 mm deep). Reprinted with permission from Lilly, L. S. (2020). *Pathophysiology of heart disease* (7th ed.). Wolters Kluwer.

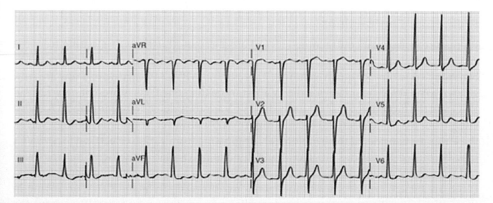

FIGURE 31.3. Left ventricular hypertrophy with deep S waves in V1–V2 and large voltage R waves in V4–V6. ST depression and T-wave inversion (strain pattern) are seen in V4–V6. Reprinted with permission from Woods, S. L., Froelicher, E. S., Motzer, S. A., & Bridges, E. J. (2010). *Cardiac nursing* (6th ed.). Wolters Kluwer.

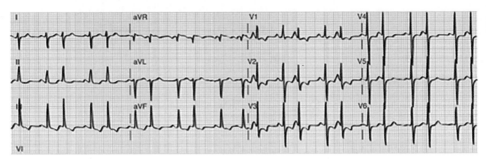

FIGURE 31.4. Right ventricular hypertrophy (RVH) in a patient with primary pulmonary hypertension. Note RAD of +120° with large R waves in V1–V3 and ST–T wave changes of RV strain. This ECG displays five of the criteria for RVH. Reprinted with permission from Woods, S. L., Froelicher, E. S., Motzer, S. A., & Bridges, E. J. (2010). *Cardiac nursing* (6th ed.). Wolters Kluwer.

LVH, such as LAE, LAD, ST-segment depression, and T-wave inversion. LVH is best confirmed by echocardiography; however, LVH is suggested when the following 12-lead ECG criteria are met:

- **Cornell voltage criteria**: Amplitude of R-wave in aVL + S-wave in V3 greater than 28 mm (male) or greater than 20 mm (female)
- **Sokolow-Lyon criteria**: Amplitude of S-wave in V1 + R-wave in V5 or V6 greater than or equal to 35 mm

Right ventricular hypertrophy (RVH) is an increase in right ventricular muscle mass and occurs primarily from pulmonary hypertension or pulmonic valve stenosis. As conduction occurs through the thickened right ventricle, R-wave amplitude in V1 and V2 is increased and S-wave amplitude is deepened in V5 and V6 (Figure 31.4). Other 12-lead ECG findings may also accompany RVH, such as RAE, RAD, ST-segment depression, and T-wave inversion. RVH is best confirmed by echocardiography.

Premature Contractions

Premature ventricular contractions (PVCs) are aberrant heartbeats originating from the ventricles and may occur randomly (isolated), in pairs (couplets), or in a pattern (i.e., bigeminy, trigeminy, or quadrigeminy). Three or more PVCs occurring in a row are considered to be ventricular tachycardia (VT). If more than one PVC is present on a 12-lead ECG and the morphology is the same, the PVCs are considered to be monofocal (originating from the same electrical focus) (Figure 31.5); however, if the morphology varies, the PVCs are considered to be multifocal (originating from various electrical foci). PVCs may be caused by various structural and functional cardiac pathologies but may also occur in a structurally normal heart and otherwise healthy patient. In general, isolated PVCs are benign and occur without symptoms; however, frequent PVCs, occurring in the setting of cardiomyopathy or bradycardia, may produce symptoms. PVCs have the following 12-lead ECG features:

- Widened QRS complex with duration greater than 120 ms

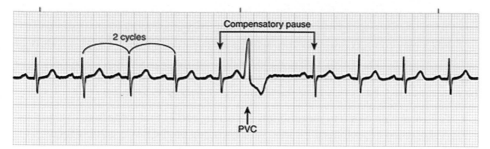

FIGURE 31.5. Normal sinus rhythm with one premature ventricular contraction (PVC). Rhythm: basic rhythm regular; irregular with PVC Rate: basic rhythm rate 88 bpm P waves: sinus with basic rhythm PR interval: 0.18 to 0.20 second QRS complex: 0.06 to 0.08 second (basic rhythm). 0.12 second (PVC) Comment: the interval from the beat preceding the PVC to the beat following the PVC is equal to two cardiac cycles and represents a full compensatory pause. Reprinted with permission from Huff, J. (2016). *ECG workout* (7th ed.). Wolters Kluwer.

- Aberrant QRS morphology
- T-wave is discordant (opposite) to the main QRS deflection
- A compensatory pause follows the QRS complex (exactly twice the R–R interval)

Premature atrial contractions (PACs) occur when there is early depolarization of the atria from an ectopic focus outside the sinoatrial node. They may occur randomly (isolated), in pairs (couplets), or in a pattern (i.e., bigeminy, trigeminy, or quadrigeminy) (Figure 31.6). Three or more PACs occurring in a row are considered paroxysmal atrial tachycardia (PAT). PACs may occur in a structurally normal heart but may also occur in the setting of acute coronary syndrome (ACS), cardiomyopathy, valvular heart disease,

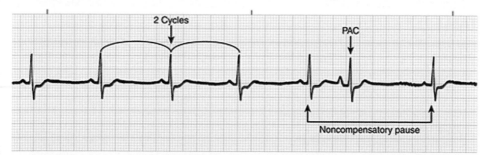

FIGURE 31.6. Normal sinus rhythm premature atrial contraction (PAC). Rhythm: basic rhythm regular; irregular with PAC Rate: basic rhythm rate 60 bpm P waves: sinus P waves with basic rhythm; premature, abnormal P wave with PAC PR interval: 0.12 to 0.16 second (basic rhythm); 0.16 second (PAC) QRS complex: 0.08 second (basic rhythm and PAC) Comment: to determine the type of pause following premature beats, measure from the QRS preceding the premature beat to the QRS following the premature beat. If the measurement equals two R–R intervals, the pause is compensatory. If the measurement is less than two R–R intervals, the pause is noncompensatory. ST segment depression is present. Reprinted with permission from Huff, J. (2016). *ECG workout* (7th ed.). Wolters Kluwer.

chronic lung disease, or other conditions that increase atrial pressure. In general, isolated PACs are benign and typically occur without symptoms or hemodynamic insult.

PACs may conduct normally through the atrioventricular node and down through the bundle branches, or they may conduct with aberration (right bundle branch block [RBBB] or left bundle branch block [LBBB]). If no QRS follows a PAC, it is considered to be nonconducted. PACs may have the following 12-lead ECG features:

- A P-wave with different morphology occurring earlier than expected
- A shortened or prolonged PR interval depending on the PAC's ectopic focus
- A conducted PAC may have a normal QRS complex or an aberrant QRS complex.
- A nonconducted PAC will have an absent QRS complex.
- A noncompensatory pause follows a PAC (less than twice the R–R interval).

BUNDLE BRANCH AND FASCICULAR BLOCKS

In a normal heart, the bundle of His divides into the right and left bundle branches. The left bundle branch is comprised of the left anterior and left posterior fascicles. Bundle branch and fascicular blocks manifest on a 12-lead ECG when there is an interruption in normal electrical flow down the His-Purkinje system. This delay in conduction (>100 ms) lengthens ventricular myocardial depolarization and will produce a widened QRS complex and axis deviation (in the direction of the block). A bundle branch block may be classified as incomplete (QRS complex duration > 100 ms but < 120 ms) or complete (QRS complex duration > 120 ms). Blocks may occur in a structurally normal heart; however, there are multiple etiologies to consider when evaluating a new bundle branch or fascicular block (Table 31.3).

TABLE 31.3 Common Causes of Bundle Branch and Fascicular Blocks

Right Bundle Branch Block	Left Bundle Branch Block	Left Anterior Fascicular Block	Left Posterior Fascicular Block
• Normal variant	• Myocardial ischemia, infarction or inflammation	• Myocardial ischemia, infarction or inflammation	• Myocardial ischemia, infarction or inflammation
• Myocardial ischemia, infarction or inflammation	• Cardiomyopathy	• Cardiomyopathy	• Cardiomyopathy
• Cardiomyopathy	• Valvular heart disease	• Valvular heart disease	• Hypertension
• Valvular heart disease	• Hypertension	• Congenital heart disease	• Hyperkalemia
• Hypertension		• Hypertension	• Acute cor pulmonale
• Congenital heart disease		• Sclerodegenerative disorders	• Degenerative conduction disorders
• Pulmonary emboli			
• Right ventricular hypertrophy			
• Pulmonary hypertension			
• Degenerative conduction disorders			
• Iatrogenic			

RBBB is present on a 12-lead ECG when the QRS complex in the precordial leads is greater than 120 ms, there is an RSR' (R prime) pattern in leads V1 and V2, there is a qRS or RS pattern in leads V5 or V6, and there is either normal axis or RAD present (Figure 31.7).

LBBB is present on a 12-lead ECG when the QRS complex in the precordial leads is greater than120 ms, there is a broad notched or slurred R-wave in leads V5 and V6, there is a widened QS in lead V1, and there is either normal axis or LAD present (Figure 31.8). It should be noted that the widened QRS complex and ST-segment changes associated with LBBB make interpretation of acute myocardial infarction difficult; therefore, any patient presenting with a new LBBB should have a thorough cardiac evaluation.

Left anterior fascicular block (LAFB) is present on a 12-lead ECG when the QRS complex is less than 120 ms, LAD is present, there is a qR pattern in leads I and aVL, and there is an rS pattern in leads III and aVF (Figure 31.9).

Left posterior fascicular block (LPFB) is present on a 12-lead ECG when the QRS complex is less than 120 ms, RAD is present, there is a rS pattern in leads I and aVL, and there is a qR pattern in leads III and aVF (Figure 31.10).

Ischemia and Infarction

Ischemia occurs when there is decreased blood flow and oxygenation to an area of the myocardium secondary to narrowing of one or more coronary arteries. As a result, conduction is delayed through this hypoperfused area, causing abnormalities in ventricular depolarization and repolarization, which can be seen on the 12-lead ECG.

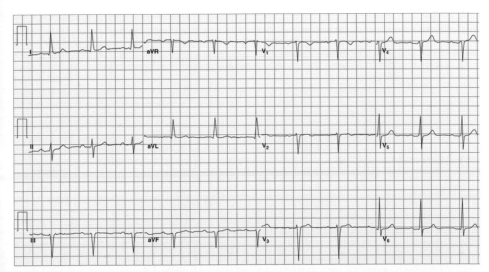

FIGURE 31.7. 12-lead ECG (abnormal). Rhythm: normal sinus. Rate: 75 bpm. Intervals: PR, 0.16; QRS, 0.15; QT, 0.42 second. Axis: indeterminate (isoelectric in all limb leads). P wave: left atrial enlargement (1 mm wide and 1 mm deep in lead V1). QRS: widened with RSR' in lead V1 consistent with right bundle branch block (RBBB). Also, pathologic Q waves are in leads II, III, and aVF, consistent with inferior wall myocardial infarction (an old one, because the ST segments do not demonstrate an acute injury pattern). Reprinted with permission from Lilly, L. S. (2010). *Pathophysiology of heart disease* (5th ed.). Wolters Kluwer.

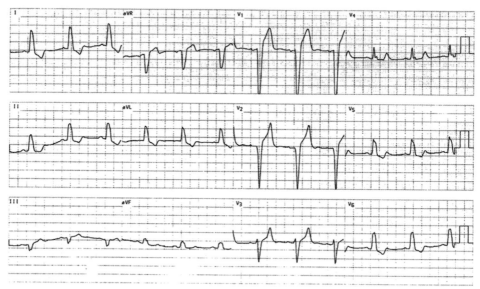

FIGURE 31.8. 12-lead ECG (abnormal). Rhythm: normal sinus. Rate: 68 bpm. Intervals: PR, 0.16; QRS, 0.16; QT, 0.40 second. Axis: +15°. P wave: normal. QRS: widened with RR' in leads V4–V6 consistent with left bundle branch block (LBBB). The ST segment and T wave abnormalities are secondary to LBBB. Reprinted with permission from Lilly, L. S. (2010). *Pathophysiology of heart disease* (5th ed.). Wolters Kluwer.

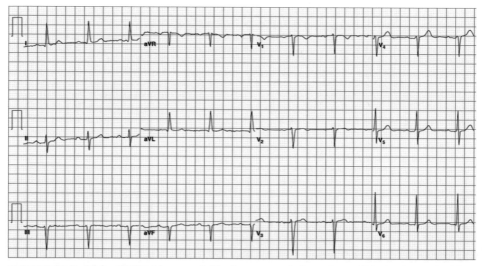

FIGURE 31.9. 12-lead ECG (abnormal). Rhythm: normal sinus. Rate: 68 bpm. Intervals: PR, 0.24 (first-degree AV block); QRS, 0.10; QT, 0.36 seconds. Axis: −45° (left axis deviation). P wave: borderline left atrial enlargement (terminal deflection of P wave in V1 is 1 mm wide and 1 mm deep—just barely). QRS: pattern of left anterior fascicular block (LAFB). The abnormally small R waves in leads V2–V4 are associated with LAFB resulting from the reduction of initial anterior forces. The ST segment and T waves are unremarkable. Reprinted with permission from Lilly, L. S. (2020). *Pathophysiology of heart disease* (7th ed.). Wolters Kluwer.

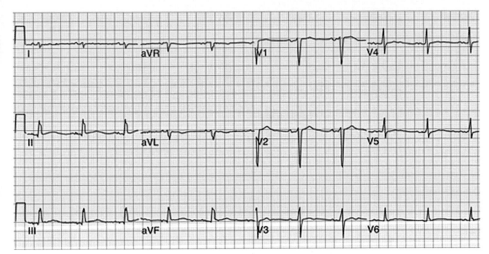

FIGURE 31.10. 12-lead ECG (abnormal). Rhythm: normal sinus. Rate: 62 bpm. Intervals: PR, 0.14; QRS, 0.10; QT, 0.52 (corrected QT, 0.53, which is prolonged). Axis: +95° (right axis deviation [RAD]). QRS: pattern of left posterior fascicular block (LPFB), with small R wave in leads I and aVL, small Q wave in leads II, III, and aVF, and RAD. The prolonged QT interval in this patient is the result of antidysrhythmic medication. Reprinted with permission from Lilly, L. S. (2020). *Pathophysiology of heart disease* (7th ed.). Wolters Kluwer.

Subendocardial ischemia refers to hypoperfusion of the inner layer of the myocardium, which may produce hyperacute T-waves, T-wave inversion, or ST-segment depression; whereas transmural ischemia refers to hypoperfusion extending through the entire thickness of the myocardium and produces ST-segment elevation (Figure 31.11).

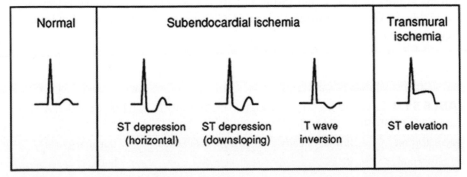

FIGURE 31.11. Common transient ECG abnormalities during ischemia. Subendocardial ischemia causes ST segment depressions and/or T wave flattening or inversions. Severe transient transmural ischemia can result in ST segment elevations, similar to the early changes in acute myocardial infarction. When transient ischemia resolves, so do the electrocardiographic changes. Reprinted with permission from Lilly, L. S. (2010). *Pathophysiology of heart disease* (5th ed.). Wolters Kluwer.

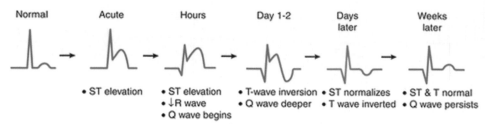

FIGURE 31.12. ECG evolution during acute ST-elevation myocardial infarction. However, if successful early reperfusion of the coronary occlusion is achieved, the initially elevated ST segment returns to baseline without subsequent T-wave inversion or Q-wave development. Reprinted with permission from Lilly, L. S. (2020). *Pathophysiology of heart disease* (7th ed.). Wolters Kluwer.

Subendocardial ischemia may be reversible or further advance to transmural ischemia and myocardial infarction. It should be noted that transmural ischemia can occur rapidly and that the T-wave and ST-segment abnormalities associated with subendocardial ischemia will not be present on the 12-lead ECG.

Infarction occurs when there is absence of blood flow and oxygenation to an area of the myocardium secondary to occlusion of one or more coronary arteries. As a result, conduction is absent through this anoxic area of myocardium, causing a lack of ventricular depolarization and repolarization. ST-segment elevation is the single most common 12-lead ECG finding during an acute myocardial infarction. It should be noted that ST-segment elevation is observed only in the acute phase of myocardial infarction and that full evolution or recovery occurs over days to weeks and involves resolution of ST-segment elevation and T-wave inversion (may also remain inverted) as well as the formation of pathological Q-waves (secondary to myocardial scarring) (Figure 31.12).

During acute myocardial infarction, review of the leads with ST-segment elevation and the leads with reciprocal ST-segment depression may help determine the anatomical area of myocardial insult and its corresponding coronary artery occlusion (Table 31.4). The following 12-lead ECGs represent acute myocardial infarction (Figures 31.13 and 31.14).

TABLE 31.4 12-Lead Electrocardiogram Correlation with Myocardial and Coronary Anatomy

Myocardium	Primary Leads	Reciprocal Leads	Coronary Artery
Anteroseptal	V1, V2	II, III, aVF	LAD
Anteroapical	V3, V4	II, III, aVF	LAD
Anterolateral	V5, V6	II, III, aVF	LAD or LCX
Lateral	I, aVL	II, III, aVF	LCX
Inferior	II, III, aVF	V5, V6, I, aVL	RCA

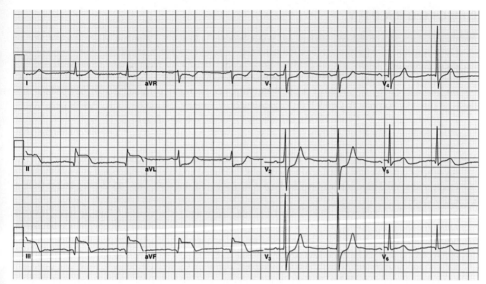

FIGURE 31.13. 12-lead ECG (abnormal). Rhythm: sinus bradycardia. Rate: 55 bpm. Intervals: PR, 0.20 (in aVF); QRS, 0.10; QT, 0.44 seconds. Axis: normal (QRS is predominantly upright in leads I and II). P wave: normal. QRS: voltage in chest leads is prominent but does not meet criteria for ventricular hypertrophy; pathologic Q waves are present in II, III, and aVF, indicating inferior wall myocardial infarction (MI), and the tall R wave in V2 is suggestive of posterior MI involvement as well. Marked ST-segment elevation is apparent in II, III, and aVF, indicating that this is an acute MI. Note the reciprocal ST-segment depression in leads I and aVL. Reprinted with permission from Lilly, L. S. (2015). *Pathophysiology of heart disease* (6th ed.). Wolters Kluwer.

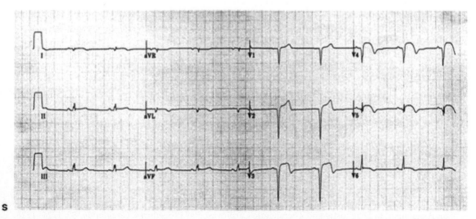

s

FIGURE 31.14. P-QRS-T Complex. There is a p before every QRS and a QRS after every p. There are no prolonged intervals or conduction delays. The rate is approximately 60 bpm. (C) Junctional tachycardia. Reprinted with permission from Ayala, C., & Spellberg, B. (2017). *Boards and wards for USMLE step 2* (6th ed.). Wolters Kluwer.

BIBLIOGRAPHY

Antman, E., Bassand, J., Klein, W., Ohman, M., Lopez Sendon, J., Rydén, L., Simoons, M., & Tendera, M. (2000, September). Myocardial infarction redefined—a consensus document of The Joint European Society of Cardiology/American College of Cardiology committee for the redefinition of myocardial infarction: The Joint European Society of Cardiology/American College of Cardiology Committee. *Journal of the American College of Cardiology, 36*, 959–969. http://dx.doi.org/10.1016/S0735-1097(00)00804-4

Bayés de Luna, A., Platonov, P., Cosio, F. G., Cygankiewicz, I., Pastor, C., Baranowski, R., Bayés-Genis, A., Guindo, J., Viñolas, X., Garcia-Niebla, J., Barbosa, R., Stern, S., & Spodick, D. (2012, September). Interatrial blocks. A separate entity from left atrial enlargement: A consensus report. *Journal of Electrophysiology, 45*, 445–451. http://dx.doi.org/10.1016/j.jelectrocard.2012.06.029

Casale, P. N., Devereux, R. B., Alonso, D. R., Campo, E., & Kligfield, P. (1987, March 1). Improved sex-specific criteria of left ventricular hypertrophy for clinical and computer interpretation of electrocardiograms: Validation with autopsy findings. *Circulation, 75*, 565–572. http://dx.doi.org/10.1161/01.CIR.75.3.565

Clochesy, J., Cifani, L., & Howe, K. (1991). Electrode site preparation techniques: A follow-up study. *Heart & Lung: The Journal of Acute and Critical Care, 20*, 27–30. https://www.ncbi.nlm.nih.gov/pubmed/1988388

Kligfield, P., Gettes, L. S., Bailey, J. J., Childers, R., Deal, B. J., Hancock, E. W., van Herpen, G., Kors, J. A., Macfarlane, P., Mirvis, D. M., Pahlm, O., Rautaharju, P., Wagner, G. S.; American Heart Association Electrocardiography and Arrhythmias Committee, Council on Clinical Cardiology; American College of Cardiology Foundation; Heart Rhythm Society, Josephson, M., Mason, J. W., Okin, P., Surawicz, B., & Wellens, H. (2007, February 23). Recommendations for the standardization and interpretation of the electrocardiogram Part I: The electrocardiogram and its technology: A scientific statement from the American Heart Association Electrocardiography and Arrhythmias Committee, Council on Clinical Cardiology; the American College of Cardiology Foundation; and the Heart Rhythm Society. *Circulation, 115*, 1306–1324. http://dx.doi.org/10.1161/CIRCULATIONAHA.106.180200

Mason, J. W., Hancock, W., & Gettes, L. S. (2007, March 8). Recommendations for the standardization and interpretation of the electrocardiogram: Part II: Electrocardiography diagnostic statement list a scientific statement from the American Heart Association Electrocardiography and Arrhythmias Committee, Council on Clinical Cardiology; the American College of Cardiology Foundation. *Journal of the American College of Cardiology, 49*, 1128–1135. http://dx.doi.org/doi:10.1016/j.jacc.2007.01.025

Panchal, A. R., Berg, K. M., Kudenchuk, P. J., Del Rios, M., Hirsch, K. G., Link, M. S., Kurz, M. C., Chan, P. S., Cabañas, J. G., Morley, P. T., Hazinski, M. F., & Donnino, M. W. (2018, December 4). 2018 American Heart Association focused update on advanced cardiovascular life support use of antiarrhythmic drugs during and immediately after cardiac arrest: An update to the American Heart Association Guidelines for cardiopulmonary resuscitation and emergency cardiovascular care. *Circulation, 138*, e740–e749. http://dx.doi.org/10.1161/CIR.0000000000000613

Peguero, J. G., Lo Presti, S., Perez, J., Issa, O., Brenes, J. C., & Tolentino, A. (2017, April 4). Electrocardiographic criteria for the diagnosis of left ventricular hypertrophy. *Journal of the American College of Cardiology, 69*, 1694–1703. http://dx.doi.org/10.1016/j.jacc.2017.01.037

Rautaharju, P., Surawicz, B., & Gettes, L. S. (2009, March 17). AHA/ACCF/HRS recommendations for the standardization and interpretation of the electrocardiogram: Part IV: The ST segment, T and U waves, and the QT interval a scientific statement from the American Heart Association Electrocardiography and Arrhythmias Committee, Council on Clinical Cardiology; the American College of Cardiology Foundation; and the Heart Rhythm Society. *Journal of the American College of Cardiology, 53*, 982–991. http://dx.doi.org/10.1016/j.jacc.2008.12.014

Schlant, R. C., Adolph, R. J., DiMarco, J. P., Dreifus, L. S., Dunn, M. I., Fisch, C., Garson, A. Jr, Haywood, L. J., Levine, H. J., Murray, J. A., Noble, R. J., & Ronan, J. A. (1992, March). Guidelines for electrocardiography a report of the American College of Cardiology/American Heart Association Task Force on Assessment of Diagnostic and Therapeutic Cardiovascular Procedures. *Circulation, 85*, 1221–1228. http://dx.doi.org/10.1161/01.CIR.85.3.1221

Sokolow, M., & Lyon, T. P. (1949). February. *American Heart Journal, 37*, 161–186. http://dx.doi.org/10.1016/0002-8703(49)90562-1

Surawicz, B., Childers, R., Deal, B. J., & Gettes, L. S. (2009, March 17). AHA/ACCF/HRS recommendations for the standardization and interpretation of the electrocardiogram Part III: Intraventricular conduction disturbances a scientific statement from the American Heart Association Electrocardiography and Arrhythmias Committee, Council on Clinical Cardiology; the American College of Cardiology Foundation; and the Heart Rhythm Society. *Journal of the American College of Cardiology, 53*, 976–981. http://dx.doi.org/doi:10.1016/j.jacc.2008.12.013

Wagner, G. S., Macfarlane, P., Wellens, H., Josephson, M., Gorgels, A., Mirvis, D. M., Pahlm, O., Surawicz, B., Kligfield, P., Childers, R., & Gettes, L. S. (2009, February 19). AHA/ACCF/HRS recommendations for the standardization and interpretation of the electrocardiogram: Part VI: Acute ischemia/infarction: A scientific statement from the American Heart Association Electrocardiography and Arrhythmias Committee, Council on Clinical Cardiology; the American College of Cardiology Foundation; and the Heart Rhythm Society. *Circulation, 119*, e262–e270. http://dx.doi.org/10.1161/CIRCULATIONAHA.108.191098

Hemodynamic Values and Parameters

Thomas Alne

Hemodynamics deals with the measurements of blood flow and circulation throughout the tissues and organs. Hemodynamic monitoring is especially important when caring for critically ill patients. The main goal of monitoring hemodynamics is to obtain an optimal level of blood flow and ensure perfusion to the body organs.

There are numerous values that we need to consider when discussing hemodynamics. First, there are several cardiovascular-related hemodynamic parameters that can be assessed invasively, including arterial blood pressure (BP), central venous pressure, pulmonary artery pressure, pulmonary artery wedge pressure, right ventricular pressure, left ventricular end diastolic pressure, cardiac output, cardiac index, venous oxygen saturation, systemic vascular resistance, peripheral vascular resistance, stroke volume, stroke volume index, stroke volume variation, pulmonary artery pulsatility index, and cardiac power output. Some non–cardiovascular-related hemodynamic parameters include intracranial pressure, cerebral perfusion pressure, and intra-abdominal pressure.

NONCARDIOVASCULAR SYSTEM–RELATED HEMODYNAMIC PARAMETERS

Intra-abdominal Pressure

Critically ill patients are at risk for developing a potentially fatal complication known as *abdominal compartment syndrome.* In order to monitor for that we measure the pressure in the abdominal compartment (Figure 32.1). Elevated intra-abdominal pressures (IAP) would be a warning sign that abdominal compartment syndrome is likely or is already occurring. Elevated pressures could also be a sign of fluid overload. Other causes of increased IAP include bowel obstructions, ileus, ascites, intra-abdominal hemorrhage, postabdominal surgery, pancreatitis, obesity, abdominal infection, severe burns, and gastric distention. Normal IAP ranges from 0 to 6.5 mmHg; however, it is typically around 3 to 7 mmHg. With obesity it is not abnormal to find IAP between 9 and 14 mmHg. Intra-abdominal hypertension is defined as IAP of 12 mmHg or higher. IAP over 20 mmHg with signs of end organ dysfunction is worrisome for abdominal compartment syndrome. IAP in excess of 25 mmHg is symptomatic of abdominal compartment syndrome. In order to measure IAP, a Foley catheter must be inserted into the patient's bladder, and a pressure system should then be connected to it. The patient must be supine for accurate measurements to be carried out.

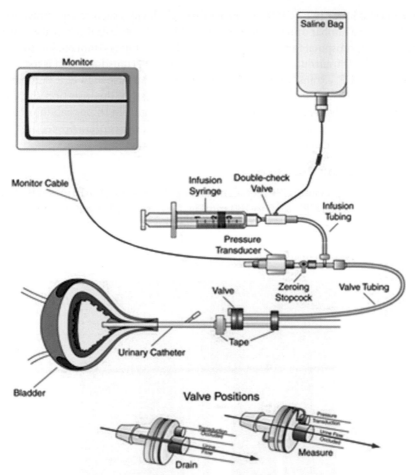

FIGURE 32.1. Intra-abdominal pressure monitoring. Reprinted with permission from Gabrielli, A., Layon, J., & Yu, M. (2011). *Civetta, Taylor, and Kirby's manual of critical care.* Wolters Kluwer

Intracranial Pressure

Numerous neurological pathologies can cause an elevated intracranial pressure (ICP). Normal ICP is about 10 mmHg. ICP should be below 15 mmHg. Increased ICP is dangerous because it could decrease cerebral blood flow. Pressures above 22 mmHg are worrisome for severe swelling and injury to the brain. Frequently, institutions set a goal for an ICP less than 20 mmHg.

Some possible causes of increased ICP include intracranial hemorrhages, tumors, cerebrovascular accident (CVA), traumatic brain injury (TBI), and fulminant liver failure. Seizures can further increase ICP in these patients. In addition, certain medical procedures such as intubation are known to increase ICP. ICP can be lowered by utilizing medications such as mannitol or hypertonic saline. Emergent neurosurgery may be necessary to lower ICP. ICP is measured through devices such as an extraventricular drain (EVD) or a lumbar drain (Figure 32.2). EVD and lumbar drains can also lower ICP by draining cerebrospinal fluid. A pressure transducer setup is connected to the EVD to monitor ICP. EVD transducers are leveled at the tragus. A transducer that is too high will give a false low ICP; a transducer that is too low will give a false high ICP. Lumbar drains can also record ICP. These drains are leveled on the basis of the insertion site. Lumbar drains are frequently used while patients are recovering from thoracoabdominal aortic aneurysms to avoid elevation of the ICP. One concern after cardiac procedures such as these is that patients can lose perfusion to the spinal nerves.

Cerebral Perfusion Pressure

Cerebral perfusion pressure (CPP) equals mean arterial pressure (MAP) minus ICP (CPP = MAP − ICP). Normal CPP is 60 to 100 mmHg. CPP is a marker for evaluating cerebral blood flow. When ICP increases without a concordant increase in MAP, it can result in a decrease in the CPP (Figure 32.3).

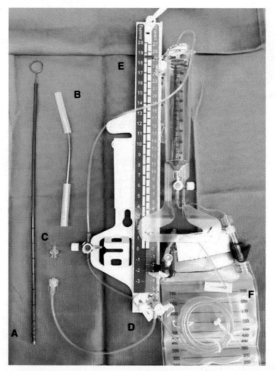

FIGURE 32.2. Extraventricular drain to measure intracranial pressure. Setup includes: ventricular catheter and stylet (A), tunneling trocar (B), connector (C), drainage system tubing and three-way stopcock (D), CSF drainage system (E), CSF collection bag (F). Reprinted with permission from Ramasethu, J., & Seo, S. (2019). *MacDonald's atlas of procedures in neonatology* (6th ed.). Wolters Kluwer.

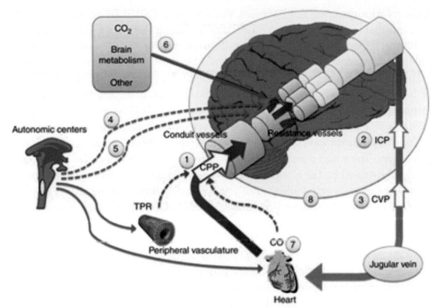

FIGURE 32.3. Device measuring intracranial pressure (cerebral perfusion pressure, CPP). The prime driving force for cerebral perfusion is cerebral perfusion pressure (1; CPP), which is determined by the difference between mean arterial blood pressure (BP) and intracranial pressure (2; ICP) under conditions where central venous pressure (3; CVP) is lower than ICP. Under steady-state conditions, mean arterial BP is determined by total peripheral resistance (TPR) and cardiac output (CO). Neurogenic control of cerebrovascular tone is controversial, but sympathetic (4) and parasympathetic (5) inputs have been implicated. Cerebral autoregulation is also under the influence of multiple modulating factors such as CO_2 and brain metabolism (6). Some controversial evidence suggests that CO influences cerebral blood flow independently of CPP (7). It is also important to note that, under conditions with elevated CVP or ICP, cerebral venous outflow (and therefore CBF) may also be "regulated" by a Starling resistor because of the enclosed nature of the cranium (8). Reprinted with permission from Bammer, R (2016). *MR and CT perfusion and pharmacokinetic imaging: Clinical applications and theoretical principles*. Wolters Kluwer. Adapted from Ainslie, P. N., & Tzeng, Y. C. (2010). On the regulation of the blood supply to the brain: Old age concepts and new age ideas. *Journal of Applied Physiology, 108*(6), 1447–1449.

CARDIOVASCULAR SYSTEM–RELATED HEMODYNAMIC PARAMETERS

Central Venous Pressure

Central venous pressure (CVP), also known as right atrial (RA) pressure, is a marker of volume status in the right atrium (RA). An elevated CVP normally means that a patient is fluid-overloaded. Other causes of an elevated CVP include cardiac tamponade and right ventricular (RV) failure. A decreased CVP means that a patient is dry and deficient in fluids. By administering fluid boluses, you can raise a CVP. By administering diuretics, you can make patients urinate more, thus lowering their CVP. An elevated CVP is above 8 mmHg. Normal CVP is between 2 and 8 mmHg. CVP is measured through a central line that is inserted either in the internal jugular vein, subclavian vein, or femoral vein. Then, a transducer is connected to the line under a pressurized system. The transducer is kept at the level of the phlebostatic axis, which is the fourth intercostal space and midaxillary line.

Although a CVP tracing on a monitor may look like a messy line, there are a few special points on those waveforms (Figure 32.4). There are three peaks, which are the *a*, *c*, and *v* waves. The *x* and *y* are two descents found on a CVP waveform. Atrial contraction is demonstrated by the *a* wave. The *c* wave signifies closure of the tricuspid valve. The v wave represents atrial filling. The *y* wave occurs when the tricuspid valve opens. The *x* wave signifies decreasing pressure in the RA. Conditions such as acute decompensated heart failure frequently lead to an elevated CVP. A falsely high CVP may be attributable to severe or torrential tricuspid regurgitation. Mechanical circulatory support (MCS) devices such as left ventricular assist devices (LVAD), extracorporeal life support (ECMO), and an Impella˚ heart pump are preload dependent. They need to have a slightly higher CVP to function, because if they are too dry then suck-down can occur when the cannulas irritate the ventricular walls, which can result in ventricular tachycardia and damage to the heart muscle. For LVADs, the CVP goal is changed to be under 12 as opposed to 8 mmHg. Optimal CVP would be 8 to 12 mmHg in the MCS population. recommends a CVP target of 10 to 15 mmHg for patients requiring the use of a CentriMag pump, which is an MCS device that can be used as an acute LVAD, right ventricular assist device (RVAD), or ECMO.

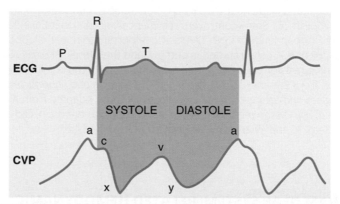

FIGURE 32.4. Normal central venous pressure waveform with atrial contraction (a peak), ventricular contraction (c peak), venous atrial filling (v peak), atrial relaxation (x descent), and tricuspid valve opening (y descent). Reprinted with permission from Connor, C. W. (2013). Commonly used monitoring techniques. In P. G. Barash, B. F. Cullen, & R. K. Stoelting (eds.), Clinical anesthesia. (7th ed.). Wolters Kluwer Health. Redrawn from Mark, J. B. (1991). Central venous pressure monitoring: Clinical insights beyond the numbers. *Journal of Cardiothoracic and Vascular Anesthesia, 5,* 163 with permission from Elsevier.

Pulmonary Artery Pressures

Pulmonary artery pressures can also be measured with a Swan-Ganz catheter, also known as a pulmonary artery catheter (PAC). A PAC is usually placed through the right internal jugular vein until it reaches the pulmonary artery but can be inserted through other veins as well. With pulmonary artery pressures we can record a systolic, diastolic, and mean pressure. PACs also provide a port that can be utilized to measure a CVP. Pulmonary artery systolic pressure (PASP) is normally between 15 and 25 mmHg. Pulmonary artery diastolic pressure (PADP) is normally between 8 and 15 mmHg. PADP can be used as a surrogate for a wedge pressure, left atrial pressure, or left ventricular end diastolic pressure. Elevated PADP can be found in mitral valve disorders and left-sided heart failure. Mean pulmonary artery pressure should be between 10 and 20 mmHg. Elevated pulmonary artery pressures can be found with pulmonary hypertension. There are numerous types of pulmonary hypertension with a variety of causes. Pulmonary embolisms and tamponade can also raise pulmonary artery pressures. There are a variety of medications that can lower pulmonary artery pressures resulting from pulmonary hypertension such as phosphodiesterase inhibitors like sildenafil, inhaled Flolan (epoprostenol sodium), and Remodulin˚ (treprostinil). For pulmonary artery pressures, the transducer is leveled at the phlebostatic axis.

Pulmonary Artery Occlusion Pressure

Pulmonary artery occlusion pressure (PAOP), also known as wedge pressure or pulmonary artery wedge pressure (PAWP), is a marker to estimate left atrial pressure (Figure 32.5). Wedge pressure is a way of estimating preload of the left side of the heart. Normal wedge pressure is 6 to 12 mmHg. PAOP greater than 18 signifies fluid overload, of the sort you may see in acute decompensated heart failure. Other causes of elevated wedge pressure include aortic and mitral valve pathologies. A decreased wedge pressure can be caused by hypovolemia. Unlike pulmonary artery pressures and CVP, which can be measured continuously, wedge pressure can be measured only as a snapshot in time when you advance the Swan-Ganz catheter and measure the waveform. Be cautious when wedging during times of severely elevated pulmonary artery pressures such as PASP greater than 70 mmHg or peripheral vascular resistance (PVS) greater than 5 Woods units. Always assess the chest x-ray prior to wedging to ensure optimal

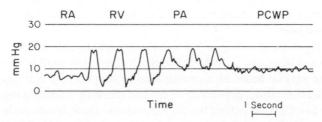

FIGURE 32.5. Pulmonary artery wedge pressure (PAWP) waveforms. Pressure tracings of right atrium (RA), right ventricle (RV), pulmonary artery (PA), and pulmonary capillary wedge pressure (PCWP). Reprinted with permission from Yao, F-S. F. (2003). *Yao and Artusio's Anesthesiology* (5th ed.). Wolters Kluwer.

placement. Do not wedge unless the PAC has been properly placed in the pulmonary artery. Also, do not force the catheter when wedging. There is a slight chance of perforating the pulmonary artery during wedging, which is an emergency situation. Look out for signs such as hemoptysis and hemodynamic instability.

Cardiac Output

Cardiac output (CO) is the volume of blood pumped by the heart every minute and that travels throughout the body. CO is measured in liters per minute (LPM). Normal CO is 4 to 8 LPM. Cardiac output (CO) = Heart rate (HR) × stroke volume (SV). CO can be measured hemodynamically in four ways:

1. Through tubing connected to an arterial line that is then connected to a special device called an EV 1000 (formerly known as a Vigileo).
2. Continuous cardiac output (CCO) Swan-Ganz catheter. It does involve a central line placement, which is more invasive than an arterial line, but because the values are coming from the pulmonary artery they are more accurate. CCO Swan-Ganz catheters are especially common in the postcardiac surgery populations.
3. There is also a method known as *thermodilution,* which can also be measured through a Swan-Ganz catheter. It is not as accurate and is open to operator error, among other challenges. It involves injecting a 10 mL syringe of saline through the CVP port during end expiration, and, depending on the time and temperature of injection, it determines the CO. Thermodilution can vary by as much as 10% every time a clinician takes a measurement.
4. The final method is using a Fick calculation. You need a complete blood count, venous blood gas, and an arterial blood gas in order to calculate a Fick. Based on the formula, a CO can be determined. It is a snapshot in time, unfortunately, so it does not give you continuous measurements like the CCO Swan-Ganz and EV 1000 platform (Figure 32.6).

Each method has its own unique benefits and challenges, and usage differs from institution to institution. A low CO can mean cardiogenic shock. Cardiogenic shock is usually caused by an acute myocardial infarction or low output heart failure. A high CO can result from septic shock. It is not unusual to have a situation where healthcare providers are not sure of the etiology of a patient's shock state; therefore, placing hemodynamic lines such as a Swan-Ganz catheter can help distinguish whether it is a cardiogenic versus a septic shock based on CO and systemic vascular resistance, which will be described later.

Notably, there are a variety of MCS devices, both durable long-term pumps and temporary devices, that also provide CO support. Clinicians need to consider that CO values obtained may be based on a certain level of support and that when devices are weaned, numbers may drop, depending on cardiac recovery. Tricuspid regurgitation can cause a falsely low CO. If a patient has an intracardiac shunt it can cause a falsely high CO measurement if the thermodilution method is used. Acute blood loss can lower CO as well. Abdominal compartment syndrome, hypophosphatemia, and hypocalcemia can also reduce CO.

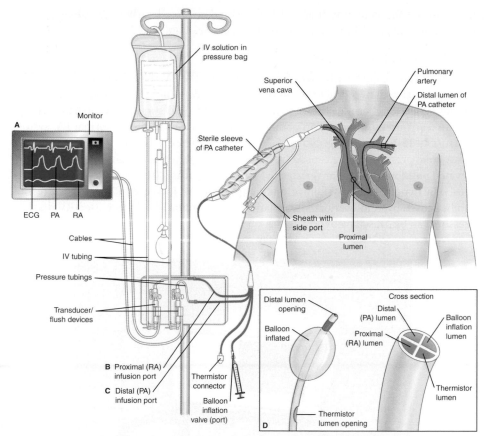

FIGURE 32.6. CCO Swan-Ganz and EV 1000 platform. (A) Bedside cardiac monitoring. (B) Right atria (RA) or central venous pressure monitoring system connected to proximal infusion lumen hub. (C) PA monitoring system connected to distal infusion lumen hub. Each system is attached to pressurized intravenous fluid, a transducer with stopcock and flush device, and pressure tubing. A cable attaches each transducer to the bedside monitor. (D) Magnified view of distal end of PA catheter with cross section of catheter lumen. Reprinted with permission from Timby, B. K., & Smith, N. (2017). *Introductory medical-surgical nursing* (12th ed.). Wolters Kluwer.

Cardiac Index

Cardiac index (CI) is CO that takes body size into consideration. People have different hemodynamic needs depending on their height and weight, so body mass index (BMI) is considered. Normal CI is between 2.5 and 4 LPM. CI = CO/ body surface area. Similarly, compared with CO, a low CI is caused by cardiogenic shock and a high CI can be caused by septic shock. In general, a CI less than 2.2 tends to be concerning. Numerous decisions such as the need for inotropes, MCS devices, and even heart transplant status upgrades can be made because of drops in CI in combination with other factors. CI can be measured the same way that CO is measured, as noted earlier (calculating a Fick, CCO Swan-Ganz, EV 1000, and thermodilution). See Figure 32.7.

Right Ventricular Pressure

As a Swan-Ganz catheter advances from the RA into the RV, the waveform changes. That helps guide clinicians to the location of invasive lines. Although a Swan-Ganz catheter cannot be left long term in the ventricle because it would stimulate ventricular ectopy, we can learn useful information about pressures in that chamber. Normal RV systolic pressure is 15 to 25 mmHg. Normal RV diastolic pressure is 0 to 8 mmHg. Elevated RV systolic pressure can be caused by pulmonary hypertension, pulmonary stenosis, or elevated pulmonary vascular resistance (PVR). A decreased RV systolic pressure can be caused by hypovolemia, RV failure, and tamponade. An increased RV diastolic pressure can be caused by fluid overload, heart failure, and tamponade. A decreased RV diastolic pressure can be caused by hypovolemia.

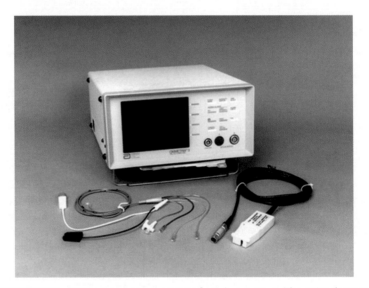

FIGURE 32.7. Measuring components of cardiac output. The mixed venous oxygen saturation (Svo2) monitoring system consists of a flow-directed pulmonary artery (PA) catheter with fiber-optic filaments, an optical mod-mule, and a co-oximeter. The co-oximeter displays a continuous digital Svo2 value; the strip recorder prints a permanent record. Catheter insertion follows the same technique as that with any thermodilution flow-directed PA catheter. The distal lumen connects to an external PA pressure monitoring system; the proximal or central venous pressure lumen connects to another monitoring system or to a continuous-flow administration unit; and the optical module connects to the co-oximeter unit. As an alternative, many facilities have cardiac monitors that also monitor Svo2. Reprinted with permission from Springhouse. (2004). *Nursing Procedures* (4th ed.). Lippincott Williams & Wilkins.

Left Ventricular End Diastolic Pressure

Left ventricular end diastolic pressure is a marker of fluid status. Wedge pressure can be used as a surrogate to measure left ventricular end diastolic pressure; therefore, normal values are 6 to 12 mmHg. Elevated values indicate fluid overload. Decreased values indicate fluid deficiency.

Systemic Vascular Resistance

Systemic vascular resistance (SVR) is a way to measure afterload on the heart. Normal SVR is between 800 and 1,200 dynes-sec/cm^{-5}. To convert to Woods units, simply divide by 80. SVR can be measured from calculating a Fick, EV 1000, or a CCO Swan-Ganz catheter. Elevated SVR is present during vasoconstricted states such as cardiogenic shock and heart failure. Decreased SVR is present during vasodilatory states such as septic shock. There are a variety of medications such as hydralazine, angiotensin-converting enzyme ACE inhibitors, milrinone, and nitroprusside that can decrease afterload and allow the heart to pump more effectively and, as a result, raise CO.

Peripheral Vascular Resistance

Normal PVR is lower than 250 dynes-sec/cm^{-5}. To convert it to Woods units, divide by 80. In order to qualify for a heart transplant, one of the listing requirements is a PVR less than 3 Woods units. PVR is the afterload of the right ventricle. In comparison, SVR is the afterload of the left ventricle. Marino describes PVR as a measure of the flow and pressure in the lungs. An elevated PVR can lead to right-sided heart failure. One of the reasons there is a PVR cutoff is that patients who have a high PVR pretransplant do significantly worse. Posttransplant atrial fibrillation occurred in 20.2% of patients with a high PVR as opposed to 10.7% of patients with a normal PVR. Thirty-day mortality postorthotropic heart transplant was 25.5% in the high PVR group and 6.4% in the normal PVR group.

Stroke Volume

Stroke volume (SV) is the actual volume of blood, measured in mL, that is ejected from the heart with every heartbeat. As SV increases, so does CO. SV is made up of three main factors: preload, afterload, and contractility. A normal SV is between 60 and 100 mL. SV can be measured by using an EV 1000. Dehydration can cause a decrease in SV. Tamponade, papillary muscle rupture, and cardiogenic shock can also cause a decrease in SV. Intra-aortic balloon pump usage can increase SV. Also, being well hydrated can increase SV.

Stroke Volume Variation

Stroke volume variation (SVV) is an indicator of how responsive a patient is to being given fluids. A normal SVV is between 10% and 15%. SVV can demonstrate whether giving fluids has helped improve the patient's clinical status. SVV is more reliable when patients are intubated. Some limitations of measuring SVV are during dysrhythmias, when IAP is elevated and the patient has an open chest. SVV greater than 15% indicates hypovolemia. SVV lower than 10% signifies myocardial dysfunction. Other factors that may increase SVV are vasodilatory medications and increasing the positive end-expiratory pressure on a ventilator.

Stroke Volume Index

Stroke volume index (SVI) is normally between 33 and 47 mL/m^2/beat. SVI is the amount of blood ejected with each beat and also takes body surface area into consideration. Therefore, the same things that increase or decrease SV will also affect SVI. In general, a low SVI indicates fluid deficiency, and a high SVI indicates fluid overload.

Pulmonary Artery Pulsatility Index

Pulmonary artery pulsatility index (PAPI) is a way of measuring how dysfunctional the RV is and whether or not a specific patient might require a temporary RVAD to be placed. PAPI is measured by subtracting PADP from PASP, then dividing that by the patient's CVP. A PAPI higher than 0.9 is considered sufficient, so an RVAD is not required. According to the National Cardiogenic Shock Initiative, if the cardiac power output (CPO) is less than 0.6 and PAPI is less than 0.9, then you should insert an RVAD to support the patient's RV.

Cardiac Power Output

CPO is the rate of energy output. According to the SHOCK trial, CPO was the strongest hemodynamic predictor of outcome in individuals with cardiogenic shock. A normal CPO is greater than 0.6. If the CPO is less than 0.6, then a PAPI score should be calculated. If the CPO is less than 0.6 and PAPI is also low, then an RVAD should be placed. If the CPO is low and PAPI is normal, then the left-sided MCS device in use should be upgraded. For example, if the patient has an Impella* cardiac pump that delivers up to 3.5 LPM of CO support, perhaps they need to be upgraded to an Impella* 5.0 or 5.5. Depending on the situation, end organ function, and oxygenation, a low CPO may be an indicator that it is time to place a patient on veno-arterial extracorporeal membrane oxygenation.

Venous Oxygen Saturation

Mixed venous oxygen saturation (SVO$_2$) represents the balance between oxygen consumption and delivery. SVO$_2$ can be measured constantly from a CCO Swan-Ganz catheter. SVO$_2$ is an important part of determining a CO and CI by using a Fick calculation. When calculating a Fick, a SVO$_2$ is obtained by drawing a venous blood gas. For optimal results a venous blood gas should be drawn from the PA port of a Swan-Ganz catheter. ScvO$_2$ is central venous oxygen saturation. Venous oxygen saturation is affected by hemoglobin, oxygenation, oxygen consumption, and CO. ScvO$_2$ shows oxygen delivery and consumption for the head and the upper body. SVO2 shows oxygen delivery and consumption for the whole body. Normal SVO$_2$ is between 60% and 80%. A low SVO$_2$ can mean a variety of things such as cardiogenic shock, hypoxia, hypovolemia, stress, anxiety, and pain. If an SVO$_2$ is above 80%, then it is advisable to assess a few factors such as lactic acid, base deficit, and oxygenation. Also, make sure that a true venous sample (not arterial) was drawn. When drawing a venous blood gas, ensure that you pull back on the syringe slowly, because if you pull back too fast it can give you an artificially high result.

Arterial Blood Pressure

BP can be measured invasively through the use of an arterial line. Most arterial lines are placed in the radial artery, but there are other potential locations such as brachial artery and femoral artery. For BP, the transducer is leveled at the phlebostatic axis.

BP includes a systolic, diastolic, and MAP (Figure 32.8). A systolic BP (SBP) is the pressure on the ventricles when the heart is contracting. Normal SBP is between 90 and 140 mmHg. Average SBP is around 120 mmHg. Diastolic BP (DBP) is the pressure on the ventricles when the heart is relaxed. Normal DBP is between 60 and 90 mmHg. MAP is an average of systolic and diastolic, but it is two thirds more weighted toward the DBP. A normal MAP is between 70 and 105 mmHg. A MAP of 65 mmHg or over is necessary to ensure adequate perfusion to other organs. An elevated arterial BP can be caused by hypertension, aortic insufficiency, and arteriosclerosis. A decreased BP can be due to shock, heart failure, cardiac tamponade, tension pneumothorax, too high a dose of antihypertensive medications, and aortic stenosis. A transducer that is leveled too low will give a false high reading. A transducer that is leveled too high will give a false low reading. Some patients with advanced heart failure live with a lower SBP; therefore, you need to determine what the baseline is before ordering any interventions. With patients who have an LVAD, only a MAP can be obtained by using a Doppler ultrasound. A normal MAP for an LVAD patient is between 70 and 90 mmHg. Shock states such as cardiogenic, septic, hypovolemic, anaphylactic, and obstructive shock pathologies can all cause hypotension in severe cases. In hemorrhagic shock (a type of hypovolemic shock), BP does not start to drop until at least Class III hemorrhages. Class III involves a 31% to 40% loss of blood volume. Giving fluids or blood products can raise a patient's preload and, thus, BP. Administering diuretics or taking too much ultrafiltration off with dialysis will lower a patient's volume state, thereby lowering BP.

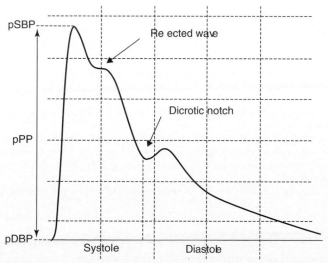

FIGURE 32.8. Arterial blood pressure waveform. Reprinted with permission from Mulholland, M. W. (2016). *Greenfield's surgery* (6th ed.). Wolter Kluwers Health.

CONCLUSION

There are a variety of hemodynamic measurements that can be obtained through the use of invasive lines such as arterial lines, Swan-Ganz catheters, EVD, and lumbar drains. The data we learn from these devices can give crucial information not only on how to diagnose a patient's problem, but also on monitoring and evaluating current treatments. We can have a better understanding of illnesses and treatment modalities if we understand the hemodynamics and physiology behind them.

BIBLIOGRAPHY

Al-Abassi, A. A., Al Saadi, A. S., & Ahmed, F. (2018). Is intra-bladder pressure measurement a reliable indicator for raised intra-abdominal pressure? A prospective comparative study. *BMC Anesthesiology, 18*(1). https://doi.org/10.1186/s12871-018-0539-z.

Colucci, W. (2020). *Treatment of acute decompensated heart failure: Specific therapies.* Retrieved March 26, 2021, from https://www.uptodate.com/contents/treatment-of-acute-decompensatedheartfailure-specifictherapies?search=milrinone&source=search_result&selectedTitle=4~65&usage_type=default&display_rank=4#H123895781.

Currie, L. A. (2020). Lumbar drains after cardiac surgery: Evidence-based solutions for safe management. *Critical Care Nurse, 40*(6), 75–80. https://doi.org/10.4037/ccn2020684.

Drugs.com (29 Compared). (2021). *Medications for pulmonary hypertension.* Retrieved March 20, 2021, from https://www.drugs.com/condition/pulmonary-hypertension.html.

Golshani, K., Azizkhani, R., & Foroutan, F. (2020). Inpatient evaluation of intra-abdominal pressure completed with a urinary catheter as compared with ultrasonographic vessel measurements. *Journal of Diagnostic Medical Sonography, 36*(1), 12–17. https://doi.org/10.1177/8756479319879072.

Henry, S. (2018). *ATLS advanced trauma life support student course manual* (10th ed.). American College of Surgery.

Hill, B., & Smith, C. (2021). Central venous pressure monitoring in critical care settings. *British Journal of Nursing, 30*(4), 230–236. https://doi.org/10.12968/bjon.2021.30.4.230.

Howells, T., Johnson, U., McKelvey, T., Ronne-Engström, E., & Enblad, P. (2017). The effects of ventricular drainage on the intracranial pressure signal and the pressure reactivity index. *Journal of Clinical Monitoring and Computing, 31*(2), 469–478. https://doi.org/10.1007/s10877-016-9863-3.

Imamura, T., Jeevanandam, V., Kim, G., Raikhelkar, J., Sarswat, N., Kalantari, S., Smith, B., Rodgers, D., Besser, S., Chung, B., Nguyen, A., Narang, N., Ota, T., Song, T., Juricek, C., Mehra, M., Costanzo, M. R., Jorde, U. P., Burkhoff, D., … Uriel, N. (2019). Optimal hemodynamics during left ventricular assist device support are associated with reduced readmission rates. *Circulation: Heart Failure, 12*(2). https://doi.org/10.1161/circheartfailure.118.005094.

Killu, K., & Sarani, B. (Eds.). (2017). *Fundamental critical care support* (6th ed.). Society of Critical Care Medicine.

Lim, H. S. (2020). Cardiac power output revisited. *Circulation: Heart Failure, 13*(10). https://doi.org/10.1161/circheartfailure.120.007393.

Liu, X., Griffith, M., Jang, H. J., Ko, N., Pelter, M. M., Abba, J., Vuong, M., Tran, N., Bushman, K., & Hu, X. (2020). Intracranial pressure monitoring via external ventricular drain: Are we waiting long enough before recording the real value? *Journal of Neuroscience Nursing, 52*(1), 37–42. https://doi.org/10.1097/jnn.0000000000000487

Marino, P. (2014). *Marino's the ICU book* (4th ed.). Philadelphia, PA: Wolters Kluwer Health/Lippincott Williams & Wilkins.

McGee, W., Young, C., & Frazier, J. (2018). *Edwards clinical education quick guide to cardiopulmonary care* (4th ed.) [PDF]. Edwards Lifesciences.

Merriam-Webster. (n.d.). *Hemodynamics.* In Merriam-Webster.com dictionary. Retrieved March 14, 2021, from https://www.merriam-webster.com/dictionary/hemodynamics.

National Cardiogenic Shock Initiative. (2017). Retrieved March 27, 2021, from https://www.henryford. com/-/media/files/henry-ford/detroit-cardiogenic-shock-initiative/national-csi---algorithm---v1-5. pdf?la=en&hash=86F6B06367AA5282D0F974134F79681A.

Pudjiadi, A. (2020). Advances of hemodynamic monitoring and the current state of fluid resuscitation in clinical practice. *Critical Care Shock, 23,* 14–22.

Ragosta, M. (2018). *Textbook of clinical hemodynamics.* Elsevier.

Rivinius, R., Helmschrott, M., Ruhparwar, A., Schmack, B., Darche, F. F., Thomas, D., Bruckner, T., Doesch, A. O., Katus, H. A., & Ehlermann, P. (2020). Elevated pre-transplant pulmonary vascular resistance is associated with early post-transplant atrial fibrillation and mortality. *ESC Heart Failure, 7*(1), 177–188. https://doi.org/10.1002/ehf2.12549

Tunstall, L. (2020). *External ventricular drains and intracranial pressure monitoring.* Retrieved March 18, 2021, from https://www.rch.org.au/rchcpg/hospital_clinical_guideline_index/External_ventricular_drains_ and_intracranial_pressure_monitoring/#Levelling.

Watanabe, K., Stöhr, E. J., Akiyama, K., Watanabe, S., & González-Alonso, J. (2020). Dehydration reduces stroke volume and cardiac output during exercise because of impaired cardiac filling and venous return, not left ventricular function. *Physiological Reports, 8*(11). https://doi.org/10.14814/phy2.14433

Pulmonary Function Test Interpretation

Janice K. Delgiorno

INDICATIONS FOR THE PROCEDURE

Spirometry is indicated to evaluate baseline lung function, causes of dyspnea, and effects of respiratory treatment.

Spirometry is an effort-dependent test that requires careful patient instruction, understanding, coordination, and cooperation. Spirometry includes the measurement of several values of forced airflow and volume during inspiration and expiration. For the most part, the purpose of spirometry is to assess the ability of the lungs to move large volumes of air quickly through the airways to identify airway obstruction. Some measurements are aimed at large intrathoracic airways, some are aimed at small airways, and some assess obstruction throughout the lungs. Measuring flow rates is a surrogate for measuring airways resistance (Figure 33.1). To a lesser extent, spirometry can also identify and quantify a restrictive pattern of pulmonary disease. Spirometry will measure the forced expiratory volume in one second (FEV_1) and the forced vital capacity (FVC), the total amount of exhaled air. The FEV_1/FVC ratio is evaluated to identify obstructive disease (Figure 33.2). Spirometry is the most common pulmonary test.

Indications for the procedure are:

1. Show the presence or absence of lung dysfunctions suggested by history or physical signs and symptoms or the presence of other abnormal diagnostic tests (e.g., chest radiograph, arterial blood gases).
2. Assess severity of known lung disease.
3. Assess change of lung function in function of time or in function of therapy.
4. Assess the potential effect of occupational or environmental exposure.
5. Assess the potential risk of surgical interventions that can affect lung function.
6. Assess impairment or disability (e.g., for rehabilitation, legal reasons, military).

CONTRAINDICATIONS FOR THE PROCEDURE

Relative Contraindications

1. Acute infection of airways or lungs because it is rarely useful to perform a lung function test in these cases, considering that the results will be affected by the acute infection.

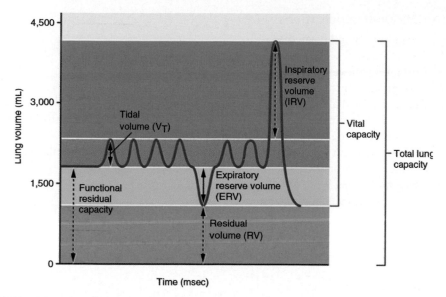

FIGURE 33.1. A spirogram. Lung volumes and capacities of an average adult female, as measured by spirometry. Upward deflections are inhalations; downward deflections are exhalations. The solid arrows indicate values that can be directly measured by spirometry. The dotted arrows indicate values that must be calculated or measured using specialized equipment. Reprinted with permission from Cohen, B. J., & Hull, K. L. (2019). *Memmler's the human body in health and disease* (14th ed.). Wolters Kluwer. Modified from McConnell, T., & Hull, K. (2011). *Human form, human function*. Lippincott Williams & Wilkins.

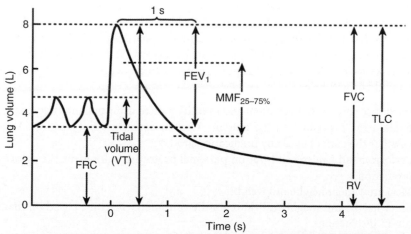

FIGURE 33.2. Spirometry and lung volumes. Reprinted with permission from Singh-Radcliff, N. (2012). *5-Minute anesthesia consult*. Wolters Kluwer.

Absolute Contraindications

1. Hemoptysis of unknown cause
2. Pneumothorax
3. Unstable cardiovascular status
4. Patients with a history of syncope associated with forced exhalation
5. Recent myocardial infarction or pulmonary embolism
6. Thoracic, abdominal, or cerebral aneurysm (risk of rupture because of the increased intrathoracic pressure during forced expiration)
7. Recent ocular surgery (within 2 weeks caused by increased intraocular pressure during forced expiration)
8. Nausea, vomiting
9. Recent thoracic or abdominal surgery

EQUIPMENT NEEDED

1. Computer
2. Spirometry device
3. Spirometry mouthpiece
4. Nose clip
5. Tissues
6. Chair for the patient to sit on

STEPS TO PERFORMING THE PROCEDURE

Two choices are available prior to testing regarding bronchodilator and medication use. Patients may withhold oral and inhaled bronchodilators to establish baseline lung function and evaluate maximum bronchodilator response, or they may continue taking medication as prescribed. If medications are withheld, a risk of exacerbation of bronchial spasm exists. If the aim of the test is to judge whether pharmacological treatment can be improved, then the patient will continue taking medication. If the purpose is to diagnose lung disease or see if there is any change in response to bronchodilators, then the medication should be withheld).

1. Introduce yourself to the patient and identify patient using patient safety identifiers.
2. Explain the procedure to the patient: Written consent is not needed. Ascertain whether the patient used any medications today.
3. Perform hand hygiene and put on personal protective equipment (i.e., gloves, eye protection).
4. Measure patient height and weight.
5. Enter height and weight and calibrate the spirometry machine based on manufacturer's instructions.
6. Attach the mouthpiece to the spirometry device.
7. Position the patient: Seated upright, ideally in a chair; however, upright on stretcher or bed may suffice.

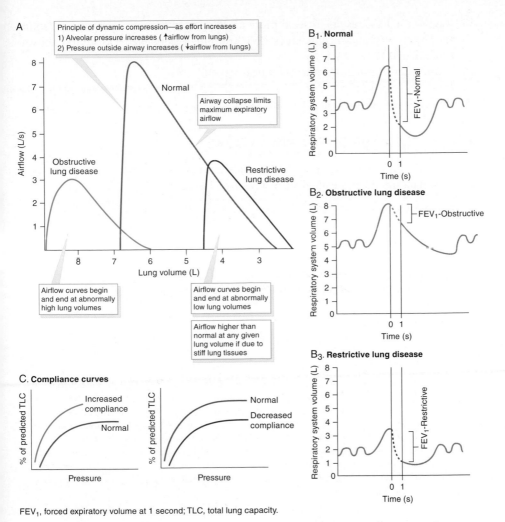

FEV$_1$, forced expiratory volume at 1 second; TLC, total lung capacity.

FIGURE 33.3. Spirometry tracings: diseased vs normal. FEV$_1$, forced expiratory volume at 1 second; TLC, total lung capacity. Reprinted with permission from Jenkins, B. (2014). *Step-up to USMLE step 1*. Wolters Kluwer.

8. Apply the nose clip to the patient.
9. Have the patient place the mouthpiece in their mouth.
10. Have the patient perform normal breathing.
11. Instruct the patient to take a deep breath in, then blow out as hard and fast as the patient is able to, and then breathe in again. Six seconds are needed for a good effort.
12. Repeat the process to ensure validity. Each patient must perform a minimum of three successful FVC maneuvers.

13. Review the FVC results to see if more assessment is needed. To ensure reliability, the largest FVC and second largest FVC from the acceptable trials should not vary more than 0.15 L.
14. Administer a bronchodilator and repeat step 10.
15. Remove the nose clip.
16. Review spirometry tracings (Figure 33.3).

COMPLICATIONS OF THE PROCEDURE

Although spirometry is a safe procedure, untoward reactions may occur, and the value of the test data should be weighed against potential hazards.

1. Pneumothorax
2. Paroxysmal coughing
3. Increased intracranial pressure
4. Contraction of healthcare-associated infections
5. Syncope, dizziness, lightheadedness
6. O_2 desaturation resulting from interruption of O_2 therapy
7. Chest pain
8. Bronchospasm

BIBLIOGRAPHY

Graham, B. L., Steenbruggen, I., Miller, M. R., Barjaktarevic, I. Z., Cooper, B. G., Hall, G. L., Hallstrand, T. S., Kaminsky, D. A., McCarthy, K., McCormack, M. C., Oropez, C. E., Rosenfeld, M., Stanojevic, S., Swanney, M. P., & Thompson, B. R. (2019). Standardization of spirometry 2019 update. An official American Thoracic Society and European Respiratory Society technical statement. *American Journal of Respiratory and Critical Care Medicine, 200*(8), e70–e88. https://doi.org/10.1164/rccm.201908-1590st

Johnson, J., & Theurer, W. (2014). A stepwise approach to the interpretation of pulmonary function tests. *American Family Physician, 89*(5), 359–366.

Kacmarek, R. M., Stoller, J. K., Heuer, A. J., Chatburn, R. L., & Kallet, R. H. (2017). *Egan's fundamentals of respiratory care* (12th ed.). Elsevier.

CHAPTER 34

Rapid Sequence Intubation

Elizabeth Tomaszewski

RAPID SEQUENCE INDUCTION

Rapid sequence induction may be utilized in those requiring intubation for mechanical ventilation or airway protection. This chapter will discuss the medications used and risks associated with rapid sequence intubation. This method provides optimal conditions for successful endotracheal intubation, while reducing the chances of pulmonary aspiration of gastric contents. Proper thorough airway assessment is essential with expectation of successful intubation, because the use of neuromuscular blockade renders the patient unable to ventilate themselves. Contingency plans for ventilation and airway support are crucial to avoid life-threatening complications.

INDICATIONS FOR THE PROCEDURE

1. Patient requires endotracheal intubation.
2. Patient has full stomach or status of intake is unknown, increasing risk of aspiration.
3. Gastric insufflation caused by bag valve mask ventilation, increasing risk of aspiration.
4. Difficulty with adequacy of procedural sedation.

CONTRAINDICATIONS FOR THE PROCEDURE

Relative Contraindications

1. Difficult airway views. Failure to successfully intubate and difficulty to ventilate could lead to negative outcomes such as cerebral hypoxia and cardiac arrest. Patients with difficult airways should be intubated by those with advanced airway training, and consideration should be given to the risk of chemically paralyzing these patients.
2. Hypotension. Sedation must be given with neuromuscular blocking agents, which can have adverse effects on marginal BP.
3. Neurologic impairments. Rapid sequence intubation medications will render a patient without a neurologic examination for minutes up to an hour after delivery of neuromuscular blockade.
4. Certain agents should not be used in those patients with degenerative neuromuscular conditions (such as myasthenia gravis), because this may worsen their condition.
5. Succinylcholine should be avoided in those with crush injuries, major trauma, or burns owing to the risk of hyperkalemia.

Absolute Contraindications

1. Total upper airway obstruction or total loss of oropharyngeal landmarks. Surgical airway is required.
2. Crash airways in patients in full arrest. The airway should be flaccid for intubation without premedications, which could limit neurologic evaluation post return of spontaneous circulation.

Rapid Sequence Intubation

The purpose of rapid sequence intubation is to provide a controlled environment in which to decrease the complications of aspiration while performing endotracheal intubation. This is achieved by providing a sedative along with a neuromuscular blocking agent to provide paralysis through muscle relaxation. The paralysis prevents gag reflex and reduces chance of aspiration of stomach contents. Care must be taken, however, in view of the possibility of passive reflux through the esophagus. Some sources promote the use of the Sellick maneuver, or cricoid pressure, to prevent passive reflux without evidentiary support.

Airway assessment is essential in determining risk versus benefit of neuromuscular blockade. Airways with high-grade difficulty are at greater risk when the patient is under neuromuscular blockade owing to the potential difficulty in ventilating once paralyzed. Patients identified as having difficult airways should be intubated only by those with advanced airway training and with multiple devices and adjuncts available. Cricothyrotomy sets should also be available in the event that oral or nasal intubation is unsuccessful. First pass success is the goal with rapid sequence intubation. The incidence of complications, such as cerebral hypoxia, increase with subsequent failed attempts; therefore, a contingency plan should be available for failed intubation attempts.

Equipment Needed

1. Intravenous (IV) catheter for IV access
2. Cardiac monitor and cardiac leads
3. Laryngoscope handle with working light
4. McIntosh blades 3, 4, 5
5. Cuffed endotracheal tubes of sizes 5, 6, 7, 8
6. Ambu bag
7. Oxygen source
8. Oxygen delivery devices: nasal cannula, BiPAP setup, ambu bag aka bag valve mask (BVM), ventilator
9. Suction source
10. Multiple visualization devices such as laryngeal scopes, video scopes, or bronchoscopes
11. Backup airway adjuncts such as laryngeal mask airways (LMA), obturator airways, nasopharyngeal airways, and oropharyngeal airways
12. Cricothyrotomy set
13. Rigid suction device should be immediately available
14. Medications as listed in Table 34.1

TABLE 34.1 Rapid Sequence Intubation Medications

	Dose/ Onset	Indications	Cautions	Notes
Adjuncts				
Lidocaine	1.5 mg/ kg IV	Head injuries, increased intracranial pressure (ICP), bronchospasm		Protection from intracranial hypertension caused by intubation
Atropine	0.02 mg/ kg IV	Bradycardia		Repeat doses of succinylcholine may cause bradycardia
Sedatives				
Midazolam				
Etomidate	0.3–0.5 mg/kg	Increased ICP	Myoclonic activity may lead to jaw clenching	Adrenal insufficiency, rare
Ketamine	1–2 mg/kg	Bronchodilator, analgesia, dissociative amnesia	May increase heart rate/BP. Associated with emergence phenomenon	Use caution in patients with hypertension
Propofol	0.5–1.5 mg/kg	Short-acting, decreased ICP	Hypotension, cardiosuppression,	Only to be given IV push by providers
Neuromuscular Blocking Agents				
Depolarizing				
Succinylcholine	1.5 mg/ kg IV	Rapid onset (<1 minute), Short duration (5–9 minutes)	Hyperkalemia, bradycardia after dosing	Do not use in patients with history of malignant hyperthermia, hyperkalemia, trauma/burns. Avoid in those with degenerative neuromuscular diseases.
Nondepolarizing				
Vecuronium	0.08–0.15 mg/kg 0.15–0.28 mg/kg (high-dose protocol)	Onset 2–4 minutes, duration 25–40 minutes High dose: duration 60–120 minutes	Not generally recommended for rapid sequence intubation owing to length of duration	

(continued)

TABLE 34.1 Rapid Sequence Intubation Medications (*Continued*)

	Dose/ Onset	Indications	Cautions	Notes
Nondepolarizing				
Rocuronium	1 mg/kg IV	Onset 1–3 minutes, duration 30–45 minutes	Tachycardia	Can be used when succinylcholine is contraindicated
Reversal of Nondepolarizing Neuromuscular Blocking Agents				
Sugammadex	16 mg/ kg for emergent reversal	Onset 3 minutes		

Data from Tintinalli, J. E., Stapczynski, J., Ma, O., Yealy, D. M., Meckler, G. D., & Cline, D. M. (2016). *Tintinalli's emergency medicine: A comprehensive study guide* (8th ed.) McGraw-Hill.

STEPS TO PERFORMING THE PROCEDURE

1. Risk stratification. Consider the risk-benefit ratio of rapid sequence intubation in the patient, given the specific circumstances. Assess resources for potentially difficult airways.
2. Preoxygenation. Increase patient's reserve by utilizing 100% FiO_2 through devices such as nasal cannula or BiPAP if able to maintain ventilation. Otherwise, provide 100% FiO_2 through bag valve mask ventilation. Oxygen via nasal cannula can be continued during the intubation procedure for passive oxygenation.
3. Assess patient's vital signs, including heart rate and BP. Begin treatment of bradycardia or hypotension at this time. May elect to give lidocaine if concern exists for increased intracranial pressure.
4. Ensure equipment availability. Multiple visualization devices such as laryngoscopes, videoscopes, or bronchoscopes should be available (Figures 34.1–34.3). Backup airway adjuncts such as LMA, obturator airways, nasopharyngeal airways, and oropharyngeal airways should be available in the event that endotracheal intubation is not successful. Cricothyrotomy set should also be available (Figure 34.4). Rigid suction device should be immediately available.
5. Timeout should be performed.
6. Optimize patient positioning.
7. Administer sedative induction agent, immediately followed by neuromuscular blocker.
8. Once blockade has been achieved, proceed with intubation (refer to Chapter 8). Direct laryngoscopy allows passage of the oral endotracheal tube through the vocal cords (Figure 34.5). If visualization is difficult, use the videoscope (Figure 34.6). Confirm placement of endotracheal tube via end-tidal CO_2 detector, absent epigastric sounds, equal chest expansion, bilateral breath sounds, and chest x-ray. Secure endotracheal tube with commercial device or tape per facility protocol.

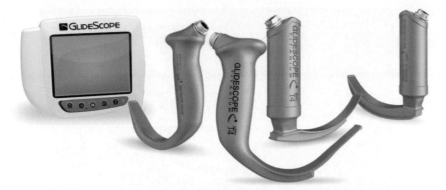

FIGURE 34.1. The GlideScope Titanium series showing both the reusable hyperangulated T3 and T4 blades, and the reusable standard geometry Mac T3 and Mac T4 blades. From Brown, C. A. III, Sakles, J. C., & Mick, N. W. (2017). *Walls manual of emergency airway management* (5th ed.). Wolters Kluwer and The Difficult Airway Course (www.theairwaysite.com). Used with permission.*

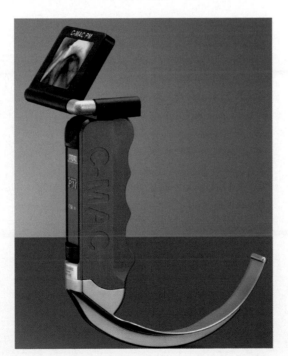

FIGURE 34.2. C-MAC. (A) The C-MAC system with both a rigid Mac blade and a flexible scope attached. (B) The portable C-MAC pocket monitor (PM). From Brown, C. A. III, Sakles, J. C., & Mick, N. W. (2017). *Walls manual of emergency airway management* (5th ed.). Wolters Kluwer and The Difficult Airway Course (www.theairwaysite.com). Used with permission.

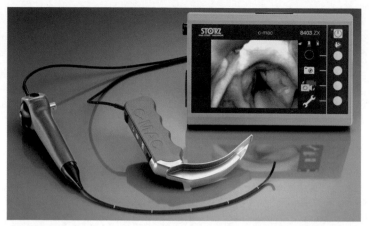

FIGURE 34.3. C-MAC. (A) The C-MAC system with both a rigid Mac blade and a flexible scope attached. (B) The portable C-MAC pocket monitor (PM). From Brown, C.A. III, Sakles, J.C., & Mick, N.W. *Walls Manual of Emergency Airway Management*, 5th Edition. Philadelphia, Wolters Kluwer, 2017 and The Difficult Airway Course (www.theairwaysite.com). Used with permission.

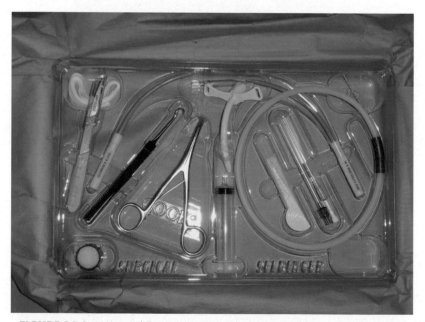

FIGURE 34.4. Universal Emergency Cricothyrotomy Catheter Set (Cook Critical Care, Bloomington, IN). Opened set containing cuffed tracheostomy tube, as well as equipment for both open surgical and Seldinger techniques. From Brown, C. A. III, Sakles, J. C., & Mick, N. W. (2017). *Walls manual of emergency airway management* (5th ed.). Wolters Kluwer and The Difficult Airway Course (www.theairwaysite.com). Used with permission.

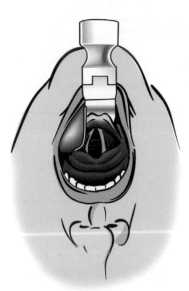

FIGURE 34.5. Direct laryngoscopy with a Macintosh blade. The mouth is opened wide, and the tongue is well controlled and kept entirely to the left by the large flange of the Macintosh blade. The epiglottis is visualized, and the tip of the blade is pushed into the vallecula to elevate the epiglottis and expose the vocal cords. Force is applied by lifting the entire blade upward, not by tilting the butt of the blade toward the upper incisors. From Brown, C. A. III, Sakles, J. C., & Mick, N. W. (2017). *Walls manual of emergency airway management* (5th ed.). Wolters Kluwer and The Difficult Airway Course (www.theairwaysite.com). Used with permission.

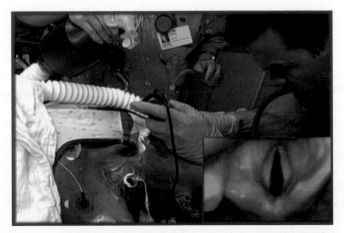

FIGURE 34.6. C-MAC in Clinical Use. The C-MAC being used to intubate a patient with penetrating trauma in the emergency department. From Brown, C. A. III, Sakles, J. C., & Mick, N. W. (2017). *Walls manual of emergency airway management* (5th ed.). Wolters Kluwer and The Difficult Airway Course (www.theairwaysite.com). Used with permission.

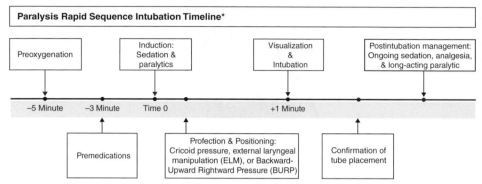

FIGURE 34.7. Rapid sequence intubation. This chart reflects details of the timed sequence of the procedure in the stable patient. It is important to note that all time intervals may be abbreviated by the clinician, when deemed necessary, owing to less than optimal or deteriorating clinical status. Reprinted with permission from Wolfson, A. B., Cloutier, R. L., Hendey, G. W., Ling, L. J., Rosen, C. L., & Schaider, J. J. (2020). *Harwood-Nuss' clinical practice of emergency medicine* (7th ed.). Wolters-Kluwer.

9. Provide long-term sedation and analgesia as indicated.
10. Timeline (Figure 34.7).

COMPLICATIONS OF THE PROCEDURE

1. **Failure to secure airway:** Manual ventilation will be required, possibly with adjunct of airway equipment such as nasopharyngeal or oropharyngeal airways. Other devices, such as LMA or obturator airways, should be readily available in the event of an emergency. In rare instances, cricothyrotomy might be required to establish airway. Failure to manage this complication could lead to death.
2. **Hypotension:** Use of IV fluid boluses or vasopressor agents (phenylephrine, norepinephrine [Levophed], epinephrine) may be required to restore perfusion.
3. **Awareness:** This may result from the use of neuromuscular blockade in the setting of too little or ineffective sedation. Significant psychological stress can occur secondary to awareness during paralysis and the procedure of intubation. Ensure proper sedation prior to and extending through the duration of neuromuscular blockade.
4. **Hyperkalemia:** Hyperkalemia can occur owing to extracellular shifting potassium when using succinylcholine. Risk of hyperkalemia is higher in those with renal failure, crush injuries, major trauma, or burns.

POSTPROCEDURE CARE

After rapid sequence intubation, long-term sedation should be provided because the paralysis will likely last longer than the initial dose of sedation. Analgesia should also be considered. If neuromuscular blockade should be continued, continuous sedation is imperative. Bispectral monitoring should be utilized to ensure adequacy of sedation during paralysis. Effectiveness of the neuromuscular blockade can be assessed with a train-of-four device (peripheral nerve stimulator used to assess neuromuscular transmission when neuromuscular blocking agents are administered to block musculoskeletal activity).

BIBLIOGRAPHY

Lafferty, K. A. (2019). *Rapid sequence intubation.* Retrieved December 16, 2019 from https://emedicine .medscape.com/article/80222-overview

Tintinalli, J. E., Stapczynski, J., Ma, O., Yealy, D. M., Meckler, G. D., & Cline, D. M. (Eds.) (2016). *Tintinalli's emergency medicine: A comprehensive study guide* (8th ed.). McGraw-Hill.

Vissers, R. J., Danzl, D. F., & Serrano, K. (2016). Intubation and mechanical ventilation. In J. E. Tintinalli, J. Stapczynski, O. Ma, D. M. Yealy, G. D. Meckler, & D. M. Cline (Eds.). *Tintinalli's emergency medicine: A comprehensive study guide (8th ed.).* McGraw-Hill. Retrieved from http://accessmedicine.mhmedical. com.ezproxy2.library.drexel.edu/content.aspx?bookid=1658&sectionid=109427490

Basics of Mechanical Ventilation

Janice K. Delgiorno

INDICATIONS FOR THE PROCEDURE

Mechanical ventilation is the process of using positive pressure devices to provide O_2 and CO_2 transport between the environment and the pulmonary capillary bed. The desired effect of mechanical ventilation is to maintain adequate levels of partial pressure of oxygen (PO_2) and partial pressure of carbon dioxide (PCO_2) in arterial blood, while also unloading the inspiratory muscles. This process should be done in a manner that avoids injury to the lungs and other organ systems.

A mechanical ventilator is a machine that takes over and/or assists the patient's breathing when a patient is unable to do so effectively on their own. There are numerous indications for the use of mechanical ventilation in the acute care setting. Mechanical ventilation is used when a patient cannot adequately protect their own airway and maintain breathing during surgical procedures requiring anesthesia or when the patient develops hypoxic or hypercarbic respiratory failure from illness or injury. A mechanical ventilator is used to decrease the patient's work of breathing until they improve enough and no longer require it. The mechanical ventilator ensures that the patient receives oxygen and eliminates carbon dioxide. Mechanical ventilation is used to provide machine delivered breaths, oxygen, and/or support to augment a patient's spontaneous breathing. The main purpose of mechanical ventilation is to allow the patient time to heal. Indications for the procedure are as follows:

1. Apnea: Apneic patients need immediate institution of mechanical ventilation
2. Airway protection in a patient who is obtunded or has a dynamic airway, for example, from trauma, burns, or oropharyngeal infection
3. Clinical signs of increased work of breathing from a disease process such as asthma, chronic obstructive pulmonary disease (COPD), pneumonia, cardiogenic pulmonary edema, and acute respiratory distress syndrome (ARDS)
4. Hypercarbic respiratory failure from a decrease in minute ventilation, e.g., from anesthesia, opiates, or trauma
5. Cardiovascular distress where mechanical ventilation can offload some of the energy requirements for breathing
6. Respiratory distress that failed to respond to noninvasive ventilation (Figure 35.1)

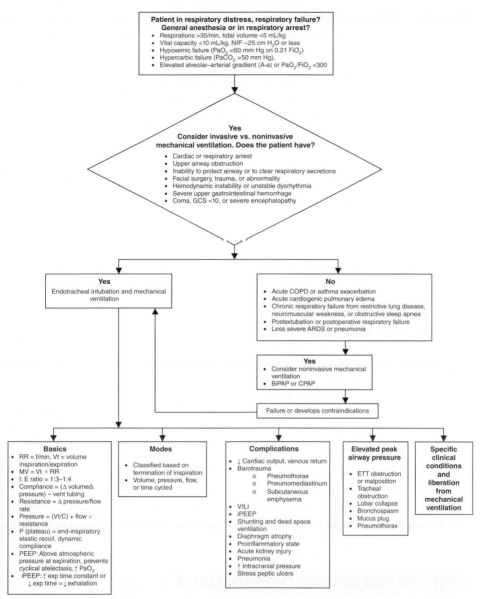

FIGURE 35.1. Decision making for ventilatory assistance. Reprinted with permission from Yunen, J. R. (2012). *5-Minute ICU Consult*. Lippincott Williams & Wilkins.

CONTRAINDICATIONS FOR THE PROCEDURE

The only absolute contraindication to mechanical ventilation is a patient's expressed request for **no intubation** as mechanical ventilation is typically delivered via an endotracheal tube. The patient with a tracheostomy may also indicate **no mechanical**

ventilation, which would contraindicate the procedure. The acute care nurse practitioner (ACNP) must know if any legal documents exist and are in the record.

Relative Contraindications

1. Noninvasive ventilation is indicated/preferred over mechanical ventilation to prevent intubation in a select group of patients, who may be difficult to wean off mechanical ventilation. Examples would include, but not be limited to, patients who are morbidly obese, have COPD, or older adults.
2. Initiation of mechanical ventilation, in addition to other life-saving measures, would be futile.
3. Mechanical ventilation is contrary to the patient's expressed wishes per the family.

Absolute Contraindications

The absolute contraindication to mechanical ventilation is the legal notification of the ACNP that the procedure should be avoided by presentation of a legal document such as a living will or physician orders for life-sustaining treatment (POLST) form (see https:// polst.org/wp-content/uploads/2020/05/2020.05.11-National-POLST-Form-with-Instructions.pdf).

EQUIPMENT NEEDED

1. Mechanical ventilator with a disposable breathing circuit: Safety check performed and circuit checked for leaks.
2. Oxygen and air sources that are 50 PSI (pounds per square inch).
3. Bag valve mask with oxygen tubing connected to an oxygen source via flowmeter. The bag should have a positive end-expiratory pressure (PEEP) valve if indicated.
4. Stethoscope.
5. End tidal CO_2 detector.
6. Suction source, suction catheters.
7. Code cart with airway equipment.
8. Prior to initiating mechanical ventilation, the patient will need to have a definitive airway. A definitive airway is a cuffed endotracheal tube or a cuffed tracheostomy tube.

STEPS TO PERFORMING THE PROCEDURE

Ventilators and modes of ventilation have become more complex. For simplicity, this will focus on getting the patient started on mechanical ventilation. Advanced modes of ventilation can be used, if needed, after initiating the patient on basic mechanical ventilator settings.

1. Perform the Standard Steps (see Preface).
2. Turn the mechanical ventilator on and select settings (see later).
3. Connect the patient to the breathing circuit.

Selecting Ventilator Settings

Anytime a clinician is considering initiating mechanical ventilation on a patient, it is important to fully understand the patient's history, reason for ventilatory assistance, anatomy, and goal of ventilation. Any of these factors can potentially dictate settings.

Prior to choosing ventilator settings, decide whether you are going to ventilate using a *set amount of volume* for each breath or *a set amount of pressure* for each breath. If you choose to deliver a set volume with each breath, the pressure required to deliver the breath will depend on the compliance of the patient's lungs. If the patient's lungs are "stiff," such as in ARDS, it will take a great amount of pressure to deliver the breath. If the patient's lungs are more elastic, such as in COPD, it will take a little pressure to deliver the breath. High airway pressures can lead to barotrauma. If you choose to deliver a set pressure with each breath, then the tidal volume will be variable based on the patient's lung compliance.

Once you decide that you are going to use a volume or pressure mode, decide whether the patient will require full support, i.e., breaths delivered by the ventilator only. The alternative, if the patient is breathing spontaneously, is that they need some assistance from the ventilator or are able to breathe on their own and can be on a spontaneous mode.

Specific ventilator settings include:

- **Mode of ventilation:** Assist control, pressure control, synchronized intermittent mandatory ventilation, pressure support (for spontaneously breathing patients). The first three modes are all appropriate for patients that require ventilatory support when mechanical ventilation is initiated. In order to choose the best mode of ventilation, it is important to understand the patient's level of consciousness, medical condition, and type of ventilator being used (Figure 35.2).
- **Tidal Volume:** 6 to 8 mL/kg (use ideal body weight for the patient's height). Most patients will require at least 500 mL tidal volume.
- **Rate:** How many breaths per minute you want to deliver: 10 to 12 breaths/minute are usually good for a start.
- **FiO$_2$:** Begin with 100% and titrate down by pulse oximeter and arterial blood gas (ABG) monitoring. The goal is an FiO$_2$ less than 60% to prevent oxygen toxicity (Figure 35.3).
- **PEEP:** PEEP increases alveolar pressure and alveolar volume. Prior to intubation, humans have approximately +5 cm H$_2$O of PEEP in their airways. After intubation, this goes away. It is standard practice to add +5 cm H$_2$O PEEP to simulate physiologic PEEP. Adding PEEP can help to recruit and distend collapsed alveoli, thus increasing oxygenation. PEEP is usually increased in increments of +2.5 cm H$_2$O.
- **Pressure Support:** Pressure support is added to augment a patient's spontaneous breaths. When a patient takes a spontaneous breath, the ventilator delivers a boost of air to enhance the patient's spontaneous volume. Pressure support of approximately +8 cm H$_2$O is needed, not required to overcome the resistance of the ventilator circuit and to assist a patient's spontaneous breathing ability. Pressure support can be titrated up to provide increased support during spontaneous breathing.

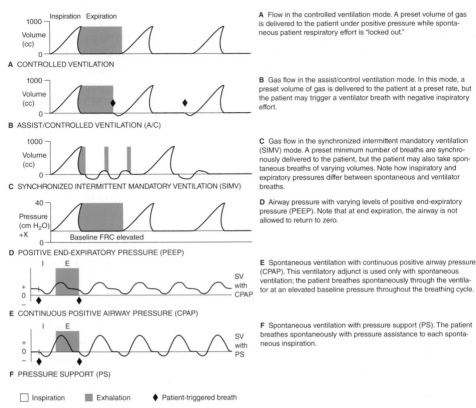

A **CONTROLLED VENTILATION**

A Flow in the controlled ventilation mode. A preset volume of gas is delivered to the patient under positive pressure while spontaneous patient respiratory effort is "locked out."

B **ASSIST/CONTROLLED VENTILATION (A/C)**

B Gas flow in the assist/control ventilation mode. In this mode, a preset volume of gas is delivered to the patient at a preset rate, but the patient may trigger a ventilator breath with negative inspiratory effort.

C **SYNCHRONIZED INTERMITTENT MANDATORY VENTILATION (SIMV)**

C Gas flow in the synchronized intermittent mandatory ventilation (SIMV) mode. A preset minimum number of breaths are synchronously delivered to the patient, but the patient may also take spontaneous breaths of varying volumes. Note how inspiratory and expiratory pressures differ between spontaneous and ventilator breaths.

D **POSITIVE END-EXPIRATORY PRESSURE (PEEP)**

D Airway pressure with varying levels of positive end-expiratory pressure (PEEP). Note that at end expiration, the airway is not allowed to return to zero.

E **CONTINUOUS POSITIVE AIRWAY PRESSURE (CPAP)**

E Spontaneous ventilation with continuous positive airway pressure (CPAP). This ventilatory adjunct is used only with spontaneous ventilation; the patient breathes spontaneously through the ventilator at an elevated baseline pressure throughout the breathing cycle.

F **PRESSURE SUPPORT (PS)**

F Spontaneous ventilation with pressure support (PS). The patient breathes spontaneously with pressure assistance to each spontaneous inspiration.

☐ Inspiration ▪ Exhalation ◆ Patient-triggered breath

FIGURE 35.2. Modes of mechanical ventilation with airflow waveforms. Reprinted with permission from Smeltzer, S. C., & Bare, B. G. (2000). *Textbook of medical-surgical nursing* (9th ed.). Lippincott Williams & Wilkins.

COMPLICATIONS OF MECHANICAL VENTILATION

Although mechanical ventilation is usually a life-saving intervention, there are many possible complications, including, but not limited to:

1. **Unplanned extubation:** This situation is urgent, and sometimes emergent. Assess the patient's respiratory status immediately. If the patient is not breathing adequately and/or unable to protect their airway, they will require reintubation. Utilize the bag/valve/mask to ventilate the patient until the patient can be reintubated.

2. **Barotrauma:** Barotrauma refers to alveolar rupture caused by elevated transalveolar pressure. This can manifest as pneumothorax, pneumomediastinum, pneumoperitoneum, and/or subcutaneous emphysema. The key to prevention is keeping the plateau pressures less than 35 cm H_2O. This can be achieved by treating the underlying cause, e.g., use of bronchodilators, lowering the tidal volume, lowering the flow rate, increasing sedation, or all of them combined. If there is suspicion of barotrauma, investigation should begin with a chest x-ray.

Arterial Blood Gas Interpretation Reference			
Normal range: pH 7.35–7.45, $PaCO_2$ 35–45 mm Hg, PaO_2 80–100 mm Hg, HCO_3 22–26 mEq/L			
Disorder	**pH**	**Primary disturbance**	**Compensation**
Respiratory acidosis	↓	↑PCO_2	↑HCO_3
Respiratory alkalosis	↑	↓PCO_2	↓HCO_3
Metabolic acidosis	↓	↓HCO_3	↓PCO_2
Metabolic alkalosis	↑	↑HCO_3	↑PCO_2

FIGURE 35.3. Arterial blood gas references. Reprinted with permission from Seffinger, M. (2019). *Foundations of osteopathic medicine* (4th ed.). Wolters Kluwer Health.

3. **Hemodynamic effects:** Positive pressure ventilation (PPV) causes decreased venous return, which results in decreased cardiac output. It also compresses the pulmonary vasculature, leading to reduced right ventricular output. PEEP also artificially elevates central venous pressure (CVP) and pulmonary capillary wedge pressure (PCWP). Fluid resuscitation usually helps to correct hypotension caused by PPV.

4. **Ventilator-associated pneumonia (VAP):** Most intensive care units have VAP prevention bundles that include things such as elevation of the head of the bed, frequent oral care, minimizing sedation/paralysis, using chlorhexidine mouth rinse, and frequent suctioning of subglottic secretions. A combination of new onset of fever (greater than 101.5), purulent sputum, leukocytosis, and decreased PaO_2 should prompt further investigation. Consolidation seen on chest x-ray in conjunction with leukocytosis and/or purulent sputum is enough to begin empiric treatment. To determine appropriate antibiotics, a bronchial aspirate lavage should be obtained from the lower respiratory tract.

5. **Respiratory distress:** The patient who is connected to the ventilator may develop respiratory distress from displacement of the endotracheal tube, obstruction of the ventilatory system, or equipment failure. The ACNP will need to troubleshoot the situation (Figure 35.4).

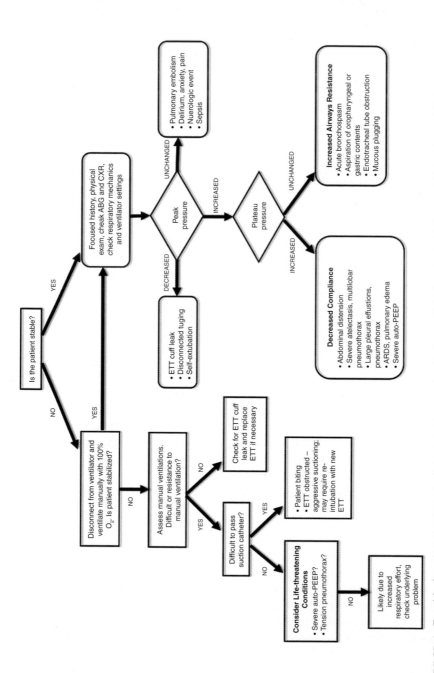

FIGURE 35.4. Troubleshooting respiratory distress in the mechanically ventilated patient. ABG, arterial blood gas; ARDS, acute respiratory distress syndrome; CXR, chest X-ray; ETT, endotracheal tube; PEEP, positive end-expiratory pressure. Reprinted with permission from Herzog, E. (2017). *Herzog's CCU book.* Wolters Kluwer.

TABLE 35.1 Ventilator Changes Based on the Arterial Blood Gases

Oxygenation	Ventilation
ABG: PaO_2 Goal 80–100 (ARDS ≥55)	PCO_2 Goal 40
Vent settings PEEP and FiO_2	Vent settings TV and RR
If PaO_2 is low, increase FiO_2 or PEEP	If PCO_2 is high >45, increase TV and/or RR
If PaO_2 is high, decrease FiO_2 or PEEP	If PCO_2 is low <35, decrease TV and/or RR

POSTPROCEDURE CARE

After placing the patient on mechanical ventilation, an ABG should be obtained after approximately thirty minutes (Table 35.1). This allows time for the patient to stabilize on the ventilator and for the clinician to evaluate the appropriateness of the settings. This ABG will help determine whether any ventilator changes are indicated. Keep in mind that the FiO_2 should be weaned to 60% or less, as able, to prevent oxygen toxicity. Adjustments to the rate and/or tidal volume will affect the PCO_2. Adjustments to PEEP and FiO_2 will affect the PaO_2.

As the patient's medical course progresses, the patient may progress to being weaned from the ventilator. The respiratory therapist will obtain weaning parameters to determine whether the patient is likely to be able to maintain a sufficient respiratory status off the ventilator.

BIBLIOGRAPHY

Barrot, L., Asfar, P., Mauny, F., Winiszewski, H., Montini, F., Badie, J., Quenot, J.-P., Pili-Floury, S., Bouhemad, B., Louis, G., Souweine, B., Collange, O., Pottecher, J., Levy, B., Puyraveau, M., Vettoretti, L., Constantin, J.-M., & Capellier, G. (2020). Liberal or conservative oxygen therapy for acute respiratory distress syndrome. *New England Journal of Medicine, 382*(11), 999–1008. https://doi.org/10.1056/NEJMoa1916431

MacIntyre, N. R., & Branson, R. D. (2009). *Mechanical ventilation*. Saunders Elsevier.

36 Oxygen Therapy

Janice K. Delgiorno

Oxygen is the most commonly used drug in the critical and acute care settings. The advanced practice nurse (APN) must review the arterial blood gas (ABG) closely (see Chapter 34) and determine the underlying cause of hypoxemia, because most applications of oxygen treat hypoxemia but not hypoventilation.

Supplemental oxygen therapy may provide the patient with extra oxygen to support vital bodily functions. Supplemental oxygen enables the delivery of oxygen concentrations of (FiO_2) of 22% to 100% depending on the type of device you are using. High-flow oxygen may supplement ventilation in addition to supplying oxygen.

INDICATIONS FOR THE PROCEDURE

Primary indications are:

1. Documentation of hypoxemia, defined as PaO_2 lower than the normal range; usually, PaO_2 is less than 60 mmHg or SaO_2 is less than 90%
2. An acute situation, such as respiratory distress, where hypoxemia is suspected
3. Low cardiac output with metabolic acidosis
4. Severe T = trauma
5. Carbon monoxide toxicity
6. Acute myocardial infarction with hypoxemia
7. Hypotension (systolic blood pressure (BP) less than 100 mmHg)
8. Postanesthesia recovery

Secondary indications are:

1. Pneumothorax
2. Acute myocardial infarction without hypoxemia
3. Sickle cell pain crisis
4. Dyspnea without hypoxemia (palliative)

CONTRAINDICATIONS FOR THE PROCEDURE

Caution should be used when administering oxygen, which has the potential to be toxic. At high oxygen concentrations, there is overproduction of oxygen free radicals that can be damaging to cells. However, with a few exceptions it is rarely contraindicated.

Relative Contraindications

1. **Chronic obstructive pulmonary disease (COPD):** In patients with COPD, they sometimes have a hypoxic drive to breathe. The use of oxygen will raise the patient's PaO_2 and decrease the patient's hypoxic drive. It is essential to monitor for decreased respirations when used in patients with COPD, because elimination of hypoxia may result in hypoventilation.
2. **High fever:** Concomitant use of oxygen in patients with high fever raises the potential for seizures.
3. **Bleomycin use:** Bleomycin is an antineoplastic agent with potential for producing pulmonary toxicity, attributable in part to its free radical-promoting ability. Anecdotal evidence and animal experimentations have suggested that the risk of bleomycin-induced pulmonary injury is increased with the administration of high concentrations of oxygen.
4. **Pregnancy:** There is nonhuman experimental evidence in animals that exposure to oxygen during early pregnancy increases the risk of congenital malformations.

Absolute Contraindications

1. **Paraquat (common herbicide) poisoning** unless the patient is suffering from severe respiratory distress or respiratory arrest, because this can increase the toxicity. Paraquat is used as a herbicide in Asia, and poisoning is rare.
2. **No patient consent:** Patient does not consent to receiving oxygen therapy.

EQUIPMENT NEEDED

1. A source of oxygen: Concentrator, oxygen tank, oxygen medical gas wall outlet (Figure 36.1)
2. An oxygen flowmeter with a nipple adapter if needed for the delivery device (Figure 36.2)
3. Extension tubing if needed
4. Humidification, if indicated for the oxygen delivery device (Figure 36.3)
5. An oxygen delivery device such as a nasal cannula (Figure 36.4A), simple face mask (Figure 36.4B), nonrebreather mask (Figure 36.4C), BiPAP/CPAP mask (Figure 36.4D)
6. A pulse oximeter to monitor the patient's response to oxygen therapy

OXYGEN DELIVERY DEVICES

Choosing an Oxygen Delivery Device

In order to effectively choose an oxygen delivery device, the APN needs to be familiar with oxygen delivery devices. Each device requires the careful consideration of the clinical status of the patient because the ability to comfortably maintain the system is of paramount importance. Additionally, the required dose of oxygen has an impact on the selection, because 1 liter of oxygen increases the percentage of inhaled gas from 21% (room air) to 24% (1 L/minute). Oxygen does not improve respiratory rate and is therefore indicated in hypoxic nonhypercarbic patients.

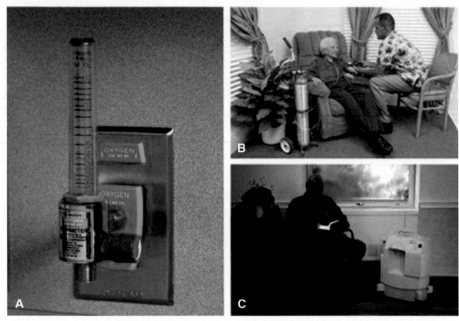

FIGURE 36.1. Oxygen sources. (A) Gas wall outlet; (B) pressurized tank; (C) concentrator. Reprinted with permission from Carter, P. J. (2019). *Lippincott acute care skills for advanced nursing assistants*. Wolters Kluwer.

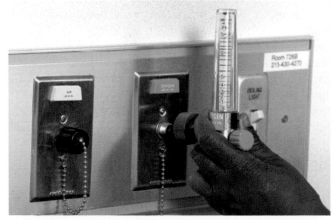

FIGURE 36.2. Flowmeter and resuscitation bag tubing that does not require a nipple adapter. Reprinted with permission from Gregory, D., Stephens, T., Raymond-Seniuk, C., & Patrick, L. (2014). *Fundamentals: Perspectives on the art and science of Canadian nursing*. Wolters Kluwer.

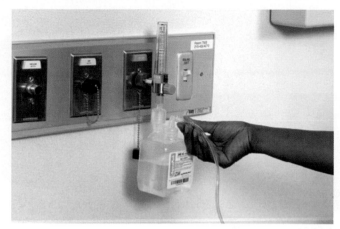

FIGURE 36.3. Humidification bottle and oxygen tubing attached to flow meter. Reprinted with permission from Gregory, D., Stephens, T., Raymond-Seniuk, C., & Patrick, L. (2014). *Fundamentals: Perspectives on the art and science of Canadian nursing.* Wolters Kluwer.

Types of Oxygen Delivery Devices

1. **Nasal cannula:** Suitable for most patients. At a flow rate of up to 2 to 6 L/minute gives approximately 24% to 40% FiO_2. Its advantages include comfort to the patient and ease of tolerance by patients *versus* simple mask, its low cost, and its nonrebreathing property. A humidifier should be added at flow rates of 4 L/minute and greater.
2. **Simple face mask:** It is a variable performance device, delivering variable FiO_2 between 35% and 60% at flow rates of 5 to 10 L/minute.
3. **Venturi/fixed performance mask:** It aims to deliver a constant oxygen concentration within and between breaths. Venturi masks are available with color-coded nozzles for desired FiO_2: 24%—blue; 28%—white, 35%—yellow, 40%—red; 60%—green. 24% to 40% venturi masks operate accurately; however, a 60% venturi mask gives approximately 50% FiO_2.
4. **High concentration reservoir mask (nonrebreather/partial rebreather):** It is a nonrebreathing reservoir mask and delivers oxygen concentration between 60% and 80%. It is effective for short-term treatment in critical illness, trauma patients, and postcardiac arrest.
5. **Tracheostomy collar for patients with tracheostomy or laryngectomy:** These are variable performance collars designed for neck-breathing patients. They fit comfortably over a tracheostomy and have an exhalation port on the front of the neck. These masks are usually a venturi device with an aerosol to provide humidity.
6. **High-flow nasal cannula:** The delivery of heated and humidified oxygen occurs. Clinical effects are mainly dependent on flow, oxygen concentration, and temperature. High flow at 50 L/minute has been shown to improve work of breathing and assist in avoiding intubation in patients with parenchymal lung disease.

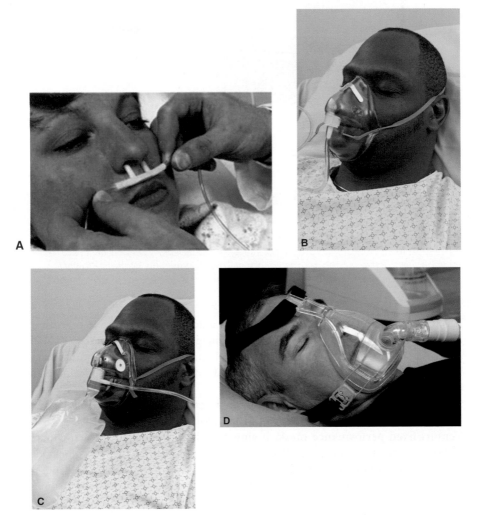

FIGURE 36.4. Devices used for oxygen delivery. (A) A nasal cannula is a two-pronged device that is inserted into the nostrils to deliver oxygen to the patient or resident. A person who has a nasal cannula in place is able to eat, drink, and speak normally. (B) A face mask fits over the person's nose and mouth. It may be used when a person requires a high level of supplemental oxygen. Face masks come in a variety of styles. A simple face mask delivers oxygen at a rate of 6 to 10 L/minute. Holes in the side of a simple facemask let room air in and carbon dioxide out. (C) A nonrebreather mask delivers oxygen at a rate of 10 to 15 L/minute. A valve lets carbon dioxide out without letting in room air. The oxygen flows through the bag. (D) A continuous positive airway pressure (CPAP) mask delivers air and oxygen under pressure. The pressure keeps the airways open and enhances gas exchange in the alveoli. Reprinted with permission from Carter, P. J. (2019). *Lippincott acute care skills for advanced nursing assistants*. Wolters Kluwer.

STEPS TO PERFORMING THE PROCEDURE

1. Assess the patient's respiratory status, including SaO_2, depth and rate of respirations, accessory muscle use, and vital signs.
2. Choose an oxygen delivery device.
3. Ensure the device is connected to the oxygen source at the appropriate flow rate.
4. Explain the procedure to the patient.
5. Place the oxygen delivery device on the patient's face or over the tracheostomy tube.
6. Monitor the patient's response to the oxygen therapy via pulse oximetry.
7. Titrate the oxygen based on the patient's response to oxygen therapy. A typical goal SaO_2 would be between 92% and 98%. Patients with COPD may tolerate SaO_2 of 88% to 92%, especially if they have a hypoxic drive that puts them at risk for type II respiratory failure.
8. High-flow oxygen may be delivered via a nasal cannula and supplies oxygen, humidification, and warmth (Figure 36.5). High flow nasal cannula eliminates nasopharyngeal dead space impediment of oxygen, increases nasopharyngeal airway pressure with a "positive end-expiratory pressure (PEEP)" effect, eliminates room air mixing, and increases oxygen delivery to the alveoli. High-flow nasal cannula should be considered for patients who require high-flow oxygen via a mask for more than one day and who do not improve with 50% oxygen via mask. Order the flow (5 – 60 mL/minute) and oxygen percentage. Titrate up the flow before the oxygen percentage to achieve adequate saturation.

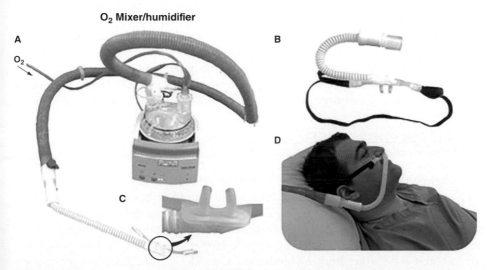

O$_2$ Mixer/humidifier

FIGURE 36.5. Apparatus for support by high-flow nasal cannula (HFNC). A: Complete circuit including humidifier. B,C: Nasal cannulae. D: Application of HFNC. Used with permission from Marini, J. J., & Dries, D. J. (2018). *Critical care medicine* (5th ed.). Wolters Kluwer Health.

COMPLICATIONS OF THE PROCEDURE

Oxygen therapy can have harmful effects, which are dependent on the duration and intensity of the oxygen therapy, such as the following:

1. **Nasal irritation:** Many patients get supplemental oxygen through a nasal cannula—a flexible plastic tubing with prongs that fit into the nose. Over time, the cannula may irritate the lining of the nose, causing soreness or occasional bleeding. Employing a nasal cannula of a different style or size or changing to a face mask oxygen delivery system alleviates this problem for most patients.

2. **Oxygen-induced hypoventilation/ hypoxic drive:** If patients with a hypoxic drive are given a high concentration of oxygen, their primary urge to breathe is removed, and hypoventilation or apnea may occur. It is important to note that not all COPD patients have chronic retention of CO_2 and that not all patients with CO_2 retention have a hypoxic drive. It is not commonly seen in clinical practice. Never deprive any patient of oxygen if it is clinically indicated. It is usually acceptable to administer whatever concentration of oxygen is needed to maintain the SaO_2 between 88% and 92% in patients with known chronic CO_2 retention verified by an arterial blood gas (ABG) test.

3. **Absorption atelectasis:** About 80% of the gas in the alveoli is nitrogen. If high concentrations of oxygen are provided, the nitrogen is displaced. When the oxygen diffuses across the alveolar–capillary membrane into the bloodstream, the nitrogen is no longer present to distend the alveoli, called a nitrogen washout. This reduction in alveolar volume results in a form of collapse, called absorption atelectasis.

4. **Oxygen toxicity:** It is caused by excessive or inappropriate supplemental oxygen and can severely damage the lungs and other organ systems. High concentrations of oxygen, over a certain period, can increase free radical formation. Free radical formation leads to damage to membranes, proteins, and cell structures in the lungs. It can cause a wide spectrum of lung injuries ranging from mild tracheobronchitis to diffuse alveolar damage. It is imperative to wean a patient's oxygen as tolerated.

POSTPROCEDURE CARE

Continue to monitor the patient's SaO_2 via pulse oximetry, and ensure you are within your desired target. Titrate oxygen as needed to achieve the desired target. Wean the FiO_2 as able to prevent oxygen toxicity. If indicated, humidify the oxygen for the patient's comfort. Patients requiring increasing doses of oxygen to maintain saturations within the desired target or those with signs of respiratory deterioration (increasing respiratory rate, drowsiness, accessory muscle use) require further assessment, including obtaining an ABG test and further studies as indicated. Consider discontinuing oxygen therapy once the patient has stable saturations (at least two consecutive recordings) within their target range on low-dose oxygen (e.g., 1–2 L/minute via nasal cannula).

BIBLIOGRAPHY

Feldman, D (2020). *Bleomycin induced lung injury. UpToDate, Topic 4316 Version 26.0.* Retrieved from https://www.uptodate.com/contents/bleomycin-induced-lung-injury

Frat, J. P., Thille, A. W., Mercat, A., Girault, C., Ragot, S., Perbet, S., Prat, G., Boulain, T., Morawiec, E., Cottereau, A., Devaquet, J., Nseir, S., Razazi, K., Mira, J.-P., Argaud, L., Chakarian, J.-C., Ricard, J.-D., Wittebole, X., Chevalier, S., … Robert, R. (2015). High-flow oxygen through nasal cannula in acute hypoxemic respiratory failure. *New England Journal of Medicine, 372*(23), 2185–2196. https://doi .org/10.1056/NEJMoa1503326

Gawarammana, I. B., & Buckley, N. A. (2011). Medical management of paraquat ingestion. *British Journal of Clinical Pharmacology, 72*(5), 745–757. https://doi.org/10.1111/j.1365-2125.2011.04026.x

Hyzy, R. (2020). *Heated and humidified high-flow nasal oxygen in adults: Practical considerations and potential applications. UpToDate, Topic 114077 Version 18.0.* Retrieved from https://www.uptodate.com/contents/ heated-and-humidified-high-flow-nasal-oxygen-in-adults-practical-considerations-and-potential- applications

Kacmarek, R. M., Stoller, J. K., Heuer, A. J., Chatburn, R. L., & Kallet, R. H. (2017). *Egan's fundamentals of respiratory care.* Elsevier.

Kane, B., Decalmer, S., & O'Driscoll, B. R. (2013). Emergency oxygen therapy from guideline to implementa- tion. *Breathe* (9), 246–253; https://doi.org/10.1183/20734735.025212

Trauma Assessment

Jennifer Schweinsburg
Salina Wydo

METHOD OF TRAUMA ASSESSMENT

Trauma assessment uses a standardized method to assess a patient and quickly develop a differential diagnosis in order to move toward effective treatment. In this way, the most life-threatening conditions are identified and handled first, followed by a more thorough assessment of the patient's traumatic injuries. This method, although classically described in the setting of traumatic injuries, can be modified and applied to any emergency to help the clinician prioritize the patient's medical needs (Figure 37.1).

STEPS TO PERFORMING THE ASSESSMENT

It is important to note that throughout the assessment, the ABCs (airway, breathing, and circulation) should be continually reassessed and intervened on if compromise is noted. Also, any life-threatening injury should take priority over performing a secondary or tertiary survey.

Primary Survey

The primary survey, also known by the mnemonic ABCDE (Airway, Breathing, Circulation, Disability, Exposure/Environmental), is a rapid, systematic approach to the assessment of the trauma patient. It prioritizes the body's most vital systems, beginning with the airway and hemodynamic stability and followed by a system-based focused assessment.

Airway

1. Assess for airway obstruction or signs of impending obstruction. Ask a simple question. If the patient is able to phonate comfortably with normal voice, the airway is patent. Signs of concern include inability to phonate, garbled speech, hoarseness, or changes in pitch/voice quality.
2. Visually inspect the oropharynx for foreign bodies.
3. Briefly assess mental status, because depressed mental status should raise concerns for the patient's ability to drive oxygenation and ventilation, as well for their ability to avoid aspiration of oral secretions or vomitus. As a general rule, if the Glasgow Coma Scale (GCS) is less than 8, proceed to intubate. (See section "Disability")

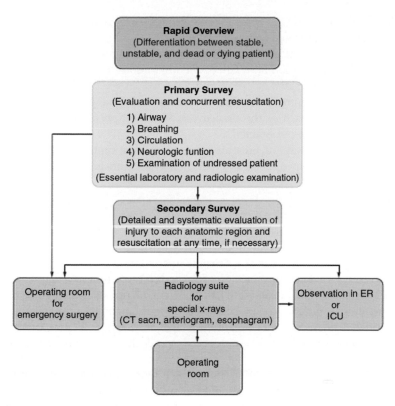

FIGURE 37.1. The general approach to evaluation of acute trauma patients includes the sequential steps of rapid overview, primary survey, and secondary survey. CT, computed tomography; ED, emergency department; ICU, intensive care unit. Reprinted with permission from Barash, P. G., Cullen, B. F., Stoelting, R. K., Cahalan, M., & Stock, M. C. (2009). *Handbook of clinical anesthesia* (6th ed.). Wolters Kluwer.

4. If concerns regarding the patency or protection of airway arise, several different techniques can be used to restore patency, culminating in the acquisition of a stable artificial airway if needed. By degrees of invasiveness/escalation:

   a. Chin lift/jaw thrust maneuver may be performed by placing fingers at the angle of the mandible and lifting the jaw anteriorly, using caution to keep the cervical spine midline and nonmobile. This serves to temporarily restore airway patency by lifting the posterior pharyngeal tissues out of the airway.

   b. Oral or nasopharyngeal airways may also be used as a bridge to obtaining a stable airway, especially in those with depressed mental status (oral airways are poorly tolerated in patients with an intact gag reflex and may increase risk of aspiration). In addition, one should apply 100% oxygen by non-rebreather. If this is inadequate to maintain oxygenation, the patient may be supported via bag valve mask until a secure endotracheal airway can be obtained.

   c. The gold standard is endotracheal intubation. Although detailed description of the procedure is beyond the scope of this chapter, it is important to note that the most reliable way to encourage oxygenation and ventilation is via appropriately placed and secured endotracheal tube.

d. If there is significant facial trauma or disfiguring injury, or if attempts at endotracheal intubation have failed, cricothyroidotomy may be performed in order to establish an airway.

e. It is critically important that in-line cervical spine precautions be maintained throughout each of the maneuvers described previously until cervical spine clearance may be obtained.

f. Note that airway and breathing issues may exist simultaneously (manifesting as hypoxia or hypercarbia) and that their evaluation and treatment may overlap.

Breathing

This is an assessment of the patient's ability to oxygenate and ventilate (exchange carbon dioxide). The patient should be connected to a monitor, including continuous pulse oximetry, and the respiratory rate should be noted. The clinician should also assess the patient's work of breathing, taking care to note intercostal muscle retractions, nasal flaring, and/or paradoxical chest wall motion (unexpected retraction of a segment of the chest wall during inspiration, indicative of flail chest/rib fractures). These signs are concerning for impending respiratory collapse caused by fatigue, and mechanical ventilation should be considered. If the patient's breathing is agonal, gasping, or slow, or inadequate to ensure oxygenation and ventilation, proceed to endotracheal intubation and mechanical ventilation.

Focused physical examination, including listening to breath sounds bilaterally and assessing for tracheal deviation, should be continued. Absence of breath sounds unilaterally may indicate a pneumothorax; in addition, if hypotension is present (with or without tracheal deviation or jugular venous distension), there is concern for tension pneumothorax. In order to immediately relieve pressure and the resulting tension physiology, the hemithorax of concern should be rapidly decompressed with a large-bore angiocatheter (needle decompression). Once decompressed, a chest tube should be placed in the affected hemithorax. (See Chapter 9 for placement of tube thoracostomy.)

Circulation

The overall goal of the circulatory assessment is to identify and treat causes of hemodynamic abnormalities and shock. Check for a pulse and assess skin color for pallor. BP and pulse should be noted. Two large-bore IV catheters (e.g., 14–18g) are inserted peripherally, and warm IV fluids are administered. Blood samples are obtained and sent to the laboratory. They include type and screen, complete blood count, basic metabolic panel, partial thromboplastin time (PTT) test, and prothrombin time/International Normalized Ratio (PT/INR). Do not delay life-saving care for the acquisition of results of laboratory studies.

If the patient shows age-inappropriate hemodynamic parameters, look for overt signs of bleeding or injuries that indicate massive blood loss. Although other causes of shock may exist in the trauma population, hemorrhage should be considered the cause until proven otherwise, because unrecognized bleeding is one of the most common causes of preventable death in the mature trauma center.

TABLE 37.1 Advanced Trauma Life Support Classification of Hemorrhagic Shock

	Class I	Class II	Class III	Class IV
Blood loss (mL)	Up to 750	750–1,500	1,500–2,000	>2,000
Blood loss (% of blood volume)	Up to 15%	15–30%	20–40%	>40%
Heart rate (bpm)	<100	>100	>120	>140
Systematic blood pressure	Normal	Normal	Decreased	Decreased
Pulse pressure	Normal or increased	Decreased	Decreased	Decreased
Capillary refill test	Normal	Positive	Positive	Positive
Respiratory rate (breaths/min)	14–20	20–30	30–40	<35
Urine output (mL/hr)	>30	20–30	5–15	Negligible
Mental status	Slightly anxious	Mildly anxious	Anxious and confused	Confused and lethargic
Fluid replacement (3:1 rule)	Crystalloid	Crystalloid	Crystalloid and blood	Crystalloid and blood

Reprinted with permission from Barash, P. G., Cullen, B. F., Stoelting, R. K., Cahalan, M., & Stock, M. C. (2009). *Handbook of clinical anesthesia* (6th ed.). Wolters Kluwer.

There are five major compartments into which the adult patient can lose enough blood volume to exsanguinate and should be considered when hemorrhage is suspected, including (Table 37.1):

1. **Chest**—e.g., hemothorax. Chest cavity should be decompressed/blood evacuated by tube thoracostomy. Urgent surgical intervention may be warranted, and timely surgical consult should be initiated.
2. **Abdomen**—e.g., hemoperitoneum
3. **Pelvis/retroperitoneum**—e.g., pelvic fractures, retroperitoneal hematoma
4. **Extremities**—soft tissue surrounding long bones (e.g., femur, humerus)
5. **Environment**—Blood loss happens external to patient (e.g., traumatic amputation, scalp laceration)

Although hemorrhagic shock is a major point of discussion in the trauma assessment, it belongs to a broader category of hypovolemic shock (Figure 37.2). There are four other categories of shock that could be responsible for unexplained hypotension in the trauma patient:

1. **Hypovolemic shock**: Loss of intravascular volume
2. **Distributive shock**: Peripheral vasodilation resulting from sepsis, severe acute pancreatitis, severe inflammatory process, etc.

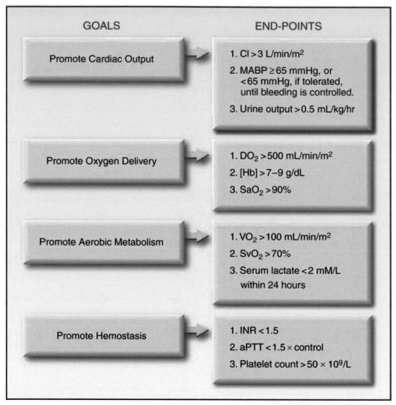

FIGURE 37.2. The general goals and associated end points of resuscitation for hemorrhagic shock. CI = cardiac index; MABP = mean arterial BP; DO_2 = systemic O_2 delivery; [Hb] = hemoglobin concentration in blood; VO_2 = systemic O_2 consumption; SvO_2 = mixed venous O_2 saturation; INR = international normalized ratio; aPTT = activated partial thromboplastin time. Reprinted with permission from Marino, P. L. (2013). *Marino's the ICU book* (4th ed.). Wolters Kluwer.

3. **Neurogenic shock:** Loss of sympathetic tone caused by spinal cord injury
4. **Cardiogenic shock:** Cardiac pump failure, which can result from massive myocardial infarction
5. **Obstructive:** Mechanical obstruction of blood flow into or out of the heart, as occurs in cardiac tamponade, tension pneumothorax.

Disability

A cursory neurologic examination is performed. The pupils should be examined for size, equality, and reactivity. Level of consciousness is assessed by using the GCS (Figure 37.3), which utilizes best eye opening, best verbal response, and best motor response to calculate a score from 3 to 15. During the motor portion of the GCS examination, note any lateralizing signs in motor function. Any alteration in sensorium should prompt a reevaluation of A, B, and C because hypoxia and hypotension can propagate

Glasgow Coma Scale	Best possible total score 15	Worst possible total score 3
Monitored performance	**Reaction**	**Score**
Eye opening	Spontaneous	4
	Open when spoken to	3
	Open at pain stimulus	2
	No reaction	1
Verbal performance	Coherent	5
	Confused, disoriented	4
	Disconnected words	3
	Unintelligible sounds	2
	No verbal reaction	1
Motor responsiveness	Follows instructions	6
	Intentional pain-avoidance	5
	Large motor movement	4
	Flexor synergism	3
	Extensor synergism	2
	No reaction	1

FIGURE 37.3. The Glasgow Coma Scale (GCS). The GCS is scored between 3 and 15, the worst score being 3 and the best score being 15. From Nath, J. (2018). *Programmed learning approach to medical terminology.* Wolters Kluwer.

secondary nervous system injury. Intoxication is on the differential diagnosis for altered mental status but should be a diagnosis of exclusion in the primary survey and can be confirmed later by serum or urine testing.

Exposure/Environmental

Special Considerations

Pregnant patients should be treated with emphasis on the primary survey and triage of life-threatening injuries of the mother. The most common cause of fetal demise in trauma is maternal demise. Fetal assessment should be done only when the mother's life-threatening injuries have been addressed. Early obstetrics consultation is strongly encouraged.

Adjuncts to Primary Survey

X-Ray

Chest x-ray is a standard part of the trauma assessment. If intubation has already occurred, it offers an opportunity to assess the position of the endotracheal tube. Several signs of pathology may be obtained from a simple chest x-ray, including mediastinal shift, pneumothorax (Figure 37.4), hemothorax, and severe displaced rib fractures. X-rays of the pelvis and extremities may also be obtained at this time if there is clinical suspicion of injury.

Extended Focused Assessment with Sonography for Trauma

Extended Focused Assessment with Sonography for Trauma (EFAST) is a quick, noninvasive, cost-effective way to assess the patient for free intra-abdominal fluid. An ultrasound is performed in four locations on the trunk (Figure 37.5): (1) Pericardial view, (2) Right

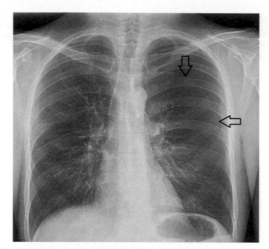

FIGURE 37.4. Use of upright chest radiograph to demonstrate presence of pneumothorax. Reprinted with permission from Daffner, R. H., & Hartman, M. (2013). *Clinical radiology* (4th ed.). Wolters Kluwer.

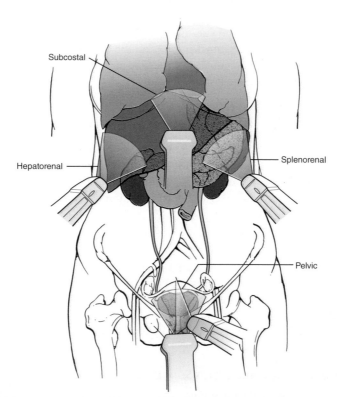

FIGURE 37.5. FAST exam locations. Four sites of focused assessment of sonography for trauma (FAST) examination: subcostal, hepatorenal, spleno-renal, and pelvic. Reprinted with permission from Berg, S. M., Bittner, E. A., & Zhao, K. H. (2016). *Anesthesia review: Blasting the boards*. Wolters Kluwer.

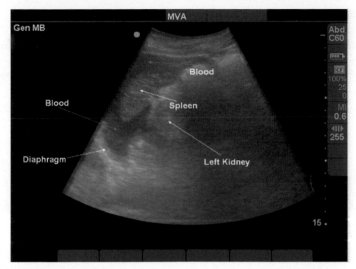

FIGURE 37.6. Photograph of left upper quadrant view with a positive FAST. This FAST examination of the perisplenic space shows significant hemoperitoneum and suggests the need for urgent laparotomy. Reprinted with permission from Bigatello, L. M., Alam, H., Allain, R. M., Bittner, E., & Hess, D. R. (2009). *Critical care handbook of the Massachusetts general hospital* (5th ed.). Lippincott Williams & Wilkins.

upper quadrant encompassing the diaphragm–liver interface, (3) Left upper quadrant encompassing the diaphragm–spleen interface and spleen–kidney interface, and (4) Suprapubic view. Given that fluid appears dark on ultrasound, a positive EFAST will show a dark area in the dependent positions in each of the above-mentioned windows (Figure 37.6).

Secondary Survey

The secondary survey is performed after stabilization of life-threatening injuries and involves a more detailed head-to-toe assessment with the intention of detecting other important but not life-threatening injuries. These include, but are not limited to:

1. Head
   a. Pupils (if not assessed in Disability step)
   b. Ears (pinnae and tympanic membranes)
   c. Dentition (broken/chipped teeth, malocclusion)
2. Neck
   a. Tracheal deviation (if not already assessed in Breathing step)
   b. Jugular venous distension
   c. For crepitus/subcutaneous air
3. Chest
   a. Chest wall deformity, flail chest (if not assessed in Breathing step)
4. Abdomen
   a. Distension, tenderness
   b. Peritoneal signs

5. Pelvis
   a. Pain on palpation, gross instability
   b. May include rectal or vaginal examination if concerned for significant pelvic trauma:
      1. The patient's clothes are removed entirely so as to expose the entire surface area of the body.
      2. Examine the patient in the supine position, from head to toe. Note any obvious injuries, abrasions, penetrating wounds, or deformities.
      3. Then, while maintaining cervical spine precautions, log roll the patient on to the patient's side and examine the back for deformities and penetrating wounds.
      4. Perform a rectal examination at this time, noting rectal tone.
      5. Examine the perineum for ecchymoses and the urethral meatus for blood because this may indicate a urologic injury, and insertion of a urinary Foley catheter should be avoided until further workup is performed.
      6. Once completed, the patient should be covered with warm blankets to prevent hypothermia.
6. Extremities
   a. Pain to palpation, deformity
7. Back
   a. Pain to palpation, step-offs

Consideration for Transfer to a Trauma Center

Patients with substantial injury or the necessity for specialized care and/or resources should be transferred to a trauma center as soon as the need is recognized. Transfer should not be delayed for further imaging or tests.

Further Diagnostic Tests

Once the patient has been stabilized (including procedures and operative intervention if necessary), and the primary and secondary surveys performed, definitive imaging may be obtained.

Computed Tomography

If the patient is hemodynamically appropriate, computed tomography (CT) scans (commonly of the head, chest, abdomen, and pelvis, or some combination thereof) can aid in identifying solid organ injury. Decision to CT scan a patient should be based on their hemodynamic appropriateness, the necessity of other procedures, and the indication for the scans.

Tertiary Survey

The tertiary survey is performed well after the patient has been initially stabilized and transferred to a definitive care setting. A comprehensive physical examination is performed, and imaging studies are reviewed for any previously undiagnosed or unaddressed injuries.

Dawn M. Specht

INDICATIONS FOR THE PROCEDURE

Rapid response systems encompass rapid response teams (RRTs), medical emergency teams, and critical care outreach teams. An RRT should be formed in settings where the early investigation of patient abnormalities may prevent cardiovascular collapse and improve the quality of care delivery. The composition of the team varies in each facility as do the roles served by the team members. There is moderate evidence linking the implementation of RRTs with decreased mortality and nonintensive care unit (ICU) cardiac arrest rates. In the inpatient setting, nurses are trained on early indicators of potential patient deterioration. A policy is developed. A team of nurses and providers typically respond to the rapid response. The nurse practitioner (NP) may function in the emergency to lead the provision of care to these patients during rapid response. The NP-led RRT is a safe and effective alternative to intensivist physician-led teams. The patients may be known or not known to the provider prior to the rapid response alert. Therefore, a uniform approach to the situation should occur. First, prior to a rapid response, the acute care NP should be familiar with the process that the bedside nurse, or even family, may use to initiate the rapid response. It is critical to know the hospital's policy! The Agency for Healthcare Research and Quality identifies the following as common triggers to call a rapid response.

Triggers:

- Heart rate over 140 bpm or less than 40 bpm
- Respiratory rate over 28 breaths/min or less than 8 breaths/min
- Systolic blood pressure greater than 180 mmHg or less than 90 mmHg
- Oxygen saturation less than 90% despite supplementation
- Acute change in mental status
- Urine output less than 50 cc over 4 hours
- Staff member has significant concern about the patient's condition (Table 38.1).

Indications for the procedure (a rapid response) are:

1. Significant vital sign abnormalities
2. Mental status change
3. Cardiac dysrhythmia

TABLE 38.1 Rapid-Sequence Intubation Induction Agents

Agent	Dose	Onset	Duration	Benefits	Caveats
Etomidate	0.3–0.5 mg/kg IV	<1 minute	10–20 minute	↓ICP	Myoclonic jerking or seizures and vomiting in awake patients
				↓Intraocular pressure	No analgesia
				Neutral BP	↓Cortisol
Propofol	0.5–1.5 mg/kg IV	20–40 seconds	8–15 minutes	Antiemetic	Apnea
				Anticonvulsant	↓BP
				↓ICP	No analgesia
Ketamine	1–2 mg/kg IV	1 minute	10–20 minutes	Bronchodilator	↑Secretions
				"Dissociative amnesia"	↑BP
				Analgesia	Emergence phenomenon

BP, blood pressure; ICP, intracranial pressure.
Reprinted with permission from Tintinalli, J. E., Ma, O. J., Yealy, D. M., Meckler, G. D., Stapczynski, J. S., Cline, D. M., & Thomas, S. H. (2020). *Tintinalli's emergency medicine: A comprehensive study guide* (9th ed.). McGraw-Hill LLC.

4. Chest pain
5. Sepsis
6. Symptomatic hypoglycemia
7. Respiratory distress
8. Seizure

CONTRAINDICATIONS FOR THE PROCEDURE

Relative Contraindications

The only relative contraindication to a rapid response would be a patient who is in cardiac arrest and requires a full resuscitation team.

Absolute Contraindications

The only absolute contraindication to initiating a rapid response would be a patient who is currently on hospice and has clearly communicated the desire to receive no further medical treatment.

EQUIPMENT NEEDED

1. Stethoscope
2. Intubation equipment/box containing endotracheal tubes, laryngeal mask airways, oral airways, stylet, bag valve mask, syringe, rapid-sequence intubation medications
3. Glucometer
4. Intravenous (IV) catheters, IV fluid, and blood draw equipment
5. Medications frequently required: respiratory treatments, antibiotics, furosemide, nitroglycerin, metoprolol, heparin and low-molecular weight heparin, naloxone, ephedrine, dopamine, glucose, glucagons

STEPS TO PERFORMING THE PROCEDURE

1. Respond to the patient's bedside and perform an across-the-room assessment noticing airway patency, breathing, skin color, and mental status.
2. Determine the critical nature of the situation and address airway, breathing, circulatory, and disability issues immediately.
3. Discuss the reason for the rapid response with the primary nurse or initiating person.
4. Investigate likely causes for the sign or symptom and treat the underlying cause.
5. Reassess the patient after each intervention.
6. Determine the need to transfer the patient to a higher level of care.

COMPLICATIONS OF THE PROCEDURE

1. **Anxiety**: In the case of an erroneous call, the NP should verbally assure the patient that they are safe.
2. **Cardiac arrest:** In the case of a patient who is in full cardiac arrest, the NP should call a code blue.

POSTPROCEDURE CARE

The acute care NP should remain with the patient until they are considered stable. At that time, a handoff report and patient note should be placed in the record. If laboratory studies have been ordered, they should be reviewed by the NP. If the patient has been intubated, a chest x-ray should be performed and reviewed at the time of intubation. If a change in level of care is necessary, then the order for the transfer should be initiated. All administered medications should be ordered and signed out. Finally, the initiating team members should receive positive enforcement for early recognition of patient deterioration.

BIBLIOGRAPHY

Agency for Healthcare Research and Quality. (2019). *Patient safety network: Rapid response systems.* https://psnet.ahrq.gov/primer/rapid-response-systems.

Davis, W., Dowling Evans, D., Fiebig, W., & Lewis, C. (2020). Emergency care: Operationalizing the practice through a concept analysis. *Journal of the American Association of Nurse Practitioners, 32,* 359–366. https://doi.org/10.1097/JXX.0000000000000229.

Hall, K., Lim, A., & Gale, B. (2020). The use of rapid response teams to reduce failure to rescue events: a systematic review. *Journal of Patient Safety, 16,* S3–S7. https://doi.org/10.1097/PTS.0000000000000748+6.

Kleinpell, R., Grabenkort, W.R., Kapu, A., Constantine, R., & Sicoutris, C. (2019). Nurse practitioners and physician assistants in acute and critical care: a concise review of the literature and data 2008-2018. *Critical Care Medicine, 47,* 1442–1449. https://doi.org/10.1097/CCM.0000000000003925.

Scherr, K., Wilson, D.M, Wagner, J., & Haughian, M. (2012). Evaluating a new rapid response team: NP-led versus intensivist-led comparisons. *AACN Advanced Critical Care, 23*(1), 32–42. https://doi.org/10.1097/NCI.0b013e318240e2f9.

Cardiopulmonary Resuscitation

Dawn M. Specht

INDICATIONS FOR THE PROCEDURE

The advanced practice provider must recognize the need for cardiopulmonary resuscitation (CPR) in any situation. The timely initiation of compressions and defibrillation may save lives. In the inpatient setting, a rapid response may be initiated prior to the loss of a pulse. Early recognition and interventions may prevent the need for resuscitation; however, cardiac monitoring and defibrillation should be readily available.

1. The primary indication for CPR is cardiac arrest.

CONTRAINDICATIONS FOR THE PROCEDURE

Relative Contraindications

1. Patient is unlikely to survive, such as a patient found who is cold and demonstrating rigor mortis

Absolute Contraindications

1. Initiation of CPR in a patient who has clearly communicated their wishes to avoid resuscitation, i.e., a Do Not Resuscitate (DNR) order

EQUIPMENT NEEDED

1. Firm surface
2. Cardiopulmonary resuscitation (CPR)-trained assistive personnel
3. Cardiac monitor with defibrillation capabilities or automated external defibrillator (AED)
4. Code cart with bag valve mask, oxygen, cardiac medications, and line supplies

STEPS TO PERFORMING THE PROCEDURE

1. Verify code status.
2. Establish unresponsiveness.
3. Check for carotid pulse for no more than 10 seconds and evaluate breathing.
4. If pulseless, immediately perform chest compression on a firm surface (may need to place headboard under the patient or hit CPR button on air mattress). Rate of 100 to

120 compressions per minute, depth of 2 inches, in the ratio of 30 compressions to two ventilations. Allow chest recoil after each compression. (If an advanced airway is in place, deliver asynchronous breaths at a rate of one breath every 6 seconds.)

5. Apply AED or cardiac monitor with defibrillation capabilities.
6. Pause compression for rhythm analysis.
7. Defibrillate shockable rhythms, i.e., ventricular tachycardia and ventricular fibrillation.
8. Resume compressions at the rate of 100 to 120 compressions per minute, depth of 2 inches, in the ratio of 30 compressions to two ventilations.
9. Ventilate with bag valve mask connected to oxygen at 10 to 15 L/min flow. Ensure chest expansion during bagging and avoid overinflation of the lungs, each breath over one second while rhythm analysis is occurring. If patient is intubated, deliver asynchronous breaths over 1 second every 6 seconds.
10. Establish intravenous line or intraosseous access. Administer epinephrine 1 mg push; may repeat every 3 to 5 minutes in all arrest states.
11. Continue compressions in 2-minute cycles.
12. Reassess rhythm and pulse after 2 minutes of compressions, while delivering two ventilations.
13. Change person performing chest compressions every 2 minutes.
14. Avoid interruptions in compressions.
15. Utilize advanced cardiac life support (ACLS) algorithms to treat pulseless rhythms until pulse returns or pronouncement occurs (Table 39.1).

COMPLICATIONS OF THE PROCEDURE

1. **Rib fractures or sternal fracture from compressions, post resuscitation:** Chest radiography is indicated. Intubation may be required.
2. **Gastric insufflation/vomiting from bag valve mask ventilation:** Turn to side for vomiting. Clear airway if not intubated; place gastric tube if intubated and connect to low wall suction.

POSTPROCEDURE CARE

Postresuscitation care is imperative when circulation has returned. Assessment of vital signs; obtaining diagnostic studies; and evaluating respiratory, hemodynamic, and neurologic status are of paramount importance. If the patient is not ventilating at a sufficient rate and depth, intubation should occur. Continuous end tidal CO_2 monitoring should occur with a goal of $ETCO_2 = 40$. Pulse oximetry should occur with a target of greater than 94%. Arterial blood gas monitoring should occur and be accompanied by avoiding hyperoxia as PaO_2 levels greater than 300 mmHg post resuscitation worsen outcomes. If the patient has a mean arterial pressure less than 65, isotonic fluids and vasopressors may be administered. If the patient is not following commands, then targeted temperature management (hypothermia) should be considered. The advanced practice provider should evaluate the 12-lead electrocardiogram to determine the need for rapid percutaneous coronary intervention as indicated by ST-elevated myocardial infarction

TABLE 39.1 Cardiopulmonary Resuscitation for Shockable and Unshockable Rhythms

Shockable Rhythms (Ventricular Tachycardia and Ventricular Fibrillation)

Steps of CPR
1. Identify the cardiac rhythm as a shockable rhythm (ventricular tachycardia or ventricular fibrillation).
2. Administer defibrillation.
   a. Biphasic (120–200 J based on manufacturer recommendation)
   b. Monophasic (300 J)
3. Begin high-quality CPR for 2 min and obtain IV/IO access.
   a. Compress at least 2 in. in depth.
   b. Compress at a rate of 100–200 compressions/min.
   c. Avoid overventilation.
   d. Monitor petCO$_2$, if available, to determine CPR quality.
4. After 2 min of high-quality CPR, recheck cardiac rhythm.
   a. If ventricular tachycardia or ventricular fibrillation, administer defibrillation, as described above.
   b. If a nonshockable rhythm without ROSC, go to Step 3 in the nonshockable rhythm pathway.
   c. If a nonshockable rhythm with ROSC, continue to post-ROSC care.
5. After second defibrillation, continue high-quality CPR, as described above, for 2 min and consider advanced airway.
6. Administer epinephrine 1 mg IV/IO every 3–5 min.
7. After 2 min of high-quality CPR, recheck cardiac rhythm.
   a. If ventricular tachycardia or ventricular fibrillation, administer defibrillation, as described above.
   b. If a nonshockable rhythm without ROSC, go to Step 3 in the nonshockable rhythm pathway.
   c. If a nonshockable rhythm with ROSC, continue to post-ROSC care.
8. After second defibrillation, continue high-quality CPR, as described above, for 2 min.
9. Administer amiodarone 350 mg IV/IO loading dose or lidocaine 1–1.5 mg/kg IV/IO loading dose.
10. Treat reversible causes of cardiac arrest.
11. Repeat the above steps until ROSC is achieved or pronouncement of death.
    a. Second dose of amiodarone is 150 mg IV/IO.
    b. Second dose of lidocaine is 0.5–0.75 mg/kg IV/IO.

Nonshockable Rhythms (Asystole and Pulseless Electrical Activity)

Steps of CPR
1. Identify the cardiac rhythm as a nonshockable rhythm (asystole or pulseless electrical activity).
2. Administer epinephrine 1 mg IV/IO immediately and then every 3–5 min.
3. Begin high-quality CPR for 2 min and consider advanced airway.
   a. Compress at least 2 in. in depth.
   b. Compress at a rate of 100–200 compressions/min.
   c. Avoid overventilation.
   d. Monitor petCO$_2$, if available, to determine CPR quality.

(continued)

TABLE 39.1 Cardiopulmonary Resuscitation for Shockable and Unshockable Rhythms (*continued*)

Nonshockable Rhythms (Asystole and Pulseless Electrical Activity)
4. After 2 min of high-quality CPR, recheck cardiac rhythm.
a. If a nonshockable rhythm without ROSC, continue high-quality CPR and epinephrine administration every 3–5 min.
b. If a nonshockable rhythm with ROSC, continue to post-ROSC care.
c. If ventricular tachycardia or ventricular fibrillation, administer defibrillation; go to step 4 in shockable rhythm pathway.
5. After 2 min of high-quality CPR, recheck cardiac rhythm.
a. If a nonshockable rhythm without ROSC, continue high-quality CPR and epinephrine administration every 3–5 min.
b. If a nonshockable rhythm with ROSC, continue to post-ROSC care.
c. If ventricular tachycardia or ventricular fibrillation, administer defibrillation; go to step 4 in shockable rhythm pathway.
6. Treat reversible causes of cardiac arrest.
7. Repeat the above steps until ROSC is achieved or pronouncement of death.

CPR, cardiopulmonary resuscitation; IV, intravenous; IO, intraosseous; ROSC, return of spontaneous circulation.
Adapted from *American Heart Association Guidelines for* CPR and ECC, 2020.

(STEMI). Additionally, the patient who demonstrated ventricular dysrhythmia will need to receive an antidysrhythmic infusion such as lidocaine or amiodarone. Consultation with cardiac and critical care experts is advised status post arrest. Laboratory analysis of electrolytes, blood counts, cardiac enzymes, and lactate levels should be obtained. Laboratory analysis may demonstrate the need for electrolyte replacement. Close monitoring of urinary output will be necessary and should be greater than 0.5 mL/kg/hr.

BIBLIOGRAPHY

American Heart Association (2018). *American Heart Association guidelines update for cardiopulmonary resuscitation and emergency cardiovascular care*. https://eccguidelines.heart.org/index.php/circulation/cpr-ecc-guidelines-2/executive-summaries/

Kleinman, M. E., Brennan, E. E., Goldberger, Z. D., Swor, R. A., Terry, M., Bobrow, B. J., Gazmuri, R. J., Travers, A. H., & Rea, T. (2015). Part 5: Adult basic life support and cardiopulmonary resuscitation quality. *Circulation, 132*(18 Suppl 2), S414–S435. https://doi.org/10.1161/cir.0000000000000259

Rittenberger, J., & Calloway, C. (2019). *Post-cardiac arrest management in adults*. https://www.uptodate.com/contents/post-cardiac-arrest-management-in-adults?search=complications%20of%20cardiopulmonary%20resuscitation&source=search_result&selectedTitle=20~150&usage_type=default&display_rank=20

Index

A

ABCs. *See* Airway, breathing and circulation (ABCs)
Abdomen, 275, 279–280
Abdominal hematoma, 108
ABG. *See* Arterial blood gas (ABG)
Abscess cavity, 124, 136–137
ACE. *See* Angiotensin-converting enzyme (ACE) inhibitors
Acidemia, 25
ACLS. *See* Advanced Cardiac Life Support (ACLS)
Acrylic nails, 148
ACS. *See* Acute coronary syndrome (ACS)
Acute asthma, 88
Acute blood loss, 235
Acute bronchospasm, 262
Acute coronary syndrome (ACS), 213, 219
Acute decompensated heart failure, 232–233
Acute kidney injury, 257
Acute myocardial infarction, 264
Acute paronychia, 139, 141, 145
Acute respiratory distress syndrome (ARDS), 49, 256, 259, 262–263
Adhesive cardioversion pads, 33–35
Adhesive disease, 58
Advanced airway training, 247–248
Advanced Cardiac Life Support (ACLS)
    12-Lead Electrocardiogram Interpretation, 213
    Cardiopulmonary Resuscitation, 286
    Cardioversion, 35–36
    Local Anesthetics, 119
    Tracheostomy, 102
    Transvenous pacing, 23
Air embolus, 17
Air entry, 17, 19
Air leak, 60, 62–63, 70–73
Airway, 95–96, 99, 102–103
    Assessment, 247–248
    Edema, 55
    Emergency, 102
    Equipment, 254, 258
    Injury, 62, 88, 92
    Management, 35, 96
    Nasopharyngeal, 50, 254, 269
    Obstruction, 50, 103, 272
    Oropharyngeal, 248, 250, 254, 256, 262
    Patency, 273, 283
    Pressure, 260, 268
    Protection, 49
    Secretions, 90, 103
    Securement procedures, 50
    Spigots, 88
    Stenting, 88
    Stimulation, 89
    Trauma, 50, 55
Airway, breathing and circulation (ABCs), 272
Alcohol, 142, 148, 194, 198
Allergic reactions, 117–118, 120
Alveolar rupture, 260
Amiodarone, 119, 287–288
Analgesia
    Bronchoscopy, 90
    Endotracheal Intubation, 51
    Lumbar Puncture, 152
    Pulmonary Function Test, 249
    Rapid response, 282
    Rapid Sequence Intubation, 254–255
    Wound VAC Application, 182
Analgesic medication, 71
Anaphylaxis, 50, 118, 121
Ancillary assistance, 96
Anesthesia, 16, 51–52, 55, 119, 134, 256–257
Angina, unstable, 117
Angiocatheter, 81, 275
Angiotensin-converting enzyme (ACE) inhibitors, 237
Antecubital fossa, 195
Anti-inflammatory drugs, 157, 172
Antiarrhythmics, 24
Antibiotics, 39, 63, 138, 141, 145, 147, 149, 261, 283
    Ointment, 127, 131–132
    Oral, 124, 127, 132
Anticoagulation, 19, 77, 84
Antidysrhythmic infusion, 288
Antimicrobial disk, 9, 19
Antimicrobial silver, 177
Antineoplastic agent, 265
Antioxidants, 117
Antiseptic, 148, 195
    Swabs, 71–72
Anxiety, 262, 283
Aortic stenosis, 215, 240
Apnea, 256, 270
Arboviruses, 157
ARDS. *See* Acute respiratory distress syndrome (ARDS)
Argon plasma coagulation, 92